BAPTIST HEALTH SOUTH FLORIDA

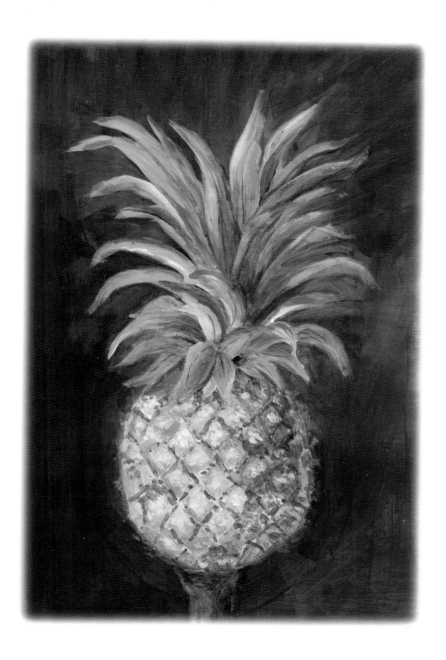

𝒜 HISTORY OF CARING FOR THE COMMUNITY

by Laura Pincus

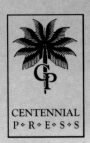

CENTENNIAL
P·R·E·S·S

Copyright © 2010
Baptist Health South Florida

Published by: Centennial Press
Miami, Florida 33129
centennialpress@bellsouth.net

By Laura Pincus

Printed in the United States
Franklin Communications

Library of Congress
Cataloging in-Publication Data
LC: 2010935901
Pincus, Laura, 1967 –

Baptist Health South Florida:
A History of Caring for the Community
1. History – Florida
ISBN: 0980226430

Historical Consultant:
Arva Moore Parks

Editors:
Jo Baxter, Corporate Vice President
    Marketing & Public Relations
    Baptist Health South Florida
Patty Shillington

Graphic Design/Production:
Rhondda Edmiston, Mixed Media, Inc.

Cover Illustration:
Eleanore Keim

Photo Credits:
Ruth Braddock: page 248
Florida Pioneer Museum Collection: pages 92, 93, 94, 95,
    98, 99, 100, 101, 103, 104, 105, 107, 108, 109, 110
Historical Museum of Southern Florida: pages 52, 53, 56,
    59, 60, 61, 97, 111, 227
Doug Jolly: pages 170, 171, 233
Joel Levin, M.D.: pages 166, 169
Dr. John T. Macdonald Foundation: page 241
The Miami Herald: pages 142, 221, 270, 271
Arva Parks & Company: pages 8, 9, 12, 13, 14,
    15, 18, 19, 57, 58, 171, 174, 224, 225, 228,
    229, 230, 231, 232
Jerry Wilkinson Collection: pages 164,
    165, 167, 168, 172, 173,
    174, 175, 176
All other photos:
Baptist Health
South Florida
and Mabel
Rodriguez

Table of Contents

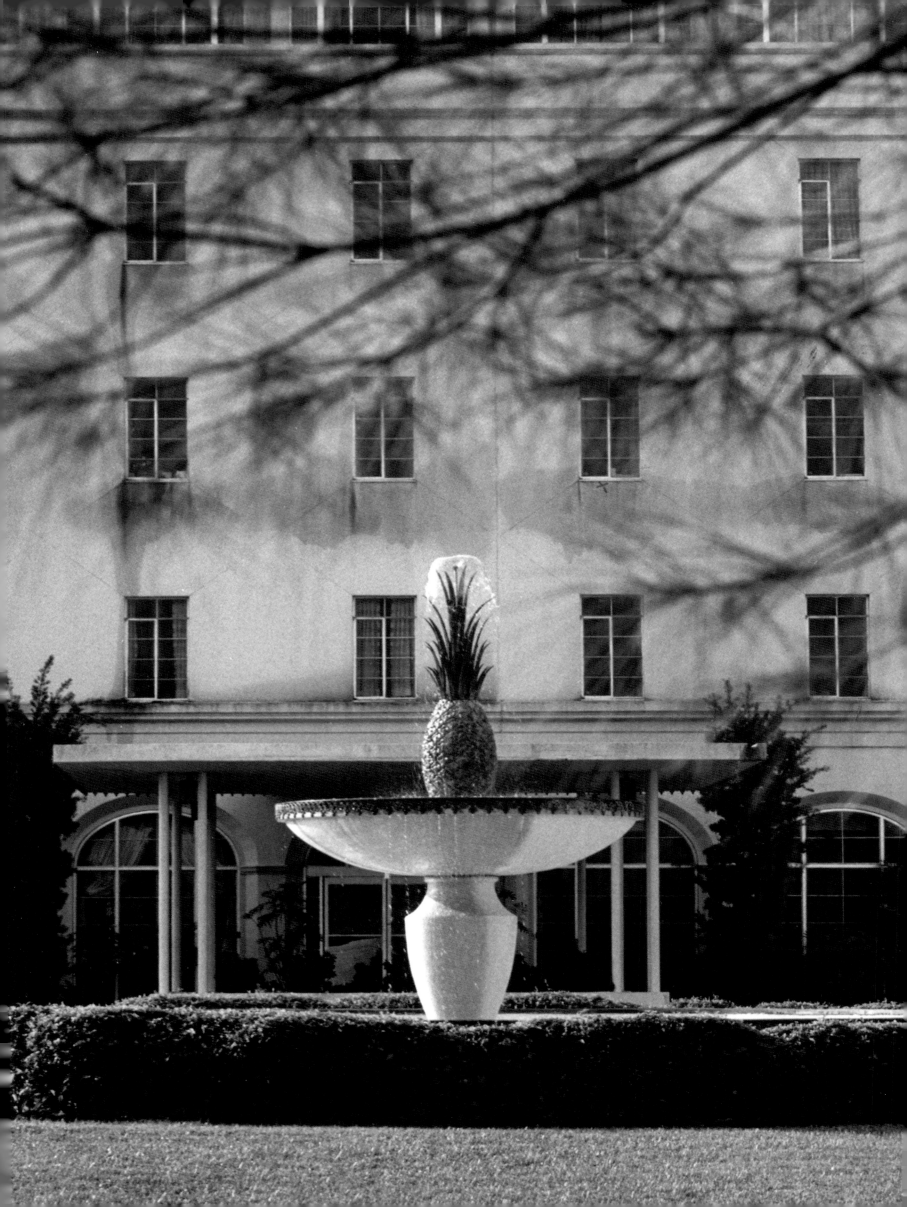

Dear Friends:

The history of Baptist Health is rich and varied and very much intertwined with the history and growth of South Florida. It all started in the late 1800s when Standard Oil magnate Henry Flagler decided to build a railroad down Florida's east coast to bring in wealthy Northern tourists. Miami was established soon after Flagler extended the railroad to what was then an isolated outpost. He continued with his dream to build a railroad from Miami to Key West. Although the legendary railroad reached Key West in 1912, it was destroyed by the 1935 hurricane. The rest is history.

As Miami transitioned from a small town to a growing, vibrant city, the local healthcare community grew with it. Baptist Hospital started out as a small, struggling community hospital on Kendall Drive — nicknamed "the road to nowhere" because it was situated in a remote location on the southern outskirts of the Dade County population. Homestead, Doctors, South Miami and Mariners were all independent community hospitals that also had sprung up to cater to the healthcare needs of their respective communities. When Baptist Health was formed with the merger and acquisition of South Miami, Homestead and Mariners Hospitals, it became one of the largest healthcare providers in Florida. Like Miami, Baptist Health also experienced growing pains during the 1990s.

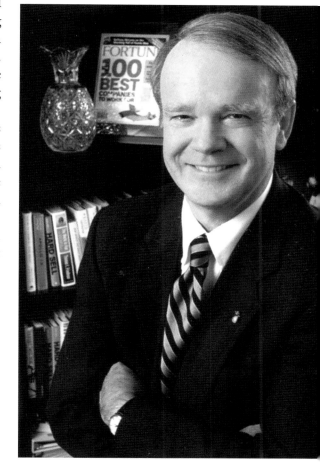

Today, Baptist Health is one of the preeminent healthcare institutions in the United States. While many attribute its many years of success to its sheer size and geographical coverage, the real answer is our passionate and continued commitment to our faith-based mission and core values — the cultural "glue" that ties us all together. While our business strategies and practices have changed to accommodate the changing community demographics and market dynamics, our core values and purpose have remained fixed and solidly entrenched in how we choose to conduct our business. It all starts with always putting our patients first.

I am sure you will find the historical photographs of the old buildings and equipment in this book interesting and fascinating, but it is the people you will see and read about — our highly skilled doctors and compassionate nurses and caregivers — who have made all the difference. So it is to this group, the Baptist Health Family — our Board members, physicians, nurses and caregivers, employees and volunteers — that we dedicate this book.

Thank you again for everything you do for Baptist Health and our patients. You are the heart and soul of Baptist Health, and it is indeed an honor and privilege to serve you.

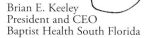

Brian E. Keeley
President and CEO
Baptist Health South Florida

The pineapple fountain at the entrance
of Baptist Hospital, c.1960

Rooted in the Community

1896
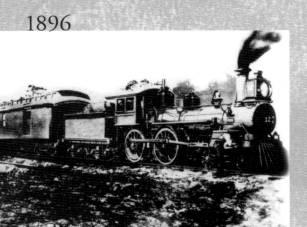

1926
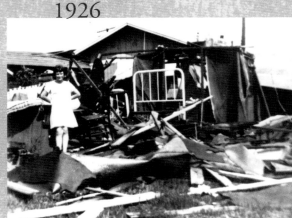

1927
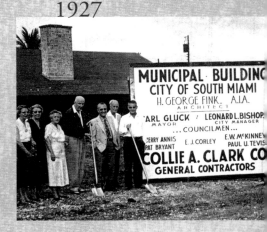

1960
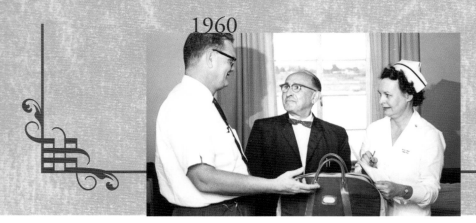

1966
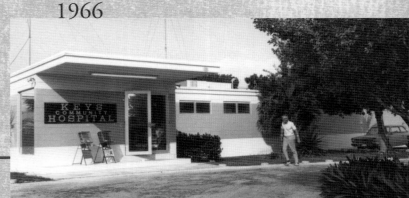

1896
Henry Flagler's East Coast Railway comes from Palm Beach into Miami

City of Miami is incorporated

1908
Daily train service begins from Miami to Marathon

1913
City of Homestead is incorporated

1925
City of Coral Gables is incorporated

1926
Major hurricane hits South Florida

1927
City of South Miami is incorporated

1935
Hurricane devastates the Upper and Middle Keys

1938
Overseas Highway is completed to link Florida Keys with a road

1940
James Archer Smith Hospital (today's Homestead Hospital) opens

1949
Doctors' Hospital opens

1960
South Miami Hospital opens

Baptist Hospital opens

1962
Overseas Hospital (today's Mariners Hospital) opens

Dadeland Shopping Center opens

1964
North Kendall Drive is widened into a four-lane road

1966
Overseas Hospital becomes Keys Community Hospital

1980
Keys Community Hospital becomes Mariners Hospital

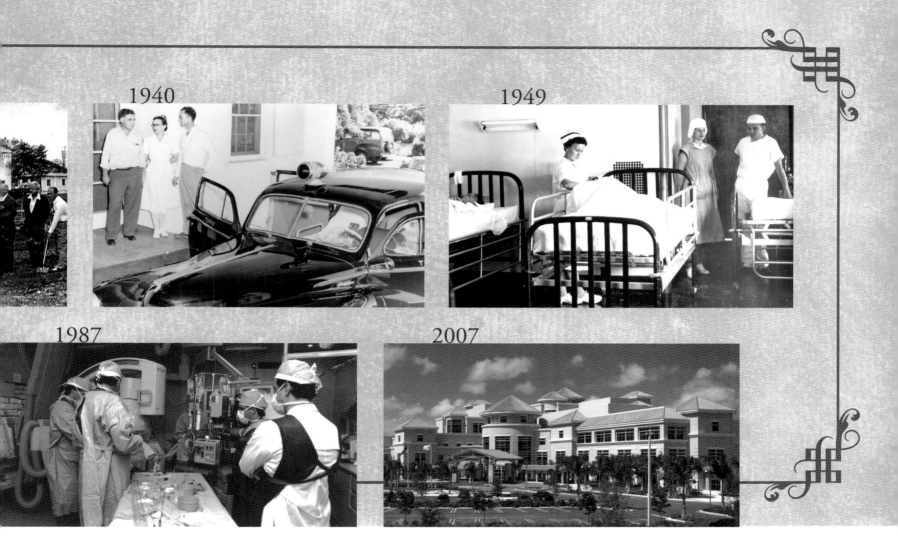

1940

1949

1987

2007

1985
Robert B. Cole takes over as chairman of the Board of Baptist Hospital

1986
Brian E. Keeley takes over as president and chief executive officer of Baptist Hospital

1987
Miami Vascular Institute (today's Baptist Cardiac & Vascular Institute) opens on the campus of Baptist Hospital

1988
James Archer Smith signs a three-year management contract with South Miami Hospital

1990
Baptist Medical Plaza at Beacon Center opens

South Miami Hospital purchases Homestead Hospital

1992
HealthSouth purchases Doctors' Hospital

Hurricane Andrew devastates South Dade

1995
South Miami HealthSystem becomes part of Baptist Health

Mariners Hospital becomes part of Baptist Health

1997
Baptist Children's Hospital opens on the Kendall campus

2003
Doctors Hospital becomes part of Baptist Health

2007
New Homestead Hospital opens

2008
West Kendall Baptist Hospital breaks ground

2009
Baptist Medical Plaza at Coral Springs opens

2011
West Kendall Baptist Hospital scheduled to open

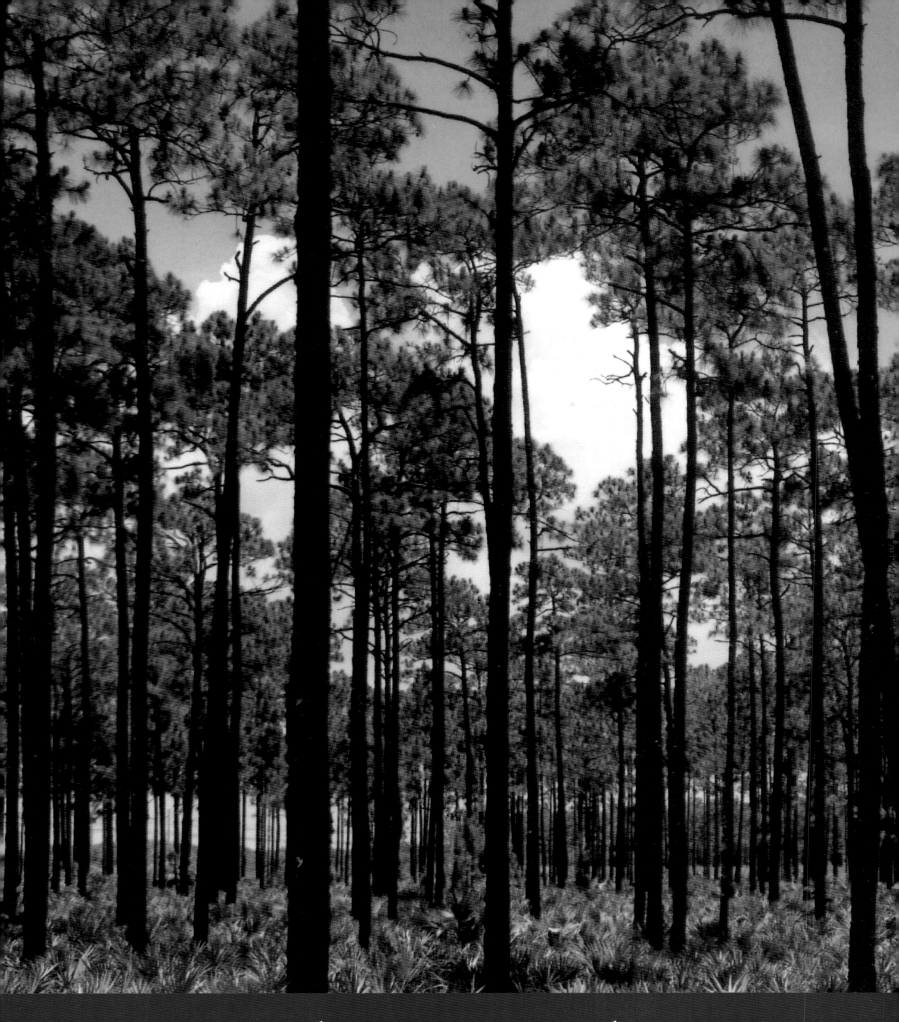

From Nowhere to Somewhere

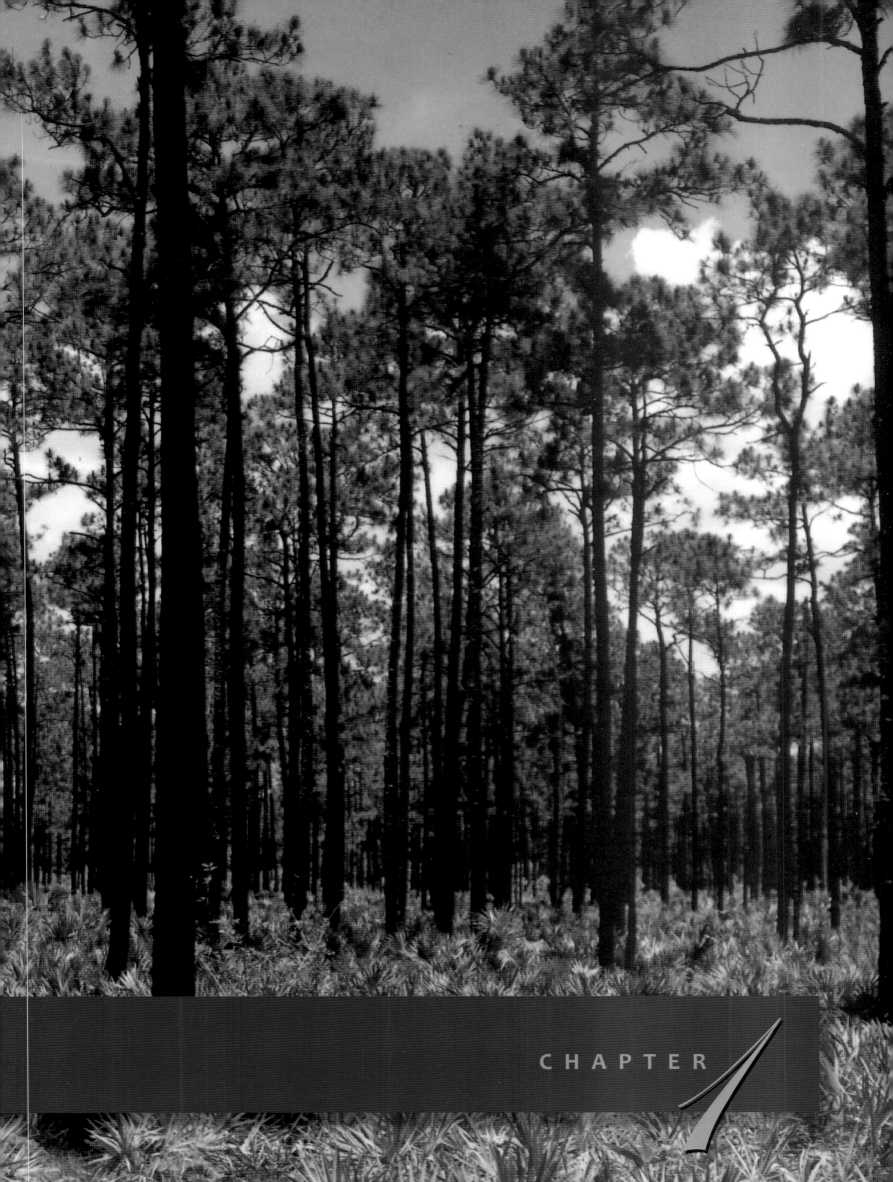

CHAPTER 1

"We have had good times and bad times, problems and lack of problems, but the one thing that has happened is that the hospital has remained open and we have continued to care for patients. This care has steadily improved since the very first day."

Ernest C. Nott Jr.
Administrator, Baptist Hospital
1964

In the 1950s, South Florida was in the throes of a post-war boom. New arrivals appeared, drawn by the sun and the promise of prosperity. Suburban communities, complete with rows of neatly landscaped homes, developed outside Miami's central core. Businesses sprouted, eager to capitalize on the new consumers. The county's population, not even 500,000 at the decade's start, would nearly double by its end.

Amid the bustling development, a pocket remained mostly undisturbed. It was home to verdant acres of palmettos and pines, a cadre of farmers and ranchers, and a fair share of rattlesnakes, opossums, horses and foxes. The wilderness had an official name, Kendall, and a primitive two-lane country road.

This road, called North Kendall Drive, was appropriately nicknamed "the road to nowhere." Running east to west off South Dixie Highway, it reached well past the fixtures of modern life. So when bulldozers began clearing land on the south side of the road in 1958, passersby watched with wonder. It was hard to imagine that anything, let alone a hospital, would be built in "the sticks."

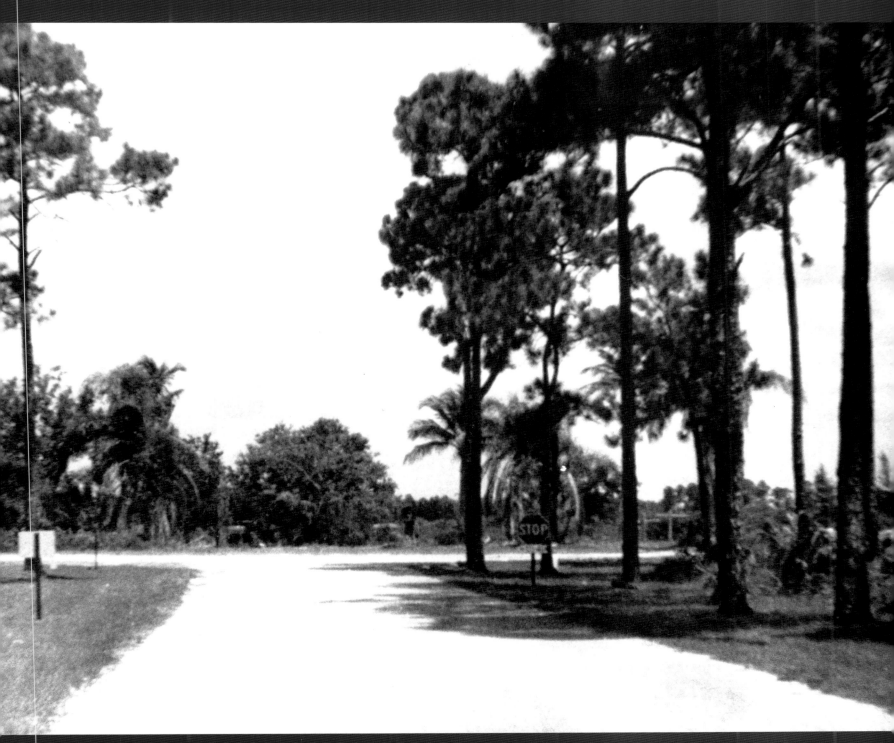

North Kendall Drive was a two-lane country road that cut through wilderness. It was nicknamed "the road to nowhere."

The Start of Nowhere

Kendall began as an official swamp. Because it flooded often, the government prohibited homesteaders from settling on it. The law did allow individuals to purchase the land, however. In 1883, the state of Florida sold four million acres, about half the area between today's North Kendall Drive and S.W. 104th Street, to a group of Englishmen. A few years later, Henry John Boughton Kendall came to South Florida to manage the holdings. Although little is known about Kendall's experience in the area, his name became his legacy.

As the new century began, a small agricultural community developed in the middle of the wilderness. Henry Flagler's East Coast Railway rolled from Miami into Homestead in 1904, making accessible the fertile lands of South Dade.

Citrus and avocado groves flourished. A small general store opened, west of the railroad and north of S.W. 100th Street. The store's proprietor relied on trade with Seminole Indians who lived near today's Baptist Hospital.

In 1916, Dan Killian moved to the rural enclave from Tennessee. He bought and ran the general store and became active in government, serving on the County Commission from 1922 until 1926. In his political role, Killian brought streetlights to the community and helped persuade the county to build a charity hospital and home for the aged, delinquent children and orphans. Killian also named various roads, including Killian Drive (S.W. 112th Street) and North Kendall Drive (S.W. 88th Street). Kendall became the area's official identity.

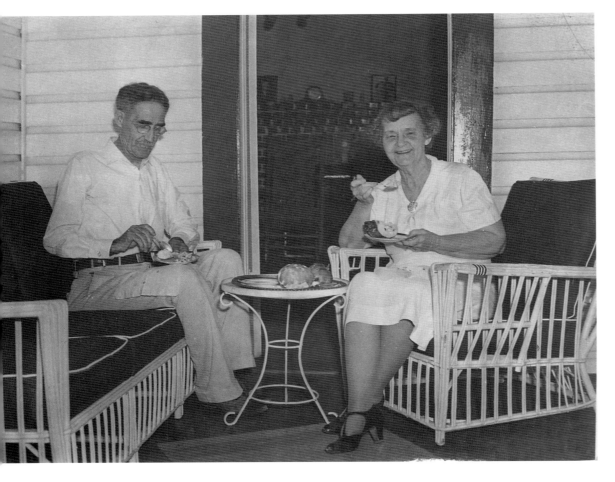

Dan Killian, county commissioner and Kendall shopkeeper, named the town's streets and helped bring electric service to the area. His wife, Mary Moore Killian, was a founder of Kendall Methodist Church.

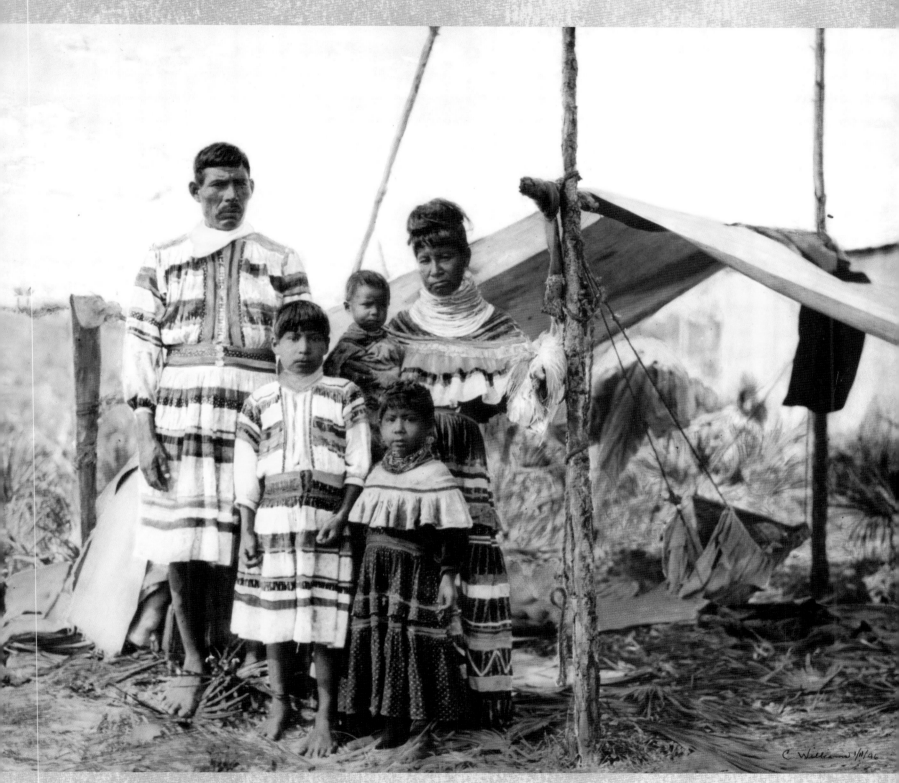

*Seminole villages were located in the area
of today's Baptist Hospital.*

Boom, Bust and Change

Dan Killian's time on the commission coincided with Miami's dizzying land boom. The early 1920s ushered in a period of dramatic growth. Real estate changed hands at a frenetic pace. Thousands bought and sold tracts of land, holding onto them just long enough to get rich. Developers built new communities, including Coral Gables, Hialeah and Miami Shores. Boom fever even reached distant Kendall — albeit on a small scale — when Coral Gables developer George Merrick purchased real estate in the area and subdivided the land.

The boom had begun to cool by 1926, when a hurricane raced through South Florida with winds blowing more than 135 miles per hour. Much of the region was left in ruins. In Kendall, the low areas flooded and the small, wooden farmhouses crumbled.

Recovery was slow, in part because Miami began to experience early the economic trials of the Great Depression. Kendall remained a gathering of small farms. In 1929, Kendall School (now Kenwood School) opened its doors to 44 students and one teacher.

Near the school, two cattlemen started a ranch, which gave the rural community its entertainment. Boyhood friends George Larkins, whose family settled South Miami, and John Pendray built the P & L Ranch in 1939 on some land south of North Kendall Drive and west of Galloway Road. A rodeo arena sat on the north side of the property, attracting locals to exciting sporting events about 500 feet south of North Kendall Drive — on the site of today's Baptist Hospital.

Over the next two decades, more people settled in Kendall. Two churches offered sanctuary and prayer. Children rode their bikes to school. Still, the neighborhood was mostly farmland, teeming with four-legged creatures.

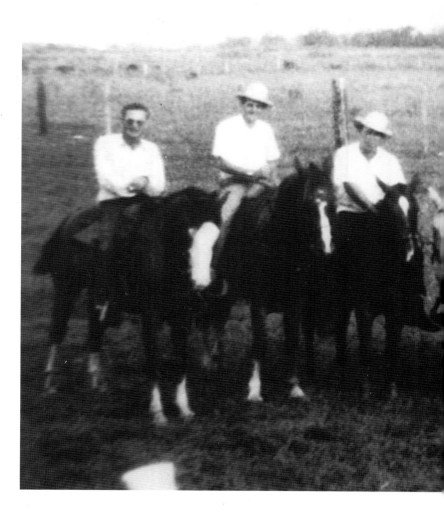

Bottom: In 1939, George Larkins and John Pendray built the P & L Ranch on land off North Kendall Drive and west of Galloway Road. The rodeo arena on the north side of the property stood on what is now Baptist Hospital.

𝓜ore and more people settled in Kendall but the area was still country. Farming was the major occupation of its residents.

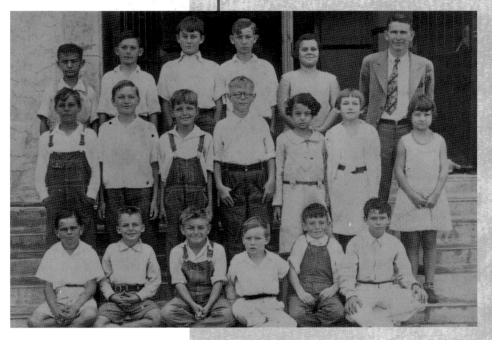

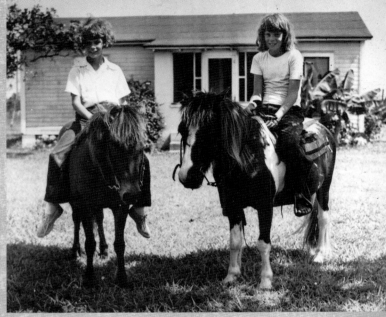

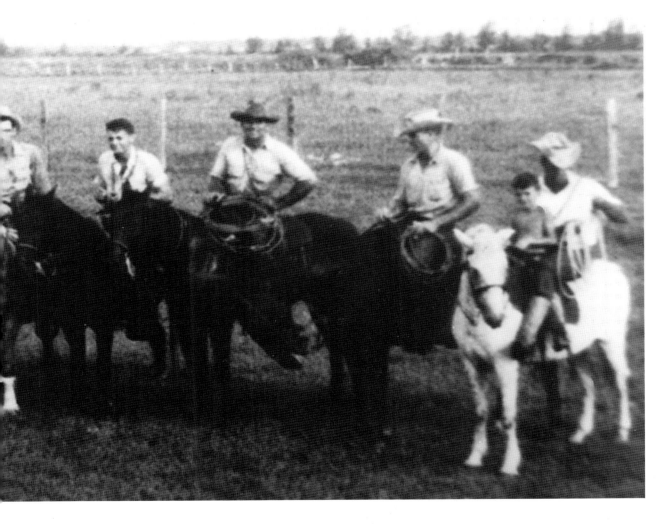

Top left: In 1929, Kendall School (now Kenwood School) opened. This photograph shows the fifth- and sixth-grade class from the 1931-1932 school year.

Top right: Kendall residents, including the Reno family, came to the community for its plentiful land and rural feel. Former United States Attorney General Janet Reno (right) and Maggie Reno embraced the area's natural surroundings.

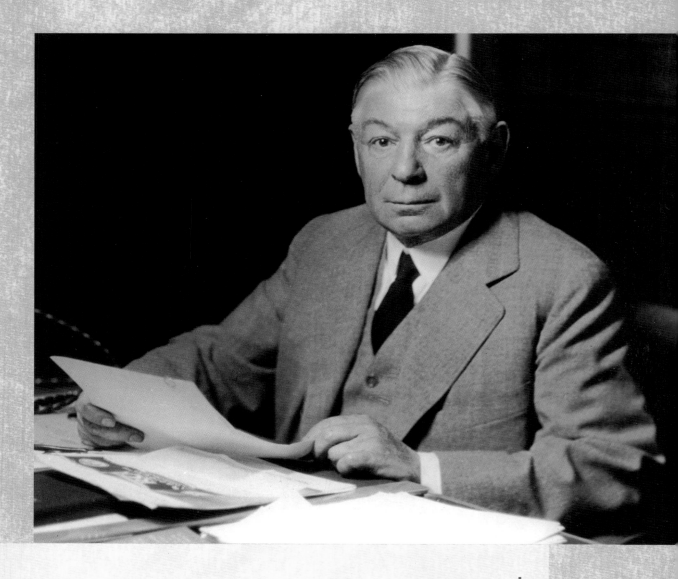

$\mathscr{A}$lcoa dominated the market, and Arthur Vining Davis became one of the nation's richest men, with a fortune estimated at well over $400 million.

An Industrialist Finds Miami

This bucolic setting would change — thanks in part to a diminutive financier whose late-in-life career brought him to Kendall. Arthur Vining Davis was born in 1867 in Massachusetts. The son of a Congregational minister, Davis excelled academically, earning the top spot in his class at Amherst College. After his 1888 graduation, he took a job with the Pittsburgh Reduction Company, a young business that was producing a new light metal called aluminum. Quickly, aluminum became the wonder metal, and Davis is credited with finding everyday uses for it, including utensils, pots and kettles. By 1920, he was president of the company, which had been renamed Alcoa (Aluminum Company of America).

Alcoa dominated the market, and Davis became one of the nation's richest men, with a fortune estimated at well over $400 million. Although he stood only five feet two, Davis had a forceful presence. He worked tirelessly, claiming in a rare interview to put in 16-hour days.

Davis moved to Miami from Pittsburgh and began a second act in real estate. In the early 1950s, he started buying land in Florida, holding 72,000 acres in Dade County alone, the largest block of private property in the area. A significant part of his holdings was south of Miami, including the area of today's Baptist Hospital.

Davis wanted to develop residential communities and industrial parks. Some of the land, however, would have a more altruistic purpose. In a merging of need and interests, 55 acres in Kendall would become home to a Baptist-run hospital.

Facing page: Arthur Vining Davis

The Arthur Vining Davis estate in Miami was named Journey's End.

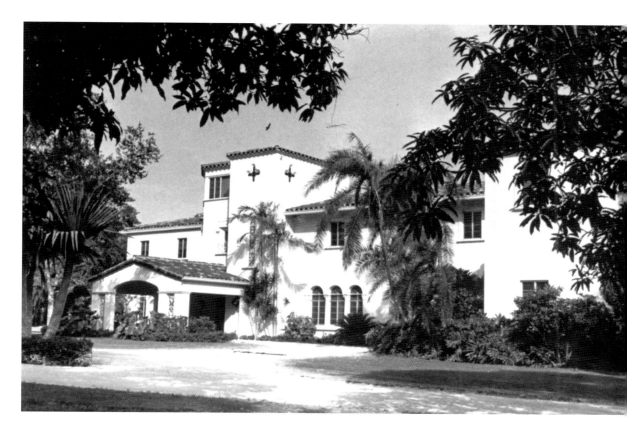

The Minister and His Dream

The Rev. Dr. C. Roy Angell joined downtown Miami's Central Baptist Church in 1936. The church, located on N.E. First Avenue at Fifth Street, had deep roots in the community. Originally called First Baptist Church, it opened two days before the city's incorporation, on July 26, 1896. In the 1930s, the church split into two separate congregations, the First and Temple Baptist Churches. When the groups decided to reunite, they chose a new name, Central Baptist Church.

Dr. Angell was the newly configured church's first minister. The native Virginian was an inspirational leader known for his meaningful sermons and big dreams for the congregation. Under his leadership, Central Baptist Church became the state's largest Baptist congregation with more than 5,000 members.

Eventually, he aspired to have impact beyond the walls of the church. As early as 1954, Dr. Angell began promoting an idea to build a Baptist hospital.

He recognized a need — Dade County's supply of hospital beds was woefully inadequate. Studies estimated that based on population, the community was short nearly 2,000 beds. "The simple fact is that hospital expansion has been unable to keep pace with Greater Miami's fabulous growth — especially when the chilly winds of mid-winter whip across the Northland to send thousands of persons fleeing toward Florida's sunshine," *The Miami Herald* wrote at the time.

Dr. Angell brought a group of Baptists together, mostly from the Central, Riverside and Allapattah congregations, to consider the idea. His enthusiasm was contagious and he was able to unite the different forces behind a single mission. "He was the human dynamo," said Miller Walton, a community leader who was active in the effort to build the hospital, "the irresistible force overcoming crisis after crisis, keeping the hospital movement alive and progressing slowly but surely to fruition."

Miami's Central Baptist Church, originally called First Baptist Church, opened on July 26, 1896. The church stands prominently in this panoramic skyline of downtown Miami, c.1930.

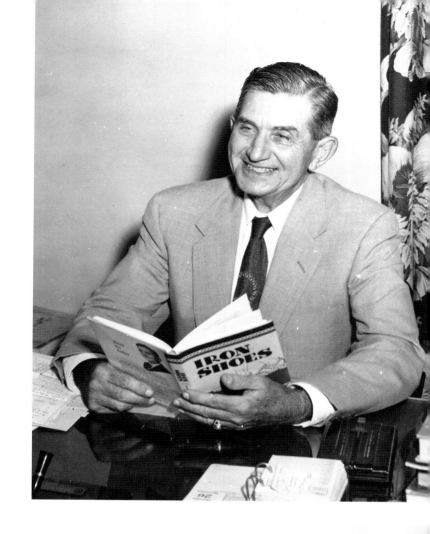

The Rev. Dr. C. Roy Angell, the minister at Miami's Central Baptist Church, led the effort to build a Baptist hospital.

The discussions turned to details. The group decided that an association of Baptist churches, dubbed the Miami Baptist Association, should build the hospital, equip it and then offer it debt-free, to be run by the Southern Baptist Convention, the national body.

With the structure in place, the Miami Baptist Association looked for a site for the hospital. The location seemed clear. Most of the churches and their members were in central or north Miami, so the hospital needed to be there. The group settled on some land — 10 acres of the golf course of the former Miami Country Club, near today's Metro government complex. In 1957, it paid the local government $1,000 for an option to purchase the land, which would ultimately cost $88,000. The agreement would last for one year. The location was set and fundraising could begin. Dr. Angell and his colleagues seemed well on their way.

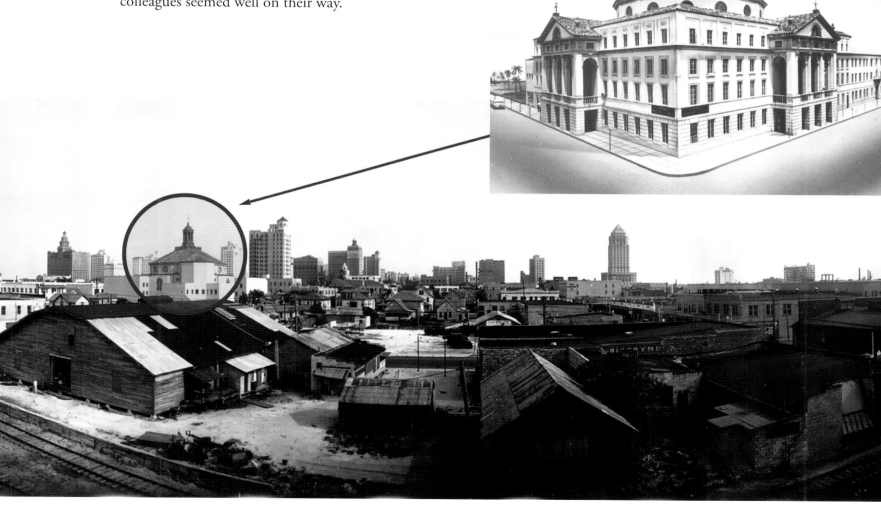

A Move to Nowhere

Exactly how the course changed is unclear. Ralph Ruhl, Arthur Vining Davis' assistant, had a personal interest in healthcare. He had lost a child to kidney disease and encouraged his boss, who had a strong sense of philanthropy, to consider hospitals a cause to support. At some point, the millionaire learned of the minister and Dr. Angell's dream fit the bill. After several meetings, Davis agreed to support the hospital. He offered one caveat: that it be built on 55 acres of his land in the rural area called Kendall. The Miami Baptist Association balked. They wanted the hospital centrally located. Like most in South Florida, they could not yet imagine that the sparsely populated, agricultural community would ever be somewhere. But Davis remained firm. He offered his land, as well as $1 million toward the hospital and another $500,000 for a cardiac wing to be named in honor of his second wife, who had died of a heart attack in 1933. The next move was up to the Baptists.

The association needed Davis' donation and the credibility it brought, but wanted the hospital downtown. The ensuing debate over what to do with the millionaire's generosity produced an unlikely compromise — the Baptists would build on the Kendall site but also on their location in downtown Miami.

With the daunting task of raising funds for two hospitals, hospital leaders began their work in earnest. They opened a small office at 1324 West Flagler Street, where a skeleton crew, including Vega Perkins, director of nursing, and Steve McCrimmon, the hospital's first administrator, planned the hospital's layout. Despite their original opposition to the site, local Baptist ministers embraced the effort. They spoke from their pulpits supporting the hospital, attended community luncheons and went door-to-door asking for donations.

By the middle of 1958, they had raised $1.2 million toward the hospital's construction. Davis pitched in another $500,000, but again the money came with certain conditions. He insisted that the hospital's size be increased and that it be built in an Italian Renaissance architectural style. He wanted it to resemble the style of the Boca Raton Club, which he had just purchased. The cost would be in excess of $5 million. Some of the Baptists with more modest sensibilities were unnerved by Davis' opulent tastes. Still, just as they had been forced to accept the hospital's location, they also had to agree to its style.

James W. Parrish, vice chairman of the campaign executive committee (center), presented plans for two Baptist Hospitals. Renderings of the two sites are in the background.

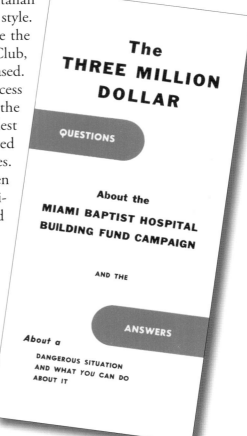

The
THREE MILLION
DOLLAR

QUESTIONS

About the
MIAMI BAPTIST HOSPITAL
BUILDING FUND CAMPAIGN

AND THE

ANSWERS

About a
DANGEROUS SITUATION
AND WHAT YOU CAN DO
ABOUT IT

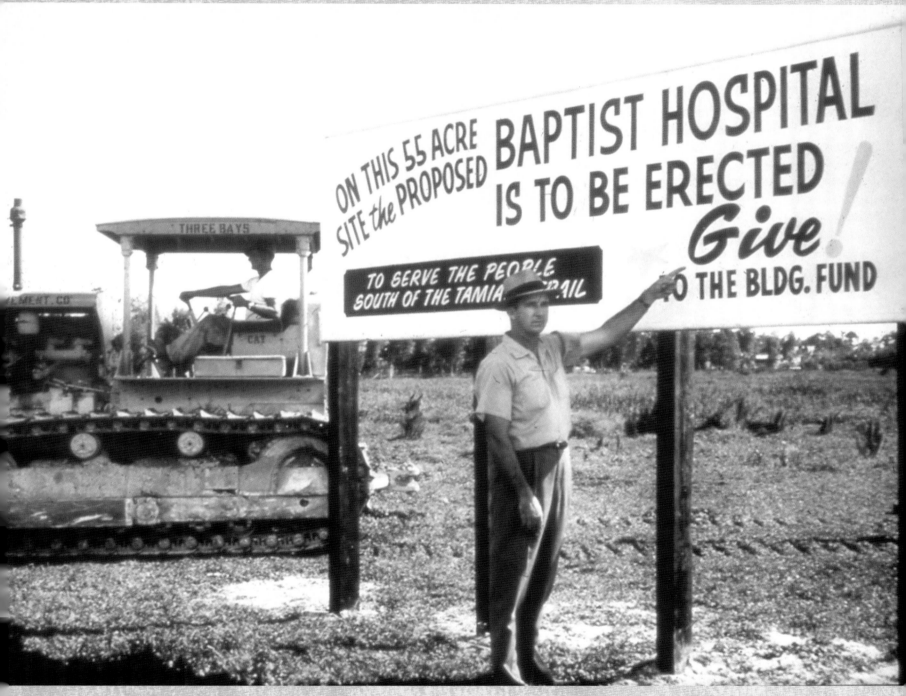

On this 55 acre site the proposed BAPTIST HOSPITAL IS TO BE ERECTED *Give!* TO SERVE THE PEOPLE SOUTH OF THE TAMIAMI TRAIL TO THE BLDG. FUND

The Miami Baptist Association looked to the community for support to build the hospital.

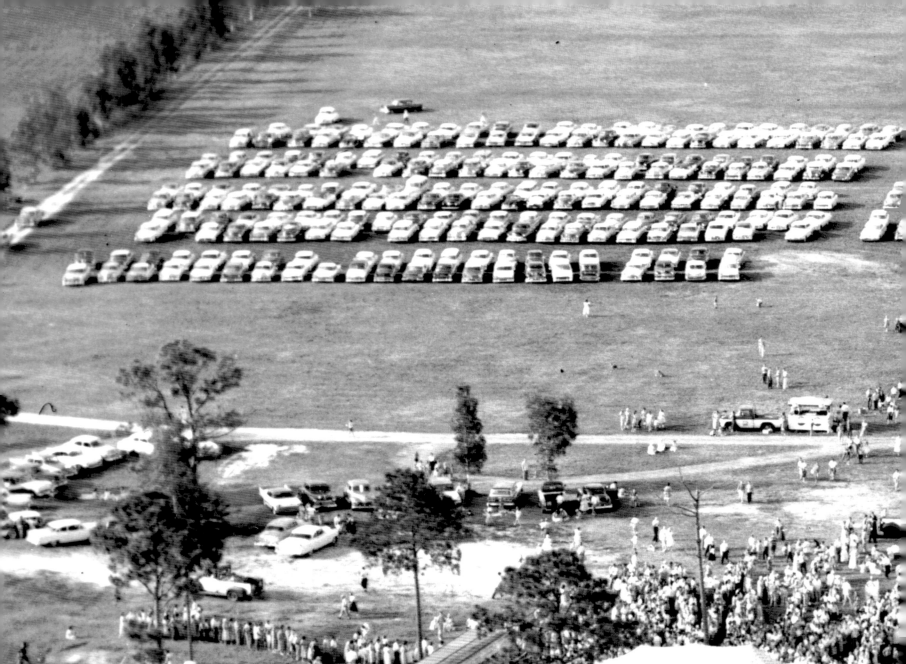

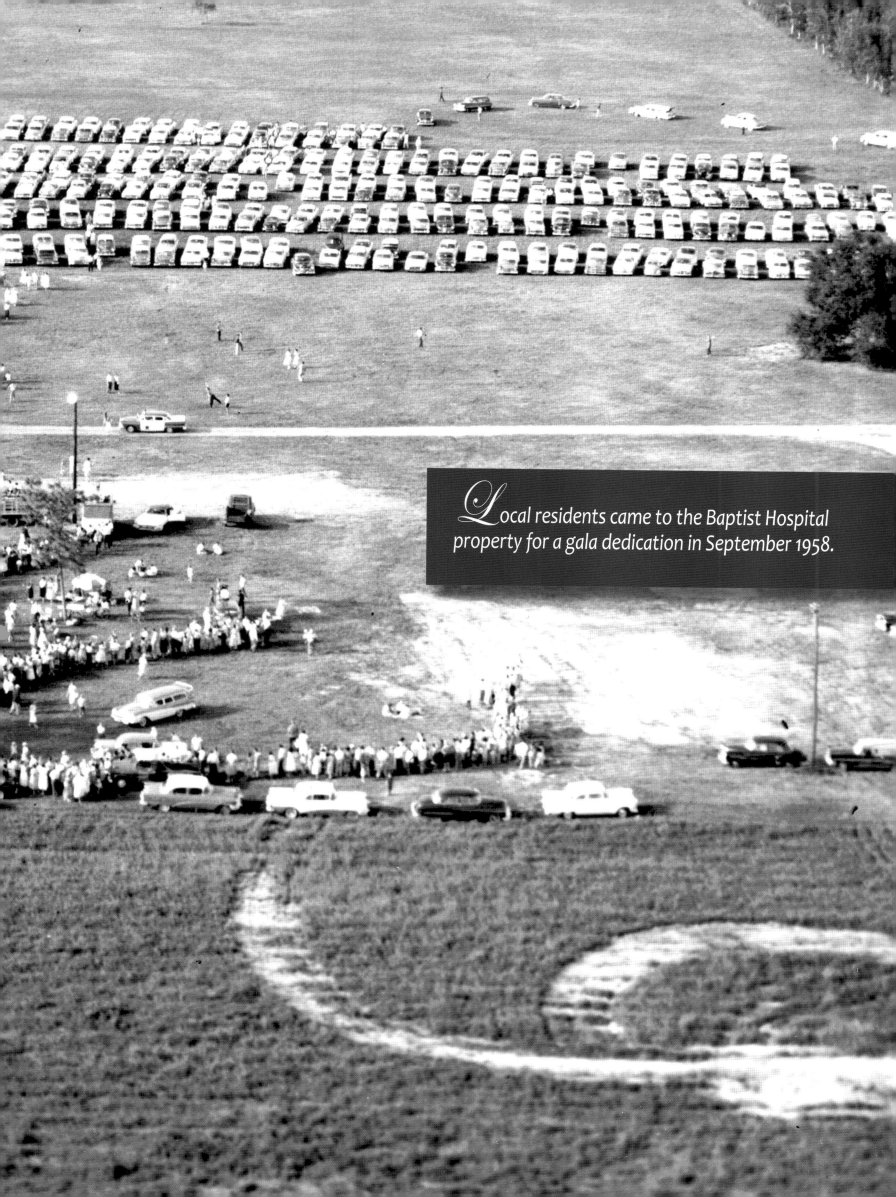

*L*ocal residents came to the Baptist Hospital property for a gala dedication in September 1958.

MOVING FORWARD

Arthur Vining Davis (far left), age 91, broke ground for Baptist Hospital on November 2, 1958. His donation of 55 acres of Kendall farmland determined the hospital's location.

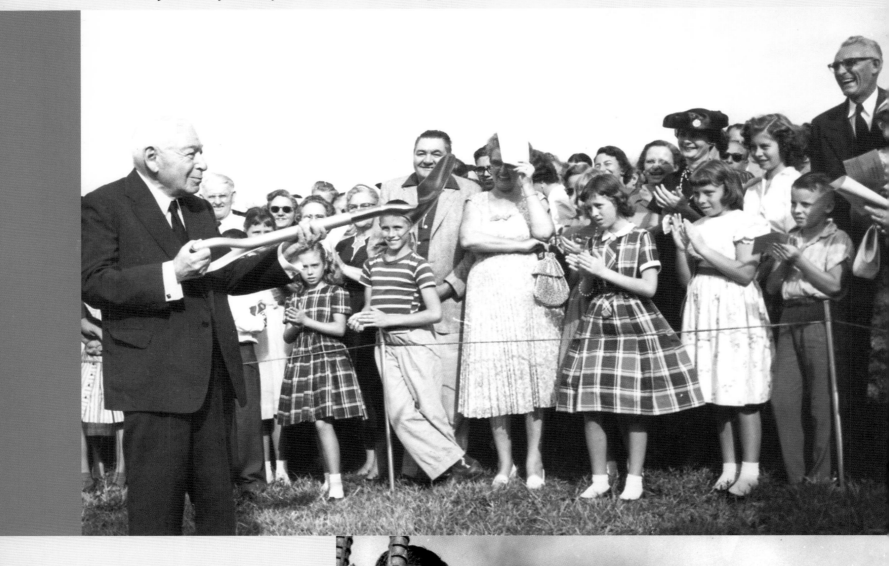

Arthur Vining Davis participated in the cornerstone-laying ceremony on April 11, 1959. He was a forceful presence in determining how the hospital should look. He insisted it be designed in the Italian Renaissance architectural style.

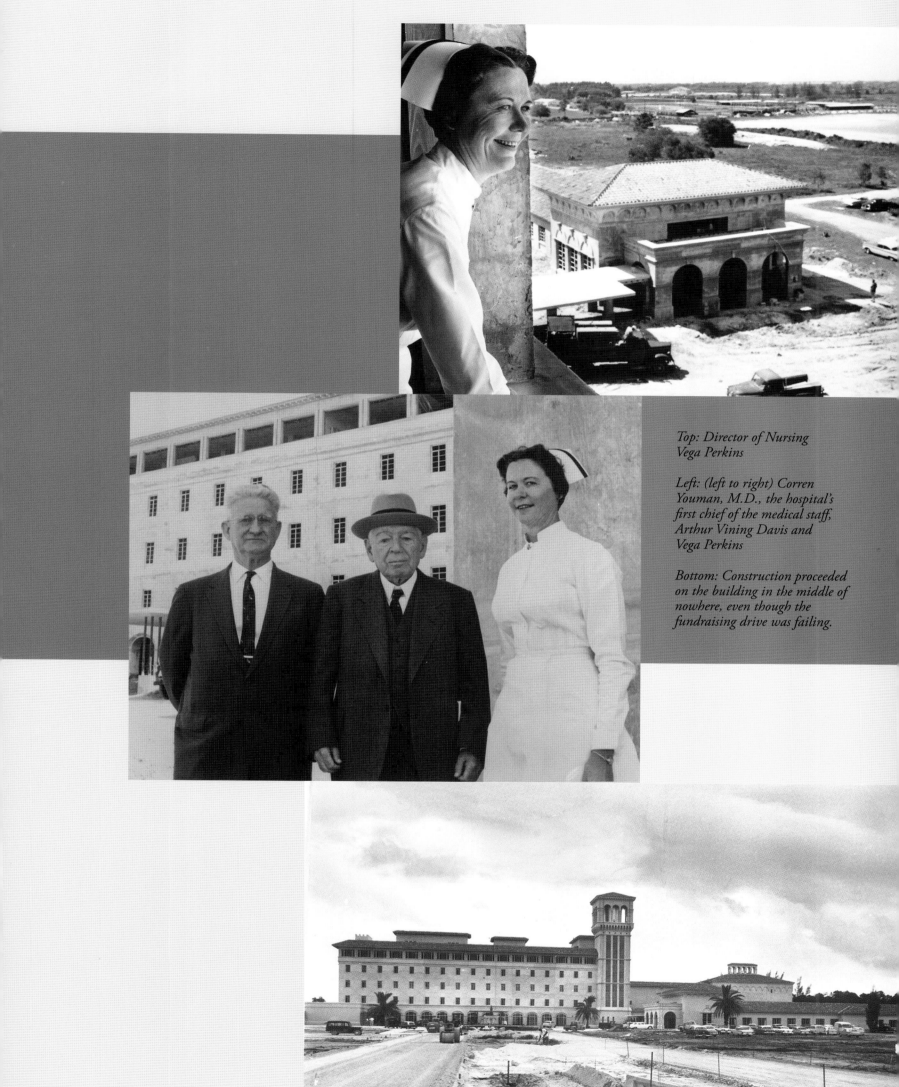

Top: Director of Nursing Vega Perkins

Left: (left to right) Corren Youman, M.D., the hospital's first chief of the medical staff, Arthur Vining Davis and Vega Perkins

Bottom: Construction proceeded on the building in the middle of nowhere, even though the fundraising drive was failing.

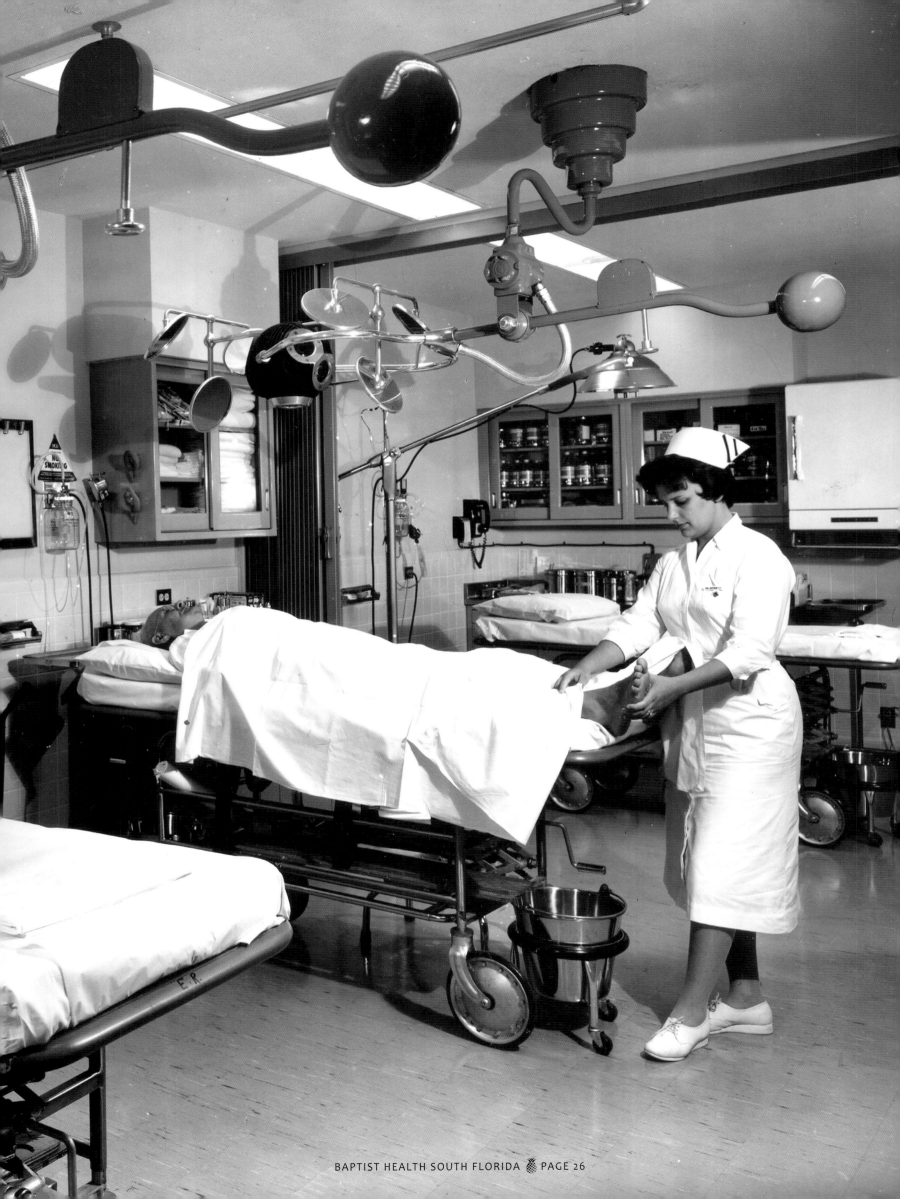

Financial Woes

The initial promise and excitement of the hospital plan were tempered by reality. The fundraising drive stalled. Pledges went unpaid. The Baptists were used to working on a small scale at individual churches and found the larger community more difficult to convince. Perhaps there was also hesitancy about the hospital's out-of-the-way location.

Whatever the reasons, some of the grand plans changed. The architects' original design included a five-story main building with a removable roof that allowed for future expansion. When the money tightened, they permanently limited the hospital to five stories. Arthur Vining Davis donated an additional 12 acres of land in May 1960, but did not increase his financial commitment. By August 1960, only about a third of the needed money had been raised. The association would have to borrow the rest.

When the hospital finally opened to its first patient, Simon Rudin, on November 21, 1960, it had a bit of a makeshift quality. While it was certainly beautiful — adorned with arches, giant windows, pink walls and a red-tiled roof, and featuring two serene lakes stocked with fish — the building was not actually finished. So many construction workers walked the halls that no one was sure who worked for the hospital and who did not. Rocks, rubble, horses and even a few snakes inhabited the surrounding campus.

For those in the trenches caring for patients, the experience was both exciting and humbling. The facility had only 55 available beds. Key equipment had not arrived, including blades for surgical knives, hospital gowns and bedpans. The specimens that doctors collected were stored in mayonnaise jars brought from home and weighed in the hospital's kitchen on food scales.

Employees carried from the hospital's lakes 1,000 gallons of water needed for cleaning. The challenges demanded improvised solutions and created camaraderie and shared purpose. "Now that I think back, there really wasn't any other way to go but up," remembered Marjorie Swenson, then associate director of nursing, on the hospital's fifth anniversary. "From the beginning there was a spirit of a spunky winning team. We scrapped a bit, got discouraged, but hung on."

Part of the problem was the hospital's location. North Kendall Drive was a two-lane, unpaved road in the middle of horse ranches and chicken farms. Patients and employees struggled to reach the hospital. The road was so bumpy that lost hubcaps and flat tires were commonplace. Some ambulance drivers even refused to come to Baptist for fear the turbulent ride would injure their patients. While the building itself was impressive, with its majestic architectural style, it sat isolated in what was still a rural neighborhood. "I thought this hospital had a beauty that gave it more of a hotel appearance," said Mary Kasprak, R.N., reflecting some years after the opening. "But I remember missing a dirt road and getting lost, and never really believing this area would ever amount to anything."

Patients did come but their arrival failed to ease Baptist's financial troubles. Leaders juggled bills and, when possible, put off paying creditors. The situation strained morale and left many wondering if the hospital was salvageable. The Baptist association realized that with the perilous situation in Kendall, any thoughts of a second hospital in downtown Miami were unrealistic. The group successfully negotiated for extensions on their option with the city, postponing action until 1966.

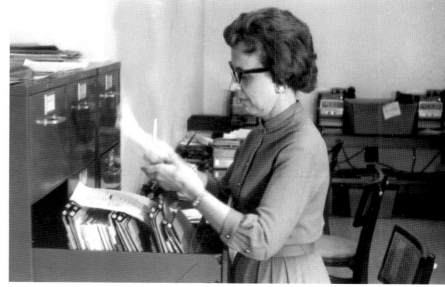

Facing page: Despite the hospital's out-of-the-way location, patients came to Kendall for medical care.

Miriam Pheasant, a coding clerk, 1963

A New Leader and New Hope

In October 1961, as the hospital neared its first anniversary, administrator McCrimmon left. After two interim leaders from Baptist Memorial Hospital in Jacksonville, Ernie Nott Jr. came aboard on March 1, 1962. Nott was an experienced administrator. He had worked at Broward General Hospital as an assistant administrator and later general administrator.

Mr. Nott arrived at a desperate time for the young hospital. During his job interview, Board of Trustees member Miller Walton told Nott that things were as bad as they could get. While Nott entered his first days determined not to be discouraged, he must have wondered what he had gotten himself into. "I lived on the fifth floor of the hospital when I first came to work, because we didn't have patients up there," he recalled years later. "It wasn't open. At night they turned the lights out and it was dark....We were beginning to think we were idiots to be in a hospital way out in the boondocks."

Fortunately for Nott, nowhere was slowly becoming somewhere. On July 16, 1961, the full 24.5 miles of the Palmetto Expressway from Golden Glades to Kendall opened. The highway snaked through some decidedly rural territory. *The Miami Herald* even reported stories of horses trotting on the Palmetto and a nighttime driver striking and killing a cow. South Dade was now more easily accessible. A year later, the 550,000-square-foot shopping mall, Dadeland, opened east of Baptist Hospital on North Kendall Drive. Although some derided the megastructure as "Deadland," its 58 stores, anchored by Burdines, drew shoppers from neighboring communities. Then, in 1964, the state widened North Kendall Drive into a modern, four-lane street. The drive from South Dixie Highway west all the way to Krome Avenue was no longer an adventure. Patients could get to Baptist Hospital quickly and easily.

With these signs of progress, the hospital's bottom line improved. In 1964, Baptist admitted more than 13,000 patients, up from fewer than 10,000 two years earlier. Its average daily patient census reached 209. "Not until this year could our nonprofit hospital corporation finish paying the architects who designed the hospital and delivered the plans and specifications back in 1958," said Miller Walton, who became chairman of the Board of Trustees in 1963. "The hospital still owes a half-million dollars for essential equipment bought on credit... And it still owes a million and a half dollars on mortgage financing... These things may sound discouraging, but there is no reason to be downhearted. Astonishing, unbelievable progress has been made."

The hospital also benefited from the able hand of Ernie Nott. Almost immediately, the young administrator (he was not yet 40 years old when he arrived at Baptist) won over employees and physicians. A Southerner with a keen sense of humor, Nott was approachable, humble and friendly. But along with this easygoing demeanor, Nott was a smart manager. "He understood that you needed to have everyone on board," said Charlotte Dison, R.N., who joined the hospital in 1966 as director of nursing. "He built a team, supported them and allowed them the autonomy to do their jobs. He was not authoritarian."

> "I lived on the fifth floor of the hospital when I first came to work, because we didn't have patients up there. It wasn't open. At night they turned the lights out and it was dark....We were beginning to think we were idiots to be in a hospital way out in the boondocks."
>
> Ernest C. Nott Jr.

Facing page: The Palmetto Expressway snaked through empty acreage west of the city. When it opened in 1961, it provided easy access to South Dade.

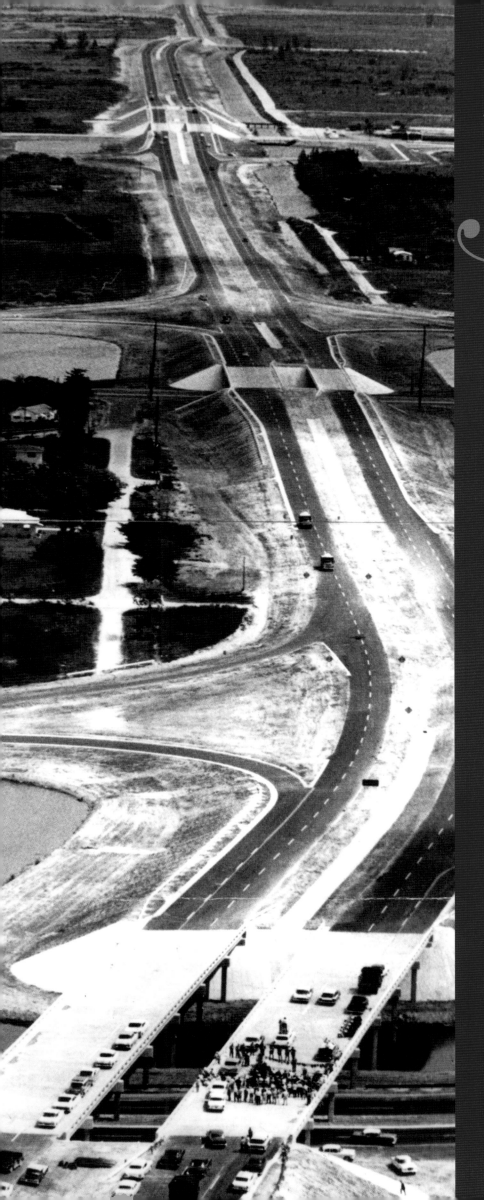

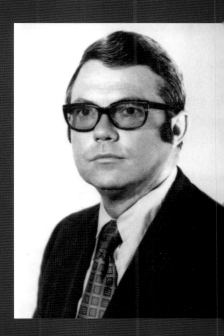

Ernest C. Nott Jr.

In its first decades of operation, one person was the undeniable representative of Baptist Hospital — Ernest C. Nott Jr. A native of Ocala, Florida, Mr. Nott earned a chemistry degree from Wake Forest University in North Carolina and a master's in hospital administration from the Medical College of Virginia. After a stint as an administrative officer during the Korean War, Mr. Nott worked at Broward General Hospital before joining Baptist in 1962. During his more than two decades at the helm, he took the hospital from infancy to maturity.

Nott was affable and charismatic — a man without airs. Each morning he would walk the halls to greet and connect with hospital workers, stopping first in the employees' cafeteria and then the doctors' lounge. The interaction produced ideas and collaboration. "Mr. Nott believed in M.B.W.A., management by walking around," said Brian Keeley, who joined Baptist as an administrative fellow in 1969. "He had a meaningful connection with employees, and I learned from him how important that was."

Mr. Nott brought an easy charm to the challenges of growing the hospital. Every bit a Southern gentleman and devout Baptist who saw his job as a calling, he could also be informal and fun-loving. With folksy warmth, Mr. Nott might break the mood of a serious discussion by uttering the catchphrase, "and that's how the cow eats cabbage."

The levity, however, did not obscure Mr. Nott's business acumen. By the time he retired in 1986, Baptist Hospital had recovered from near bankruptcy and matured into a thriving medical center. Mr. Nott died in 2001 in Ormond Beach, Florida.

Under the popular Nott, the situation at Baptist Hospital stabilized. The hospital leadership was confident in Baptist's viability and turned its attention to developing the downtown Miami site. The task proved difficult and controversial. The land, initially optioned for $88,000, could now garner in excess of $500,000 on the open market. If Baptist exercised its option, the county stood to lose several hundred thousand dollars.

In a tension-filled meeting on November 30, 1965, the County Commission voted to cancel the hospital's right to the 10-acre tract. It justified the action by a loophole — Baptist paid the county $1,000 for the initial option but never for the additional extensions. Miller Walton received word of the commission's action and quickly sent a cashier's check via registered mail for the total land price. But the county attorney ruled that the check was only good if it had been mailed before the vote was taken. It turned out that Walton was about 30 minutes too late. Baptist Hospital no longer had a claim on the downtown Miami site.

The loss of the second location, although disappointing, especially given the strange circumstances, strengthened the Kendall campus. The Baptist Association and hospital team could turn their attention and talents to the existing hospital.

The leaders focused on building up Baptist Hospital. In early 1966, the hospital took a tentative step toward expansion with a 90-seat chapel. The Women's Auxiliary worked for three years to raise the $110,000 needed to build the sanctuary. The Pink Ladies, as they were called, ran a hospitality shop and gift cart, offered cradle pictures and signed up more and more members.

As the hospital completed its sixth year of operation in a growing community, Ernie Nott and the Board began to look to what was next.

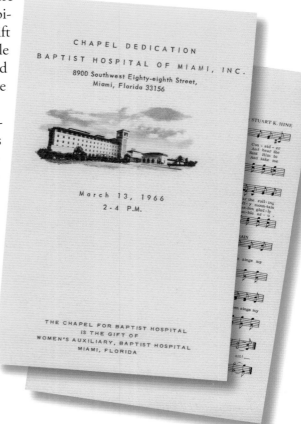

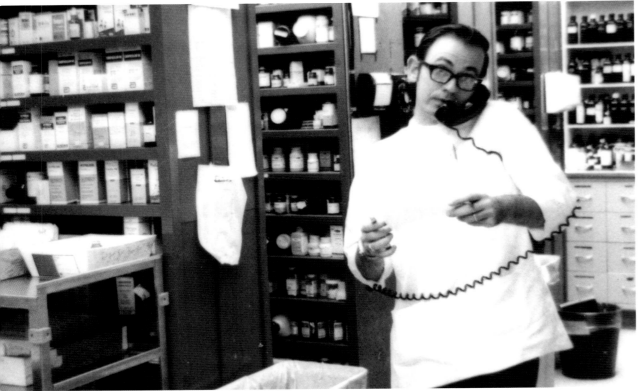

Above: The Baptist Hospital Chapel opened in March 1966. The Women's Auxiliary raised the funds for its completion.

Left: The Baptist pharmacy handled the medicines for the hospital.

1964

Baptist Hospital...
LOOKING BACK

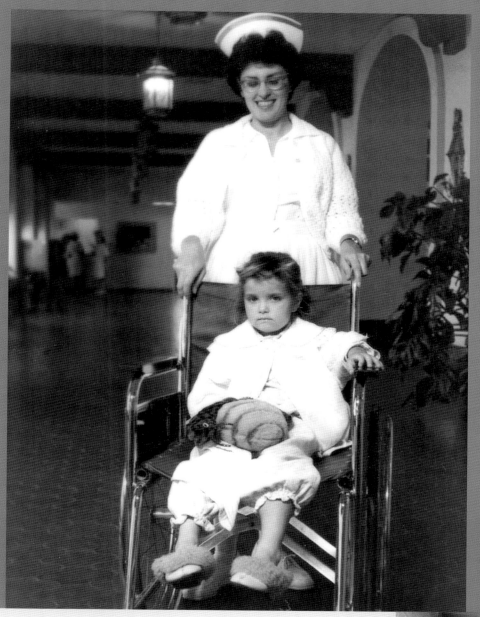

Excellence in Pediatrics

Baptist Hospital's second patient was a young girl who broke her arm playing kickball. Her arrival signaled a lasting focus for the hospital — pediatric care. By 1964, countless children with broken bones, inflamed tonsils and ruptured appendixes had come to Baptist Hospital for treatment.

The tradition continues today with Baptist Children's Hospital, founded in 1997. In 2009, the team at the hospital within a hospital performed more than 1,100 inpatient and outpatient surgeries. There were more than 22,000 visits to the Emergency Department. With more than 200 pediatricians and pediatric specialists on staff, the hospital handles most everything, from the minor injuries and illnesses of childhood to life-threatening cancers.

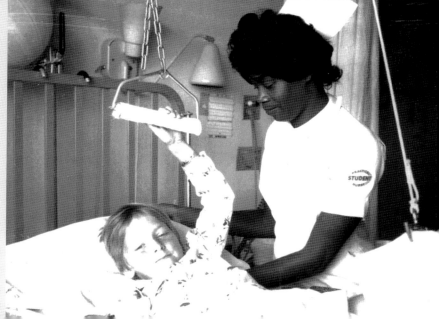

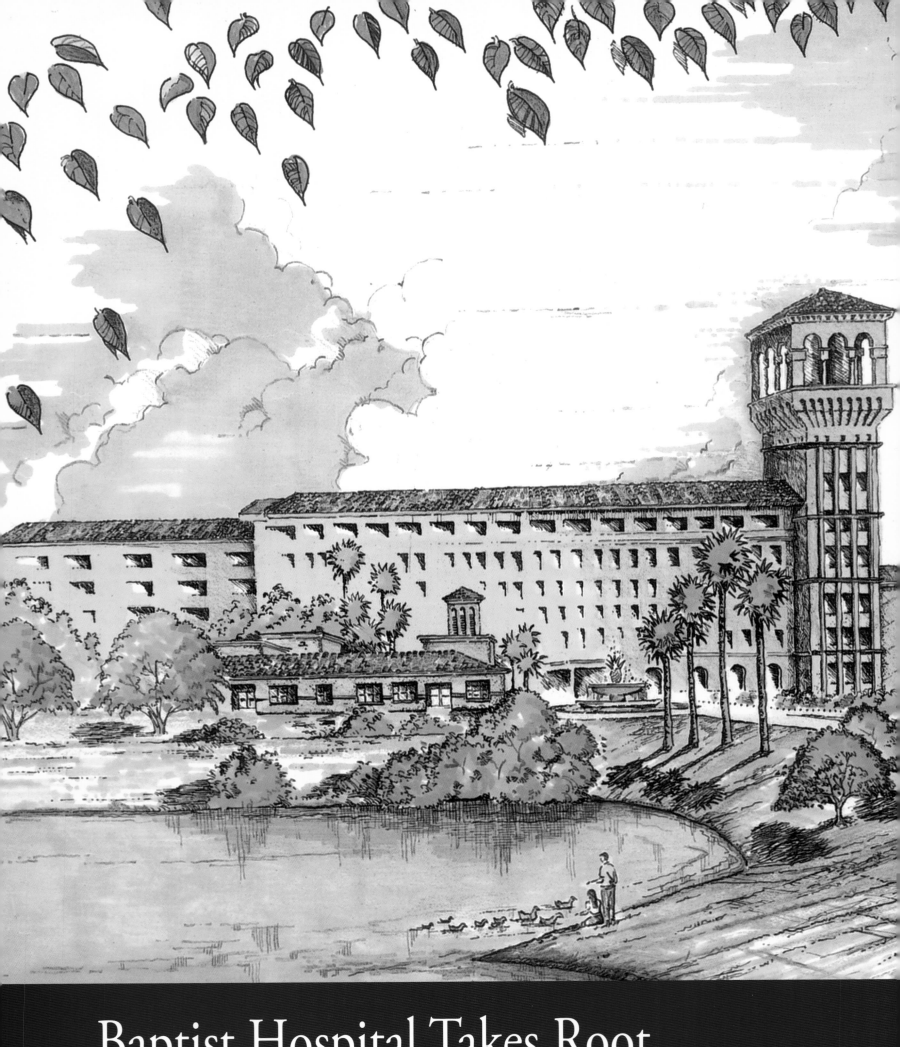

Baptist Hospital Takes Root

This artist's rendering showed the Baptist Hospital campus.

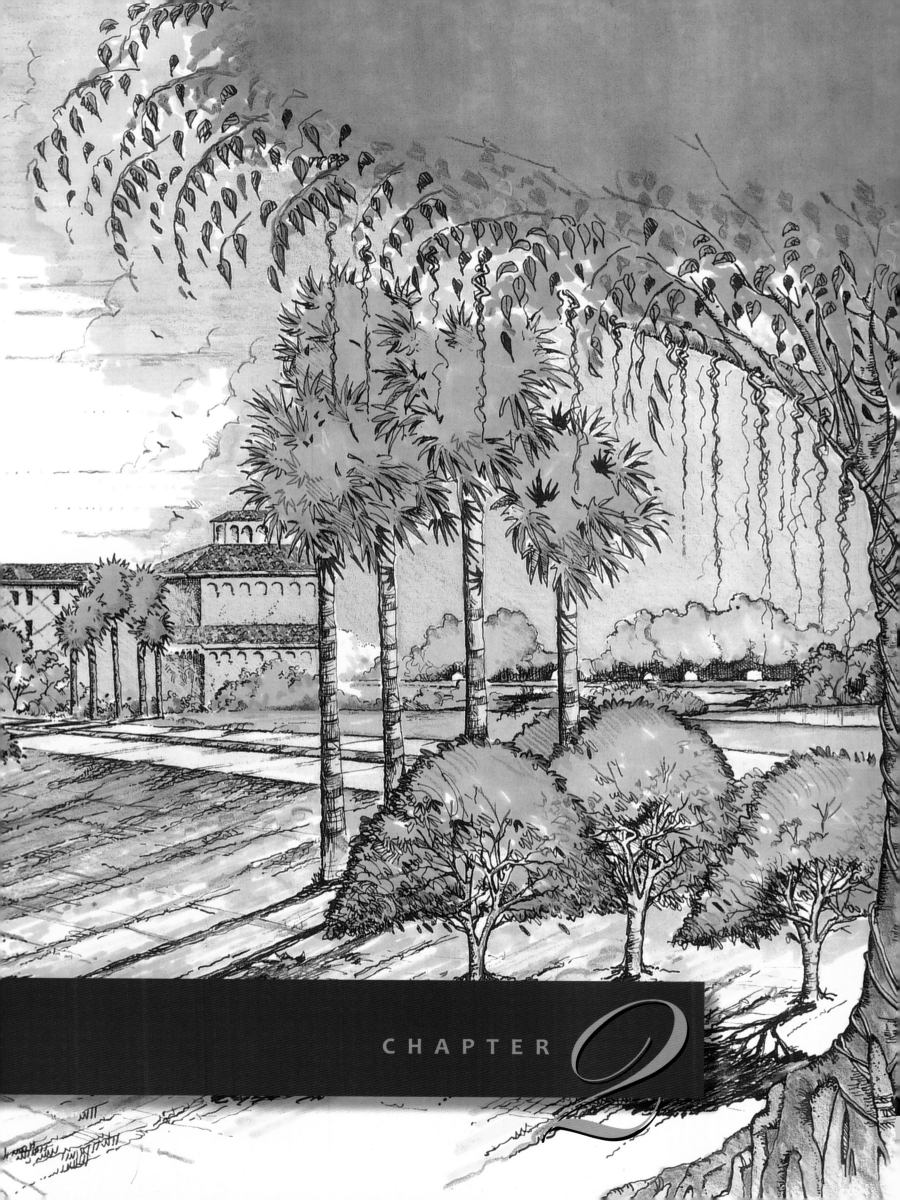

CHAPTER *2*

"Still but a youth and immature in many ways with a young staff and young administration, Baptist Hospital suddenly found itself with a new crisis. The sudden, explosive-like growth in the community posed heavy burdens for such a youth to shoulder. The problem at first was too large a facility, too small the demand. Reversed, the crisis became too large a demand, too small the necessary space to meet that demand."

The Rev. Dr. George W. Miller
Chaplain, Baptist Hospital
1970

South Florida's dramatic growth, particularly in the Kendall area, proved to be both a blessing and a problem for the young hospital. The everyday struggle for survival was over. With 306 beds, the hospital often operated at more than 90 percent capacity, but the demand stretched personnel and resources thin. The issue was not unique to Baptist Hospital. Throughout Dade County, hospitals overflowed with patients. Newspaper accounts described corridors lined with beds, emergency rooms flooded with people needing care and limited equipment. In fact, county officials estimated that by 1975, the community would need at least 1,000 additional beds to adequately serve residents.

The leaders at Baptist Hospital recognized they had to expand. For a hospital inching its way into the black financially and with some leftover debt from its first days, the question became one of money. Just how would the hospital, and its governing Miami Baptist Association, fund the expansion?

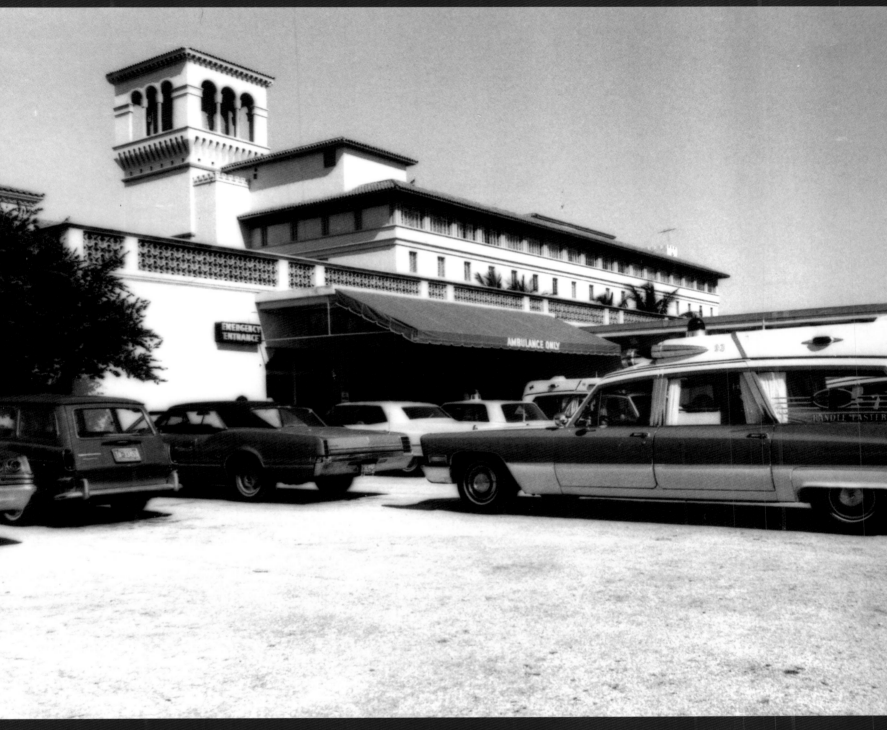

By 1968, the Kendall area was a thriving community. The residents looked to Baptist Hospital for all their healthcare needs. It became one of the busiest hospitals in South Florida.

A Change in Structure

The Miami Baptist Association started and supported the hospital through donations. As a religious organization, it worked independently of government and believed strongly that any connection with government finances would violate the principle of the separation of church and state. With Baptist Hospital considering a major building project, hospital leaders were in a bind. Because of its ties to the Baptists, the hospital could not seek federal funds, and the Association did not have the money to finance the expansion.

The next step was necessary but painful — especially for those pastors who nurtured the hospital from its infancy. In a 1967 meeting of the Miami Baptist Association, the group, after prolonged debate and an earlier failed attempt at separation, allowed the hospital to become independent. "Baptists have frowned on receipt of federal funds by organizations they sponsor and are legally

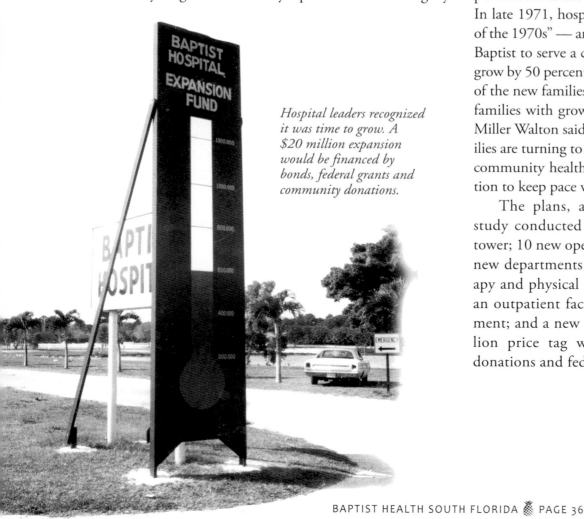

Hospital leaders recognized it was time to grow. A $20 million expansion would be financed by bonds, federal grants and community donations.

bound to," said the Rev. Dr. Conrad Willard, who had succeeded Dr. Angell as pastor at Central Baptist Church. "But it was also felt that further expansion would be needed by the hospital. This would mean the need for more funds, which the Association could not provide."

The separation left hard feelings. During the debate, the Rev. Jim Silver suggested turning the hospital over to Dade County, believing "it can give more public service than a private institution." Another pastor wanted to remove the name "Baptist" from the hospital, permanently distancing it from any religious origin. The ideas never gained traction but they did indicate how contentious the issue was. Ernie Nott, a Bible teacher and deacon at Wayside Baptist Church, remembered the bitter issue almost splitting the Association.

However difficult the separation was, the independent status allowed the hospital to move forward. In late 1971, hospital leaders announced "Progress of the 1970s" — an expansion that would transform Baptist to serve a community that was predicted to grow by 50 percent within the next 10 years. "Many of the new families moving into this area are young families with growing children," Board Chairman Miller Walton said at the time. "Most of these families are turning to Baptist Hospital as their primary community health facility, and we have an obligation to keep pace with their needs."

The plans, an outgrowth of a long-range study conducted in 1967, included a new bed tower; 10 new operating rooms; a new laboratory; new departments for radiology, respiratory therapy and physical therapy; an ICU with 16 beds; an outpatient facility; a new emergency department; and a new pharmacy. The nearly $20 million price tag would be financed by bonds, donations and federal grants.

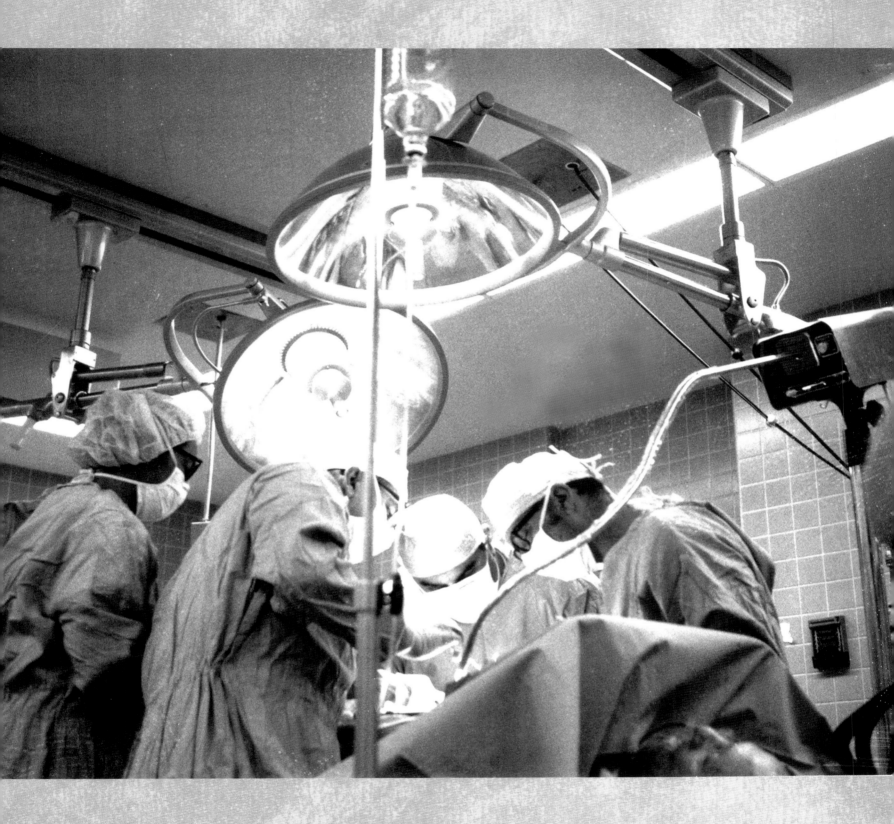

"*Many of the new families moving into this area are young families with growing children. Most of these families are turning to Baptist Hospital as their primary community health facility, and we have an obligation to keep pace with their needs.*"

Miller Walton
Chairman of the Board
Baptist Hospital

PROGRESS

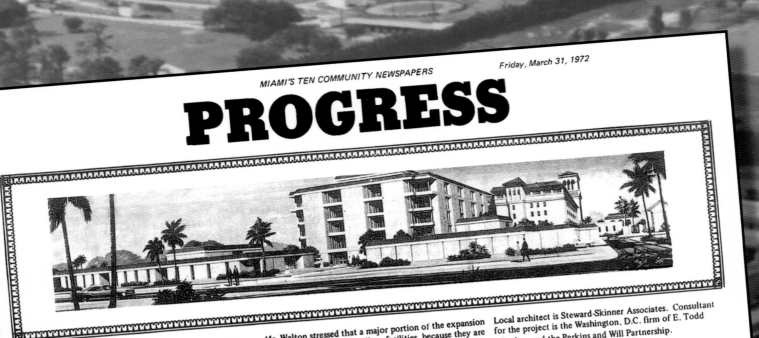

A $16,000,000 expansion and renovation program that will almost double the size of Baptist Hospital of Miami has been announced by Miller Walton, Chairman of the Board of Trustees. The hospital is located at 8900 Southwest 88th Street.

A new four-story patient tower with 216 new beds will be located to the east of the existing hospital bringing the total bed capacity to 510. The Baptist Hospital program will help fill a shortage of beds that the Hospital Planning Council of South Florida has found to exist in the fastgrowing South Dade area.

Mr. Walton stressed that a major portion of the expansion will be involved with the ancillary facilities, because they are overworked now and cannot support the additional beds. Ten new operating rooms will be provided, in addition to new facilities for recovery, laboratory, radiology, respiratory, therapy, emergency, outpatients, physical therapy, pharmacy, electrocardiology and anesthesia. Space vacated in the existing building will be used to expand and renovate maintenance, administrative and food service facilities.

Hospital Administrator Ernest C. Nott, Jr. said site preparation is under way, and construction will start early in 1972.

Local architect is Steward-Skinner Associates. Consultant for the project is the Washington, D.C. firm of E. Todd Wheeler and the Perkins and Will Partnership.

Mr. Walton said $14,700,000 of the total needed for the program will be made available through long-term financing, a federal grant, and annual improvement and replacement funds. A public campaign will be undertaken to raise the remaining $1,300,000, he said.

"In 1970, we admitted more than 15,000. Every category of service that we perform has climbed just as dramatically."

SOME INTERESTING FACTS ABOUT 1971

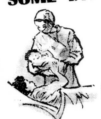

Births—2,013
Average per day—6

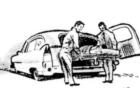

Emergency Dept. Visits—31,865
Out Patient Vists—13,728

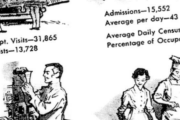

Admissions—15,552
Average per day—43

Average Daily Census—272
Percentage of Occupancy—90%

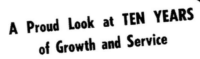

Radiological Exams.—60,535
Isotope Exams.—3,202

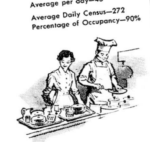

Medications Dispensed—
(Doses) 900,100

Meals served to patients—267,000

BAPTIST HOSPITAL

Proud of the Past

Looks to the Future

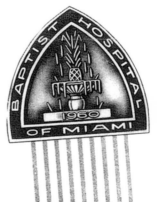

QUEST
FOR
QUALITY

1960

A Proud Look at TEN YEARS of Growth and Service

Another milestone in the growth of the South Dade area was reached in mid-November, 1960 with the opening of Baptist Hospital of Miami. This modern, life-preserving facility featured modern concepts in patient care skillfully blended with personalized attention.

Growth of Baptist Hospital has been tremendous and the list of accomplishments impressive—the addition of a physical therapy department, a medical/surgical intensive care unit, a chaplaincy program with two full-time chaplains, a hospital chapel-auditorium, a six-bed intensive coronary care unit, a respiratory therapy department, expanded radiology facilities and others.

Besides new facilities and services there have been other noteworthy achievements—full three-year accreditations by the Joint Commission on Accreditation of Hospitals; affiliation with the Miami-Dade Junior College, South nursing program; development of hospital staff members through special inservice training and management courses, just to name a few!

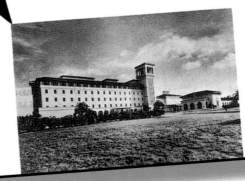

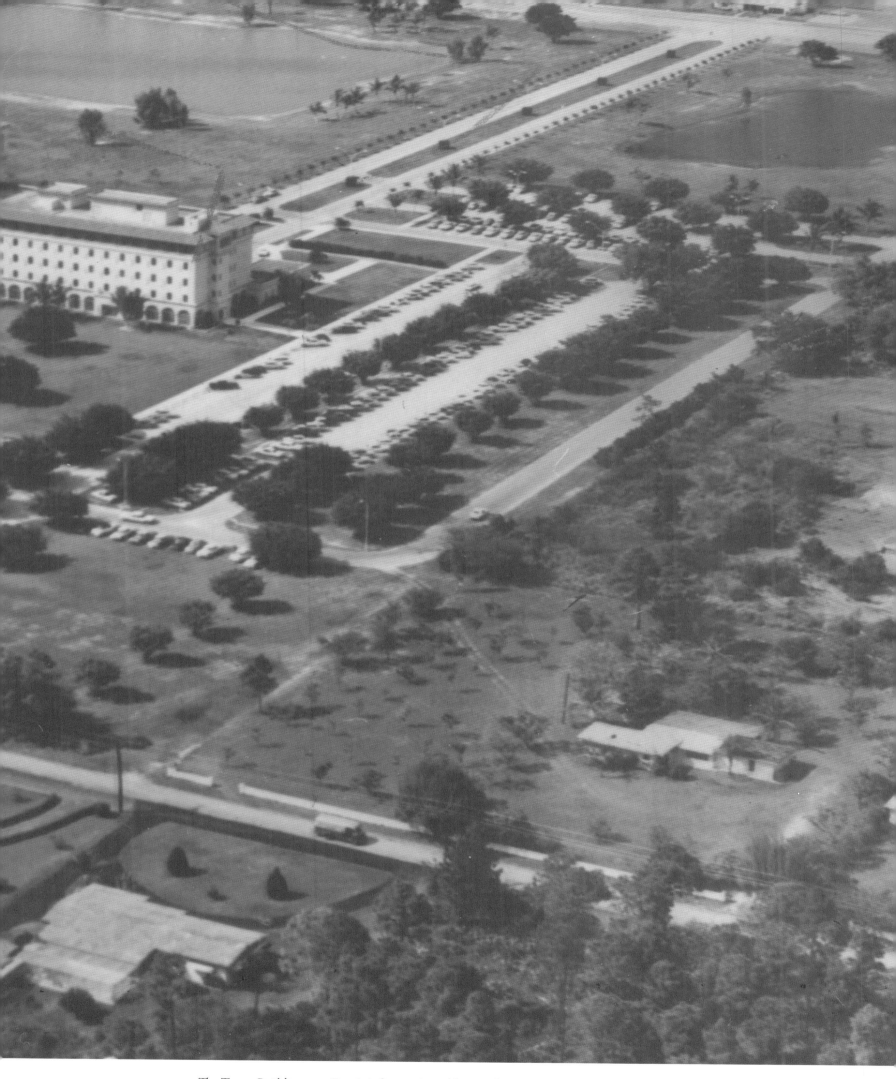

The Tower Building was Baptist's first major addition. Controversy arose over its original design, which the Board felt was too plain and not in harmony with the more elegant original hospital building. The design was ultimately changed.

The sights and sounds of progress — jackhammers, bulldozers and construction workers — became as much a part of the scene as patients and medical tests. The employee newsletter featured regular updates about area closures and department relocations, but the hospital continued to thrive. "Our dust, noise and confusion is a pathway to progress," Ernie Nott reassured.

The employees were among the hospital's biggest boosters and felt the impact of construction more than others. "A solid show of support from [the Baptist family] will demonstrate to others that those closest to the hospital believe the program is worthwhile," Nott said. "There is no better endorsement." During the initial stages of the fundraising drive, employees rallied behind the cause. Within three months, they donated nearly $100,000, more than 80 percent of their goal. The response was so strong that the usually lighthearted Ernie Nott struggled to express his appreciation. During a fundraising meeting in the Chapel, his voice broke with emotion when he reviewed the total.

On August 25, 1974, more than 500 people toured the new patient tower at an open house. The crowd feasted on a cake — a sweet replica of the expanded hospital. The addition's 156,000 square feet doubled Baptist's size. The bed total reached 326 with plans to grow to 525 within four years. Private room rates hit $85 a day, with semi-private rooms costing between $67 and $75.

Hospital leaders were careful to celebrate the growth with an eye toward the patient. They understood that while the hospital could get bigger, it could not lose its personal feel. "Surely we have the finest of equipment and accommodations.... But now comes the dedication, the skill, the concern, the personal touch of people who, in the final analysis, will determine to what extent we shall be better," said Rev. Miller. "If being bigger does not guarantee being better, then it also is true that being small and cramped for space and needed equipment does not make for better service."

With that in mind, Baptist began tangibly measuring the quality of patient care. Patients received questionnaires asking them to evaluate everything from food to nursing to housekeeping. The purpose, Assistant Administrator Fred Messing explained in the employee newsletter, "was to pinpoint problem areas and implement changes where indicated."

As the patient tower opened, more improvements followed. The new surgical area created a roomier and more cheerful environment, and featured an updated paging system and the latest equipment. As a result, the number of surgical cases increased by 1,000 patients, reaching nearly 8,000 in 1975. The next year, the Center for Rehabilitation Services opened in the renovated Davis Pavilion. With the model of integrated patient care as its foundation — from medical needs to vocational and family counseling — it offered a broad range of services. Improvements came to other areas as well, including the nursery and obstetrical suites, dining room and pediatrics.

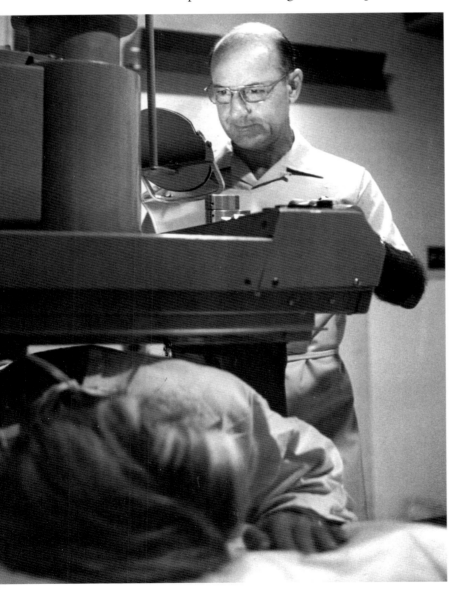

Radiology department head Oliver Winslow, M.D., is pictured fluoroscoping a patient's stomach, looking for a possible ulcer.

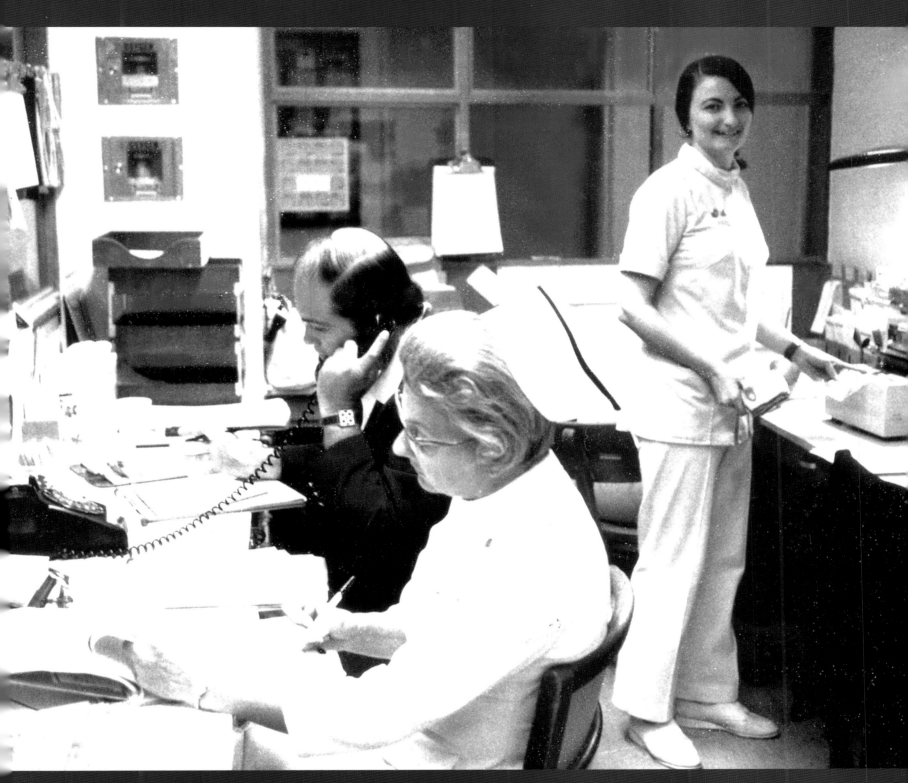

The nurses' station was the center of activity.
Barbara Russell, R.N., (standing) worked alongside
Mary Davis, R.N., and Richard Glatzer, M.D.

The Baptist Way

It was certainly boom-time conditions for the hospital, and the atmosphere was markedly different from just a decade earlier. In February 1969, Brian Keeley came to Baptist Hospital as an administrative fellow. The Ohio native had earned his bachelor's degree from Miami University in Ohio and was working toward his master's degree in health administration at George Washington University. As part of his graduate studies, Mr. Keeley came to Baptist for a year to work with Ernie Nott and observe the ins and outs of running a hospital. More of an internship than a job, he earned $2.50 an hour during his 12-month residency.

Mr. Keeley remembered arriving in South Florida and driving up North Kendall Drive for the first time. "There was really very little beyond S.W. 107th Avenue," he said. "Here was Baptist — a big building in the middle of a huge piece of property with very little landscaping — and it felt almost like we were in the Sahara Desert. I remember see-ing signs advertising Kendale Lakes and thinking, who was going to live out there?"

Keeley returned to Baptist in 1973 as an assistant administrator and noticed the transformation. "It was obvious then that this was a booming area," he said. "The hospital was right in the middle of it and there was an opportunity to really grow. We were attracting more doctors and developing more services. It was exciting."

Along with the expansion, a discernible Baptist culture emerged — salient features of a place that was beginning to mature. With its deep Baptist roots, the hospital was a disciplined organization. Mr. Keeley remembered arriving at a meeting with Board Chairman Miller Walton and member Robert B. Cole a few minutes late. The two men, both known for their quiet strength and the power of their unspoken words, glared at the young administrator, making clear their expectations. "I remember almost immediately being struck by the formality of the Board," Keeley said. "There was a clear understanding that those at the hospital needed to be prepared and disciplined. Someone did not offer an opinion unless he knew what he was talking about. Every idea went through a rigorous process before moving forward."

Perhaps owing to the precarious nature of its founding, hospital leaders acted very conservatively when it came to money. "We had some superb business leaders on the Board. Both Miller Walton and Robert Cole were extremely successful lawyers and we had business owners, bankers and real estate developers," Keeley said. "They all kept an eye on the bottom line."

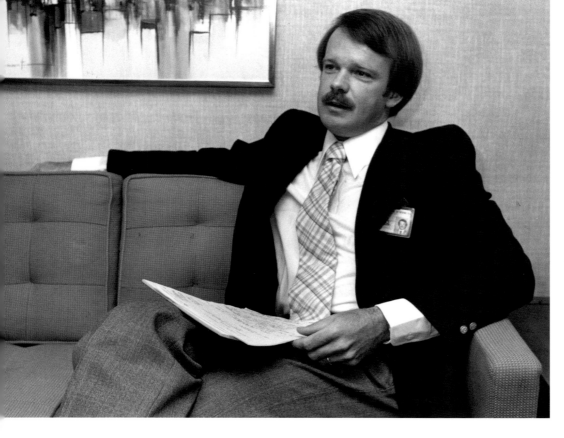

Brian E. Keeley came to Baptist Hospital in 1969. He served as an administrative fellow while working toward his master's degree in health administration.

While the Board set the tone for fiscal responsibility and discipline, Ernie Nott used his considerable people skills to create an employee-friendly workplace. He valued the bedside caregivers for their integral role in developing and maintaining the hospital's reputation. Baptist became known as a progressive workplace. Employees received financial incentives to further their training. Suggestions were rewarded with cash bonuses, and promotions were an important part of career paths. "There was a real sense that Baptist was a place to stay at as an employee," said Diane Bolton, R.N., who was hired in 1969. In fact, Ms. Bolton was on her way to working at Mercy Hospital in Coconut Grove when she stopped by an open house at Baptist. "I was immediately attracted to how favorable the environment was to nurses. There was an employee nursery, and it was open until midnight, so we could work the 3 p.m. until 11 p.m. shift. This was great because I had twin babies. Nurses were given a priority." The nursery had opened in 1964 and, at the time, Baptist was one of the few businesses offering such a benefit.

Nott also recognized that alongside the employees, the physicians were key to running a successful hospital. Physicians were in a unique position. They were not employed by the hospital but had to be integrated within it. They needed to be satisfied with its day-to-day operations. "Ernie Nott believed that the doctors were our customers. They brought us our patients," Keeley said. "We had to collaborate with them. He was always responsive to the physicians. He had an open door and was available to hear their concerns. It was the art to the science of medicine."

The attitude paid off for the administrator, hospital and surrounding community. The doctors were on the front line, supporting and promoting Baptist. Naturally, they were drawn by demographics, the impressive physical plant and new technology. But they also found a supportive leadership team. "We had a cohesive medical staff," said Sol Colsky, M.D., who arrived at Baptist in 1960 and served as chief of staff from 1974 to 1977. "We required the best in equipment and services and the Board of Trustees and administration gave us that. If we presented Ernie with an idea, he was receptive. It was a very collegial environment."

Beyond the tangibles — workplace benefits and a satisfied medical staff — the employees had fun. Activities promoted camaraderie. There were bowling leagues, picnics, softball teams and annual lawnmower races where employees raced their home machines across Baptist's sprawling grounds. Departments engaged in spirited competitions to raise money for community causes and celebrate holidays. "We enjoyed an atmosphere of togetherness," said JoAnn Crebbin, R.N., a nurse who cared for the first patient and worked at Baptist for 32 years. "We were close, more like brothers and sisters. It was a fun place to go to work every day."

Resource magazine, produced by the Marketing & Public Relations Department, premiered in 1975. Three years later, Jo Baxter took over as the magazine's editor. She has continued overseeing the award-winning publication for more than three decades. In 2010, the quarterly magazine reached 425,000 South Florida homes.

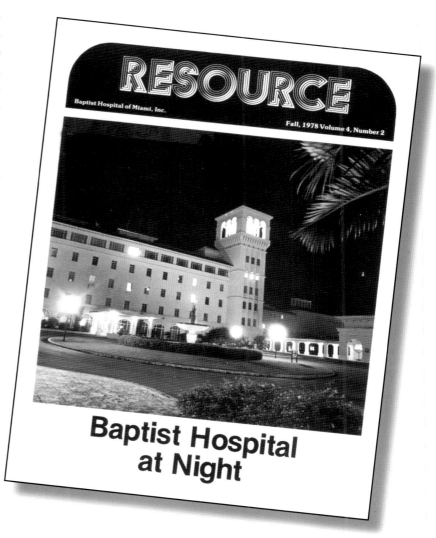

RESOURCE

Baptist Hospital of Miami, Inc.

Fall, 1978 Volume 4, Number 2

Baptist Hospital at Night

Groundbreakings Galore

As the 1970s ended, the hospital Board of Trustees approved a long-range plan, dubbed "Project 1980." The study examined current healthcare trends, including patient census fluctuations, inpatient and outpatient numbers and treatments, as well as demographic data such as population and residential building. The resulting plan would guide the hospital through the next decade and ensure that the future growth fit in with community needs.

One groundbreaking after another occurred as the hospital added services, buildings and technologies. The study predicted a dramatic increase in the demand for outpatient services. Due in part to advances in medical technology and changes in insurance payments, physicians began performing more procedures in an outpatient setting. From 1976 to 1977, Baptist's general surgery numbers grew by several percentage points, while the outpatient surgery load increased 96 percent.

To handle the shifting numbers, phase one of the plan called for a new outpatient procedure suite that included endoscopy services, ambulatory surgery and a minor surgery treatment area for "lumps and bumps." In addition, phase one would replace an outdated and inadequate critical care area with a new 40-bed Concentrated Care Center that would also house a cardiac catheterization laboratory, cardiovascular diagnostic center, cardiac rehabilitation, and a community and health education area. The total cost of the building was more than $9 million.

In April 1982, the 63,000-square-foot, two-story South Building opened. Beyond the variety of outpatient services, the building completely transformed how Baptist cared for the critically ill. The old setup was crowded with 24 beds and narrow hallways. "We were constantly playing musical beds," said Andrew Piergeorge, M.D., the coordinator of critical care medicine. "We would have to

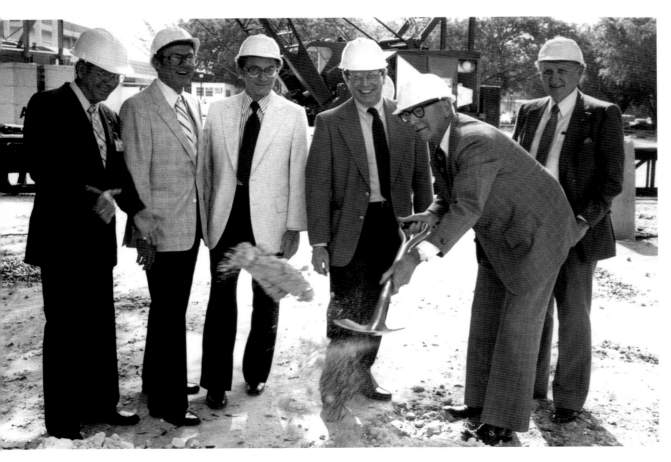

More than 200 people attended the groundbreaking ceremony on June 18, 1980, for the Concentrated Care Center. Board of Trustees Vice Chairman Robert B. Cole ceremonially tossed some dirt on the site with the same gold shovel used for the hospital's groundbreaking in 1958. Other hospital leaders who participated in the event were (left to right) Chaplain George W. Miller; Ernie Nott, executive director; Andrew Piergeorge, M.D., coordinator of critical care medicine; Eugene Bloom, M.D., chief of staff; and Board member William Scharrer.

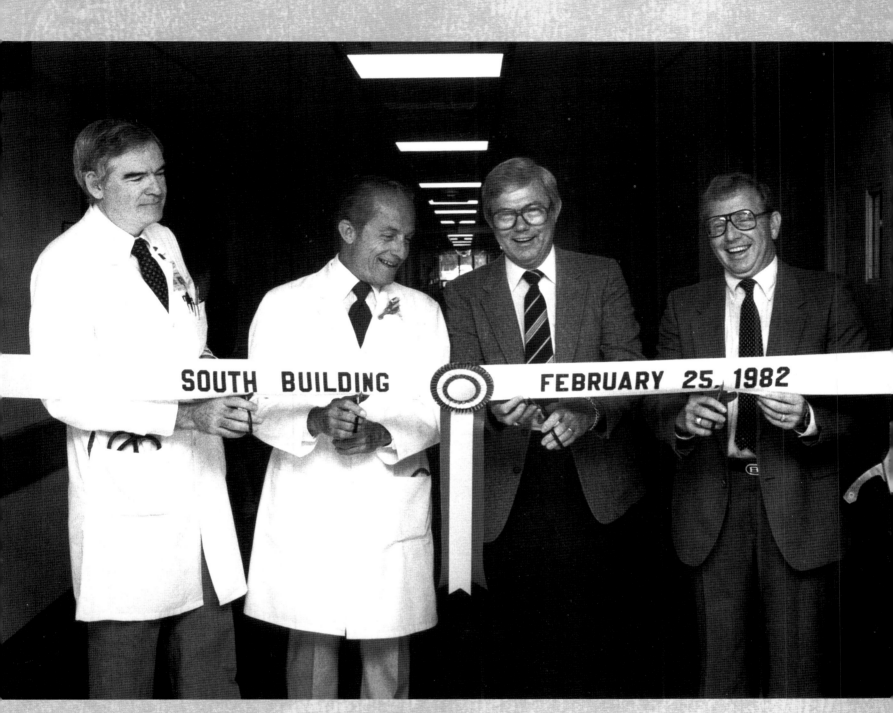

SOUTH BUILDING ⬤ FEBRUARY 25, 1982

With sharpened scissors and skillful hands, (left to right) Thomas Noto, M.D., medical director of the Cardiovascular Lab, Dr. Piergeorge, Ernie Nott and Dr. Bloom cut the ribbon for the open house of the Concentrated Care Center and South Building.

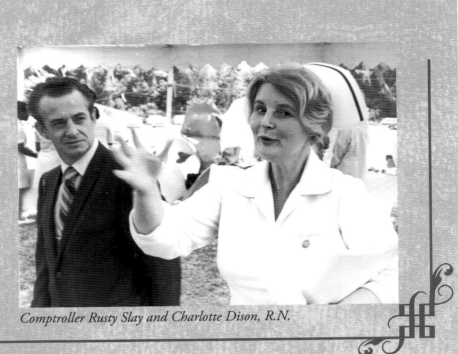

Comptroller Rusty Slay and Charlotte Dison, R.N.

move patients out of critical care to make room for sicker patients." The new center solved the issue of space with 40 beds equipped for a range of care, large rooms measuring 15 square feet (replacing the old 11-square-foot rooms) and a pod-like arrangement that allowed the medical staff to move freely and efficiently. In another design improvement, the bed was placed in the center of the room to provide access to the patient from all directions.

The new building exemplified the careful planning that characterized Baptist Hospital. It reflected both the current trends in medical care and future demands. It was "oriented less to what is happening today and tomorrow and more to the healthcare services that will be needed by our community throughout the 1980s," Mr. Keeley said at its opening.

The organization grew thoughtfully and purposefully in other ways. In May 1982, the hospital opened a new Cancer Treatment Center, the only radiation therapy facility between Mercy Hospital and Key West. A year later, workers put the finishing touches on a 7,400-square-foot child care center, complete with skylights and an Italian Renaissance facade. The building almost tripled the capacity of the older facility, a testament to a workforce that was more than 80 percent women.

Construction also began on an expanded Emergency Department, which doubled the size of what had become one of Baptist's most active areas. In 1980, more than 30,000 patients visited the emergency room, ranking it second busiest in the county behind Jackson Memorial Hospital. Planners predicted that the number could reach 40,000 within a few years. Completed in May 1985, the $2.3 million center included 20 treatment rooms, an X-ray room and a communications room with two-way radios. The same year, the hospital renovated the South Building by enlarging its second floor and adding a third story.

During the 1980s, Baptist enjoyed a renaissance. What was once a community hospital burgeoned into a thriving medical center, with state-of-the-art buildings and a range of sophisticated services, including cancer treatment and a newly created Diabetes Care Center. The decade brought innovation as well. Baptist became the first hospital in South Florida to offer home visits for rehabilitation and maternity patients after they left the hospital. "There was a real sense that we were on the cutting edge," said Charlotte Dison, R.N., chief nursing officer. "We were proud of all that was happening. We were eagerly looking to the future and what it would bring."

Facing page: Ernie Nott had some help at the June 30, 1982, groundbreaking for the hospital's new child care center. The $700,000 building — complete with skylights and classic Italian Renaissance features — opened a year later.

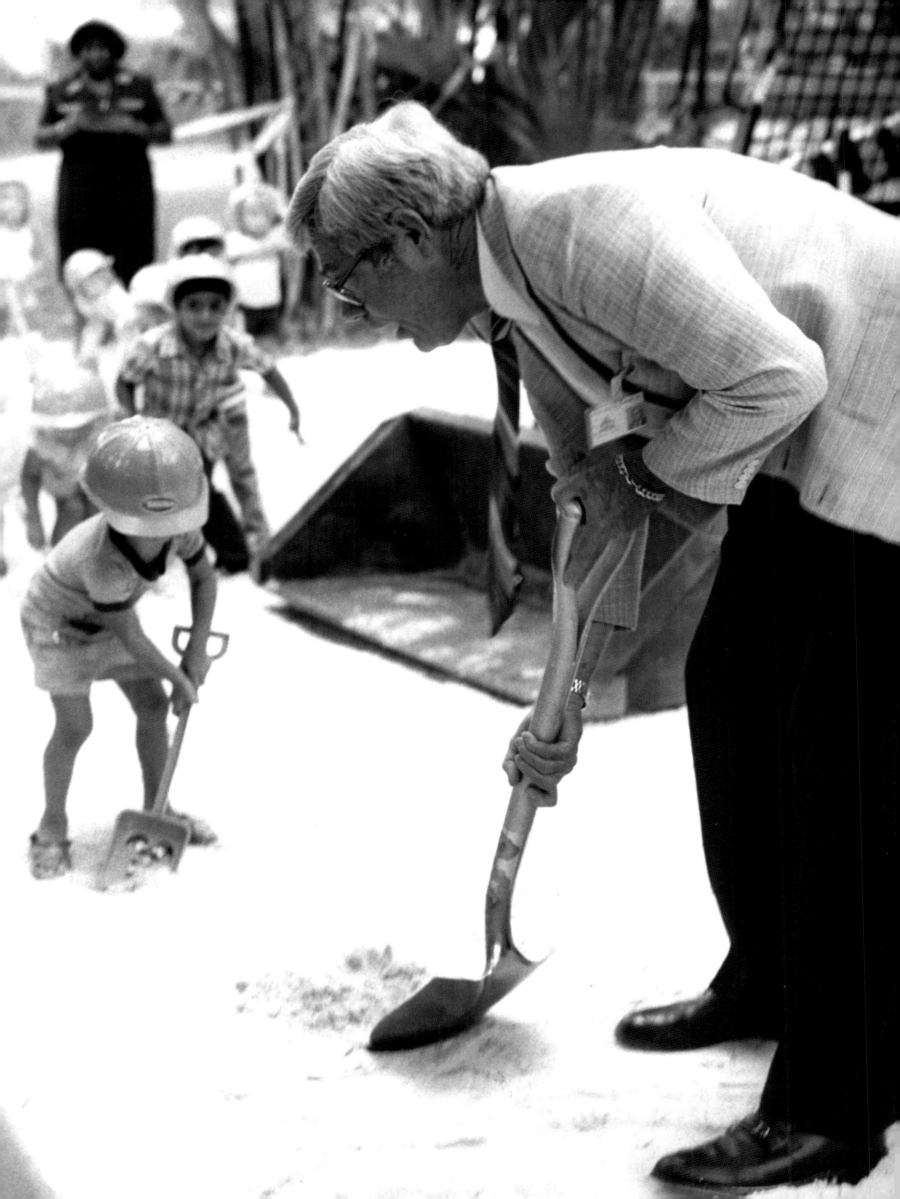

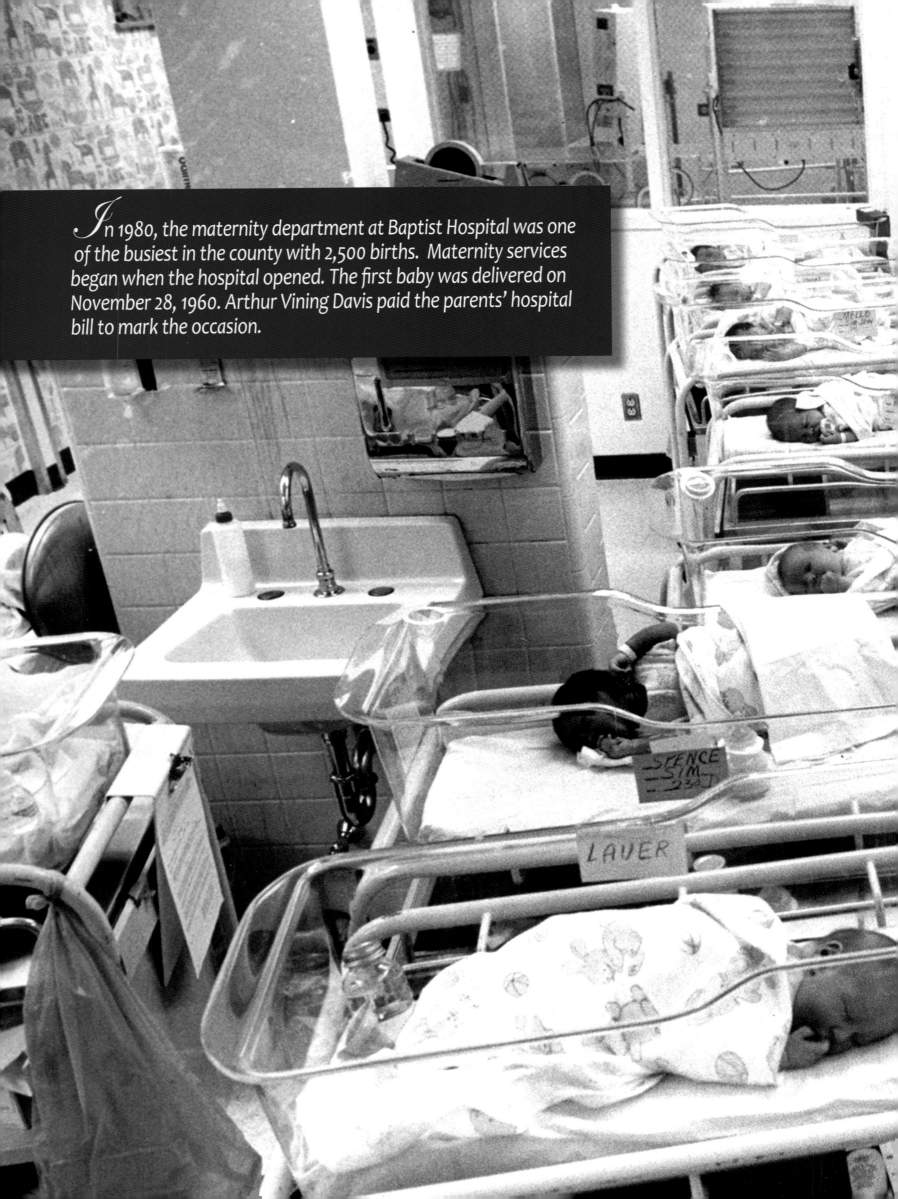

In 1980, the maternity department at Baptist Hospital was one of the busiest in the county with 2,500 births. Maternity services began when the hospital opened. The first baby was delivered on November 28, 1960. Arthur Vining Davis paid the parents' hospital bill to mark the occasion.

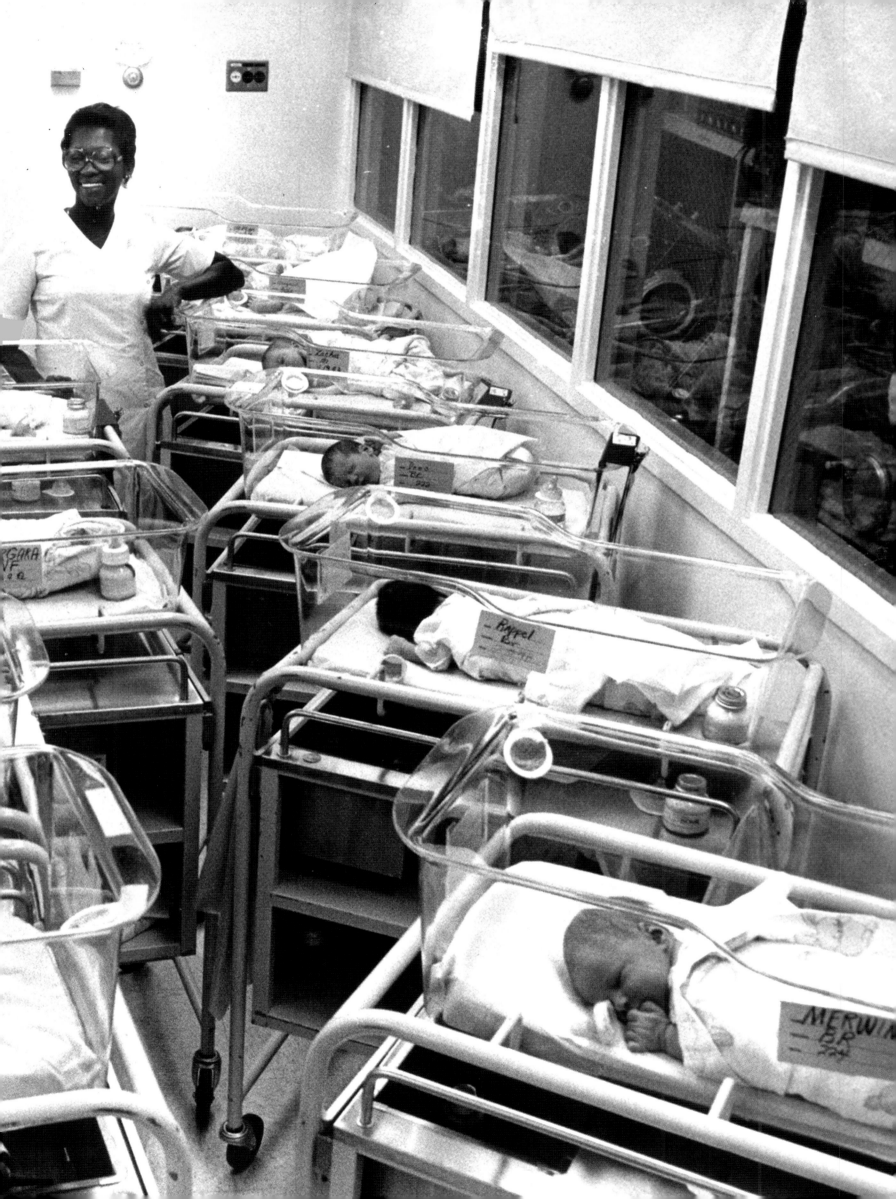

Troubling Trends

In the middle of this exciting time at Baptist Hospital, the national medical community was in a state of upheaval. Managed care with its accompanying acronyms, HMO (health maintenance organization) and PPO (preferred provider organization), was becoming part of the landscape. The public was digesting the changes, including an increase in insurance premiums. The government added to the confusion by overhauling the Medicare system in 1983. Enacted in 1965, Medicare traditionally paid hospitals and doctors for the cost of the services delivered to enrolled patients, typically citizens over the age of 65. As costs began to spiral, reaching $70 billion for Medicare payments alone in 1983, the government adjusted the reimbursement formula. With the change, Medicare paid the hospital a flat amount for a particular treatment or procedure, regardless of the hospital's cost for treating the patient.

The intent of the government's move was admirable. By attempting to limit payouts, the program hoped to encourage efficiency and economy in healthcare. But clearly a hospital's bottom line would be affected. "Because we offer so many types of healthcare services, and because 40 percent of our revenue comes from Medicare, there's no doubt that we will feel the impact," Nott said. "As we have for some time, we'll continue to cut our hospital's expenses wherever we can without sacrificing our commitment to quality and excellence in healthcare."

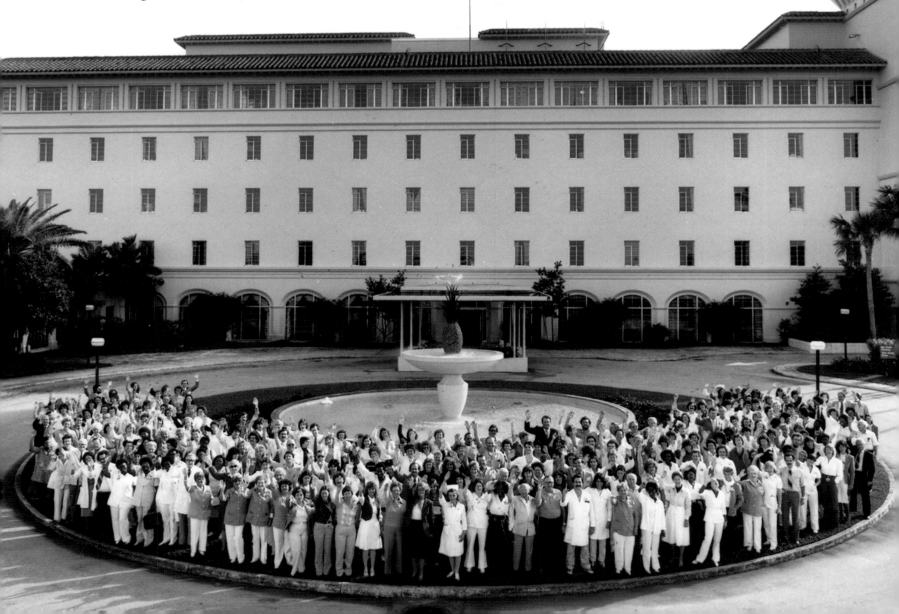

Facing page: In this 1983 photograph, employees gathered in front of what was now a modern medical center. The familiar pineapple symbol still welcomed patients.

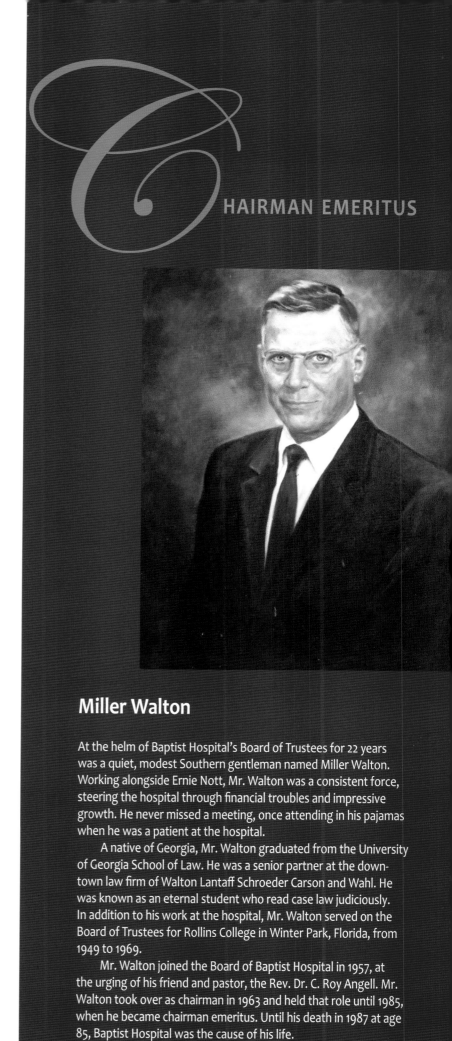

Baptist Hospital grappled with the challenges and uncertainty amid a dramatic change in leadership. In 1985, when the hospital was celebrating its silver anniversary, Board of Trustees Chairman Miller Walton resigned. Mr. Walton, whose health had been declining, joined the Board in 1957 and had served as its chairman since 1963. He had shepherded Baptist Hospital from its infancy. He directed more than 200 Board meetings, monitored patient censuses, watched the financials and planned for the future. The hospital, he once described, "was a regular part" of his life. While it must have been bittersweet to step aside, Walton knew the hospital's foundation was strong.

To succeed him, the Board looked to prominent attorney Robert Cole. Mr. Cole had been a Board member for 23 years and was vice chairman for 17 years, working closely with Miller Walton. He had been head of the Finance Committee for the past five years and seemed particularly well-suited for the task of adapting to the changes in insurance and government regulations.

Five months after Cole became head of the Board, Ernie Nott resigned. Nott had suffered a minor heart attack in February 1985, and his physicians urged him to simplify his life. He took an early retirement, and Brian Keeley, a longtime presence at the hospital and Nott's right hand, took over in April 1986.

The team that had guided the hospital for more than two decades was gone. And the men who stepped in, Brian Keeley and Robert Cole, faced a new era of medical care.

They took over a thriving hospital in a time of transition. The first years of their tenure would be spent handling the changes and navigating the world outside North Kendall Drive. It would be a world of physician groups and insurance companies, outpatient centers and, most surprisingly, alliances with competing hospitals. Keeley and Cole did not know it at the time, but South Miami Hospital, four miles down the road, would play a key role in Baptist Hospital's next decade.

Miller Walton

At the helm of Baptist Hospital's Board of Trustees for 22 years was a quiet, modest Southern gentleman named Miller Walton. Working alongside Ernie Nott, Mr. Walton was a consistent force, steering the hospital through financial troubles and impressive growth. He never missed a meeting, once attending in his pajamas when he was a patient at the hospital.

A native of Georgia, Mr. Walton graduated from the University of Georgia School of Law. He was a senior partner at the downtown law firm of Walton Lantaff Schroeder Carson and Wahl. He was known as an eternal student who read case law judiciously. In addition to his work at the hospital, Mr. Walton served on the Board of Trustees for Rollins College in Winter Park, Florida, from 1949 to 1969.

Mr. Walton joined the Board of Baptist Hospital in 1957, at the urging of his friend and pastor, the Rev. Dr. C. Roy Angell. Mr. Walton took over as chairman in 1963 and held that role until 1985, when he became chairman emeritus. Until his death in 1987 at age 85, Baptist Hospital was the cause of his life.

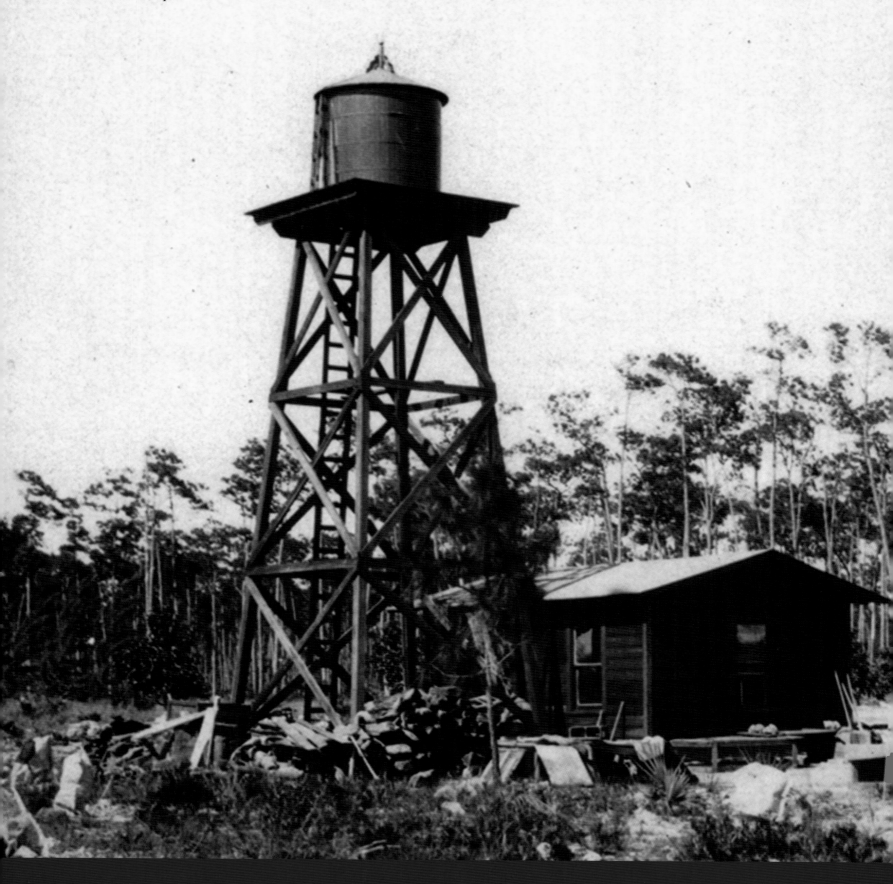

This 1917 photo shows the homesite of Dr. and Mrs. Sigmund Graenicher, between today's Sunset Drive and S.W. 68th Avenue, near the site of today's South Miami Hospital.

South Miami Comes Together

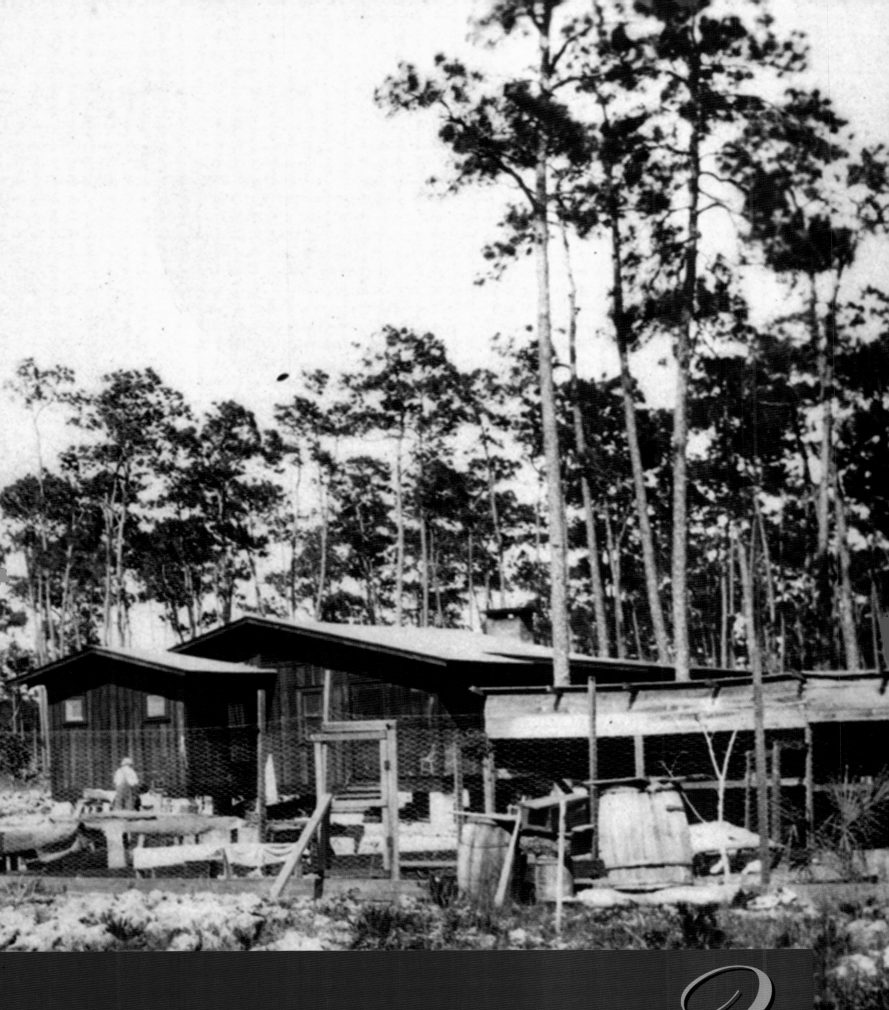

"Each organization very quickly develops a personality. Our hospital's personality is rather unique. In the sometimes cold, impersonal atmosphere of clinical medicine, we have been successful in developing a warm, kind, friendly atmosphere... What we may lack in an impressive physical plant, we more than make up for in genuine interest and kindness to the people we serve."

Ray Poore
Administrator, South Miami Hospital
1966

As Miami's Baptist community was envisioning a hospital in Kendall, a group of neighboring doctors and community leaders started their own journey. In early 1959, residents of South Miami watched as construction progressed on a building just off South Dixie Highway at 62nd Avenue. Located in the center of the small community, it was to house professional offices. The enterprise was the brainchild of James F. Lyons, M.D., a local surgeon with an entrepreneurial spirit.

Dr. Lyons had ambitious plans for what he called the South Dade Professional Building. With 45,000 square feet of rentable space at four dollars a foot, he hoped to gross $180,000 per year. "This will be the finest office building in South Dade," he wrote in a 1958 prospectus. He wanted to attract doctors, dentists, engineers, architects and accountants, and even planned for an apothecary shop.

Lyons' choice of location was well-timed: South Miami was on the cusp of major development. The small community was lined with post-war starter homes and rows of apartments, as well as a small shopping district. An enclave of farmland, ranches and open fields sat on the fringes. Locals described South Miami as a bit of both city and country.

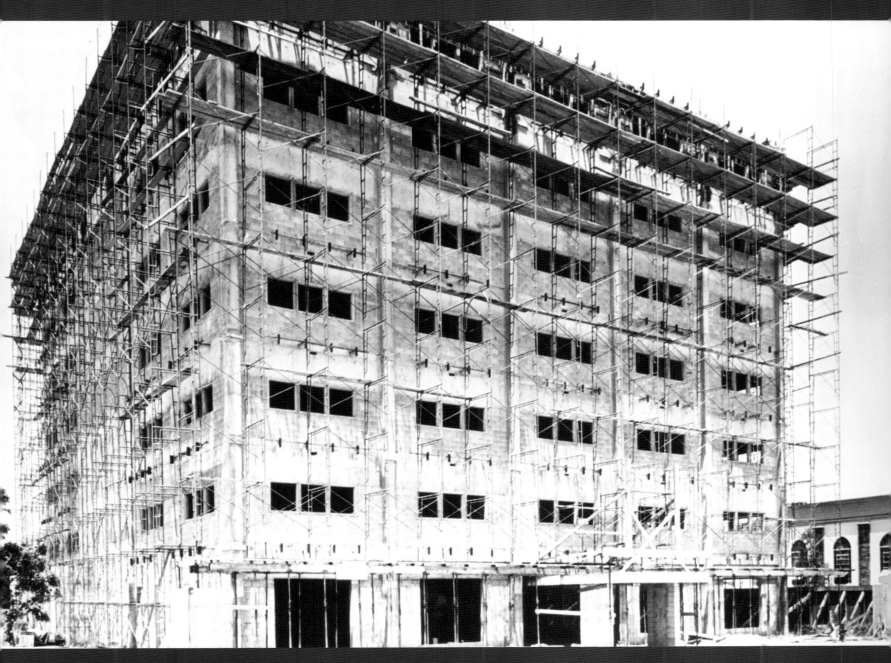

The 1959 construction of an office building in South Miami provided an opportunity for community doctors to build a hospital. Five decades later, South Miami Hospital is a thriving medical center.

In the Beginning

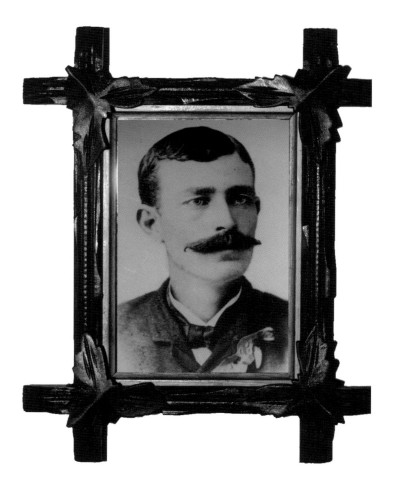

Wilson A. Larkins, a Tennessean with a love of horses, cows and farming, arrived in the vicinity of today's South Miami in January 1897. He moved his wife, Essie, and five children south to join his in-laws, the Burtashaws, who had established some citrus groves in the area. Drawn by the prospect of vast wilderness, Larkins built a dairy farm, grew crops of tomatoes, peppers and eggplants, and cultivated grapefruit, guava and orange groves. A quiet and persevering man, Larkins delivered the fruits of his land on a large bicycle fitted with storage containers. One of his best customers was downtown Miami's famed Royal Palm Hotel — the epicenter of the community's high society.

Larkins endured the challenges of pioneer life. Supplies were often hard to come by, and early residents had to travel into Miami for necessities. The enterprising businessman opened a general store near today's Cocoplum Circle.

The nascent settlement became known as Larkins with the general store as its headquarters. It served as the post office and Wilson Larkins filled the role as postmaster. When Henry Flagler's Florida East Coast Railway extended from Miami to Homestead in 1904, more development followed. Larkins became a regular railroad stop and stores and packing houses sprouted up by today's Sunset Drive and U.S. 1 to handle the shipping of citrus and vegetable crops.

By 1917, the population of Larkins reached 350. The community enjoyed telephone service, a sewing club called the Cocoplum Thimble Club (today's Cocoplum Women's Club), a school and a drugstore.

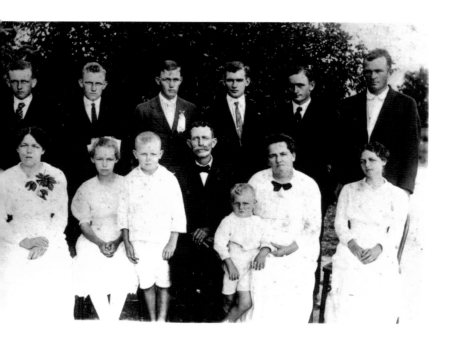

Top: Wilson Larkins

Bottom: In 1920, Wilson Larkins (center) posed with his extended family. They were pioneer settlers of today's South Miami.

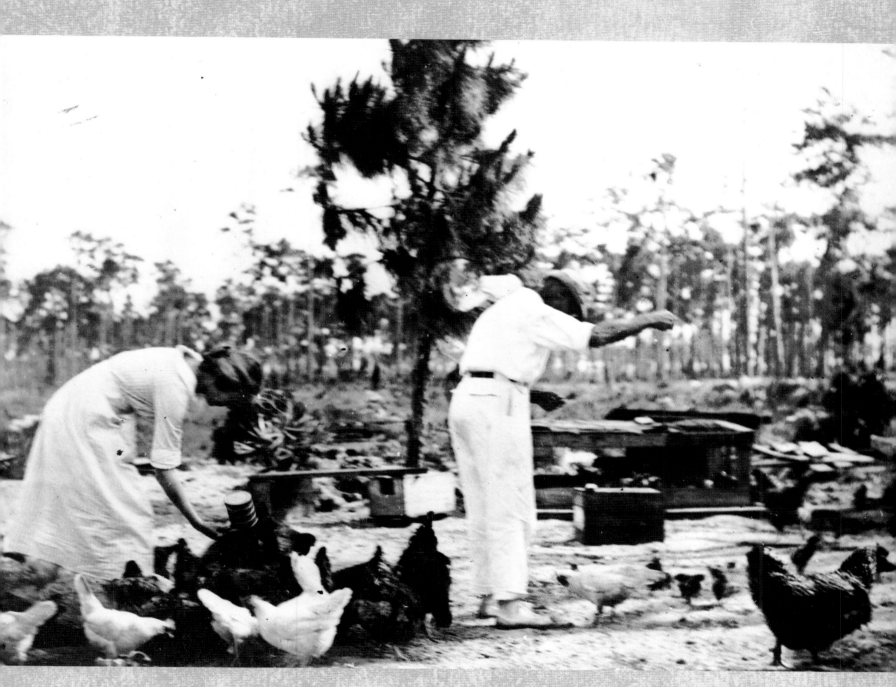

Life in the Larkins community revolved around agriculture.
The residents cultivated the land and farmed.

From Settlement to City

The new decade heralded change. World War I ended and social mores loosened. Women shortened their hemlines and bobbed their hair, and South Florida became home to flappers, bootleggers and master salesmen. A land boom swept Miami, peaking in 1925, when building permits totaled over $15 million for one month alone.

The sleepy wilderness of Larkins was not immune to the building and speculation. It was reported that one 10-acre tract of land sold for $100,000.

In response to the growth, the pioneers of Larkins pushed for incorporation. On March 2, 1926, citizens voted to incorporate six square miles from today's Bird Road on the north to one mile south of North Kendall Drive on the south; from Red Road (57th Avenue on the east) to Palmetto Road (77th Avenue on the west) as the Town of South Miami. They elected Judge W.A. Foster as mayor and seven men as aldermen. Within weeks, the group established a town seal, formulated a town code, purchased the first fire truck and appointed a health officer.

The Town of South Miami was short-lived. On September 17, 1926, a great hurricane blew through South Florida, battering the South Miami area. Days after the storm, the Florida East Coast Railway station, the town's economic lifeblood, burned to the ground. In the wake of the challenges, South Miami's leaders looked to the state and federal government for relief, but felt dissatisfied with the response. They concluded that the area's status as a "town" diminished its importance in the eyes of outsiders. On June 24, 1927, the Florida Legislature approved a new charter and the City of South Miami was born.

In the 1930s, growth was slow and tentative. South Florida, like the rest of the nation, experienced economic hardships. In 1933, South Miami's population reached approximately 1,500 residents. In the hopes of greater government efficiency, the city's area was reduced from six square miles to less than four. Among the 30 or so businesses was Fuchs Baking Company, which moved from Homestead to the Riviera Theatre building on South Dixie Highway west of Red Road in 1934. The building became home to Holsum Bakery — South Miami's most noteworthy business. Longtime residents still remember the aroma of freshly baked bread wafting through the mostly rural community.

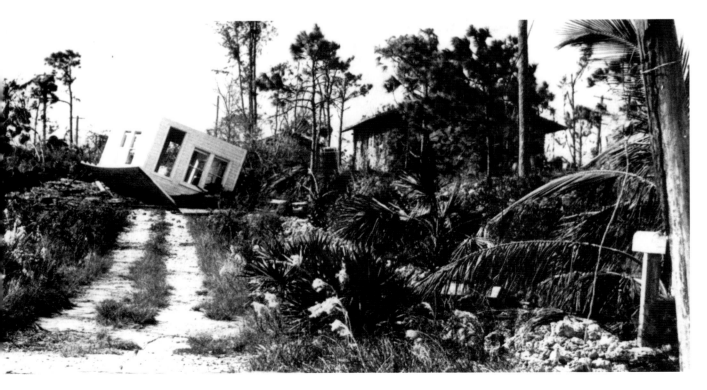

The 1926 hurricane brought massive destruction not only to the coastal area, but well inland where wooden farm houses were particularly hard hit.

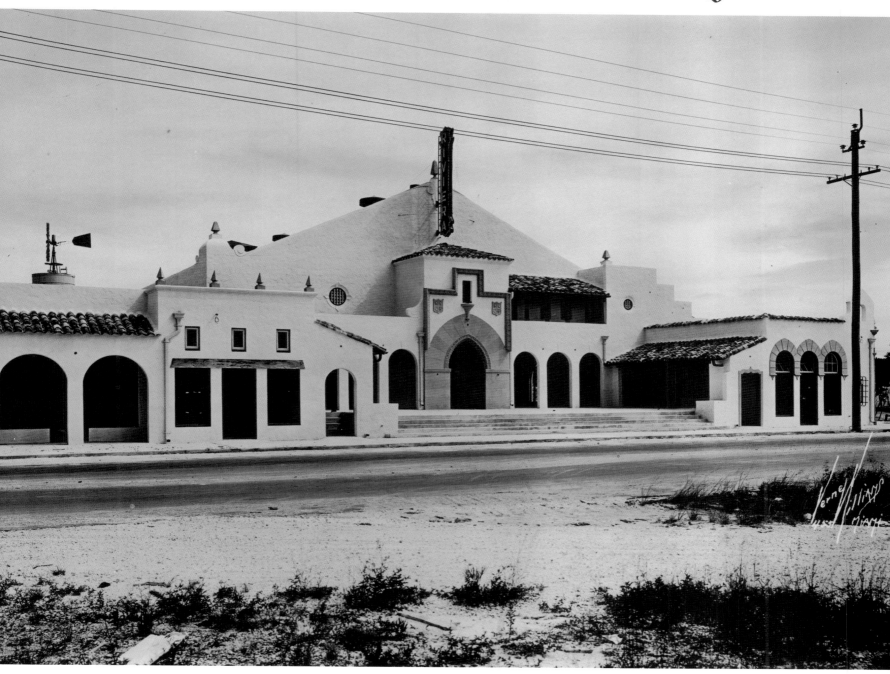

Fuchs Baking Co.

The Fuchs Baking Company, known by most as the
Holsum Bakery, moved into the old Riviera Theatre building
on South Dixie Highway in 1934. Holsum became the
centerpiece for South Miami's business community.

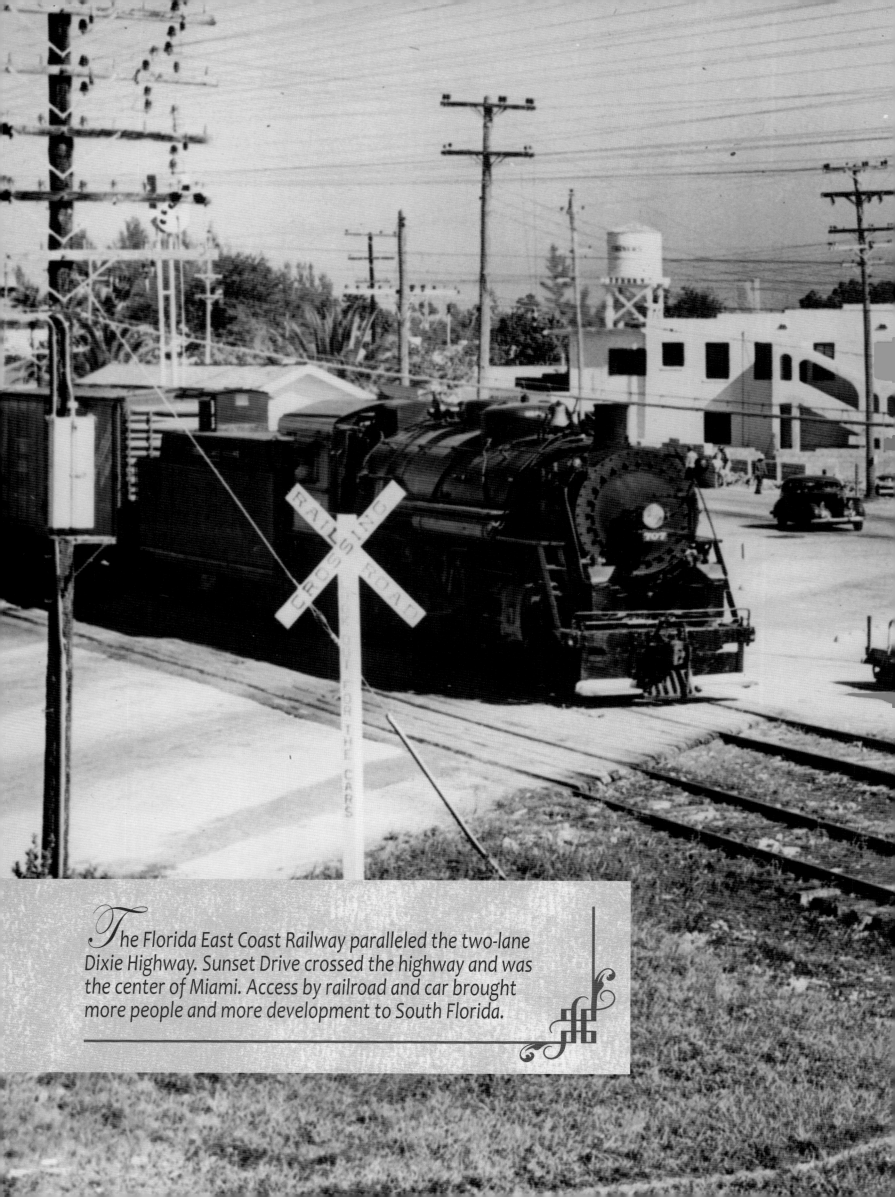

The Florida East Coast Railway paralleled the two-lane Dixie Highway. Sunset Drive crossed the highway and was the center of Miami. Access by railroad and car brought more people and more development to South Florida.

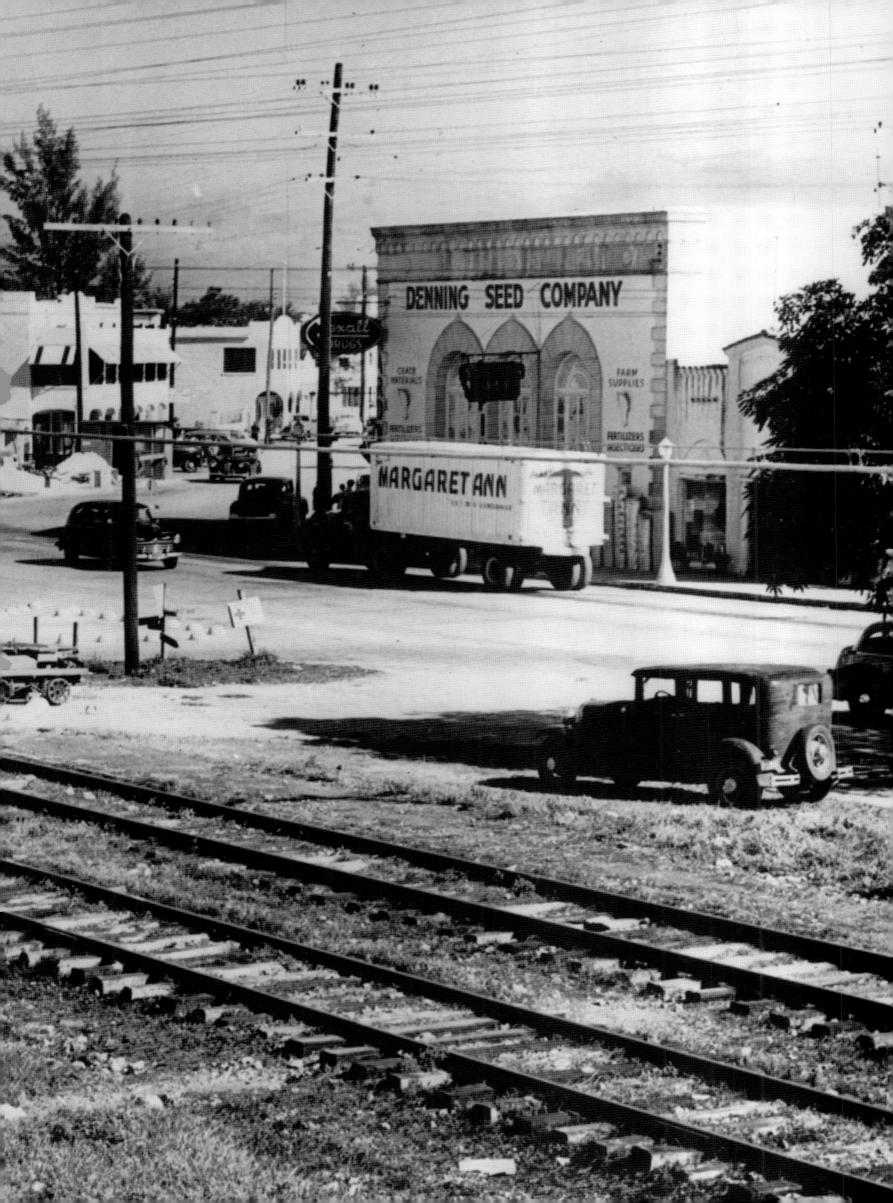

A City Develops

James Lyons arrived in South Florida in 1941. The Illinois native had attended medical school at St. Louis University and, like so many others, came south for sunnier skies. He completed his internship at Jackson Memorial Hospital and built a medical practice in Coral Gables.

The young physician established a reputation as a skilled and methodical surgeon. His bustling career notwithstanding, Lyons developed other interests, notably real estate investing. "When he came to this part of Miami, it was pretty open," said his son, James Lyons II. "I think there were a lot of tomato fields and other farms. But he recognized pretty early that U.S. 1 had to develop. He had a knack for seeing possibilities and what could be."

Tall, handsome and impeccably dressed with finely tailored suits, he fit easily into the business world. Though he came from modest beginnings, the son of a secretary and railroad brakeman, he learned the value of financial independence. "He was a real sharp guy," said David Hallstrand, M.D., one of the founding members of South Miami Hospital. "I think that he had heard or read somewhere that the center of Miami would one day be at 62nd Avenue, so he bought some land there and started to build an office building." Dr. Lyons went on to purchase other property in Florida and developed timeshares, condominiums and golf courses in North Carolina.

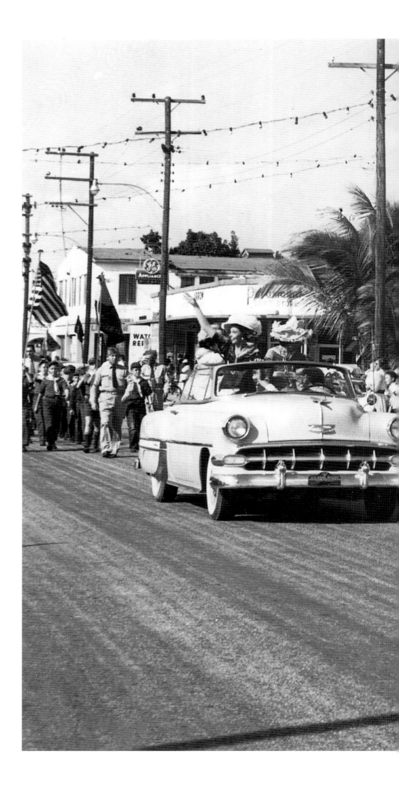

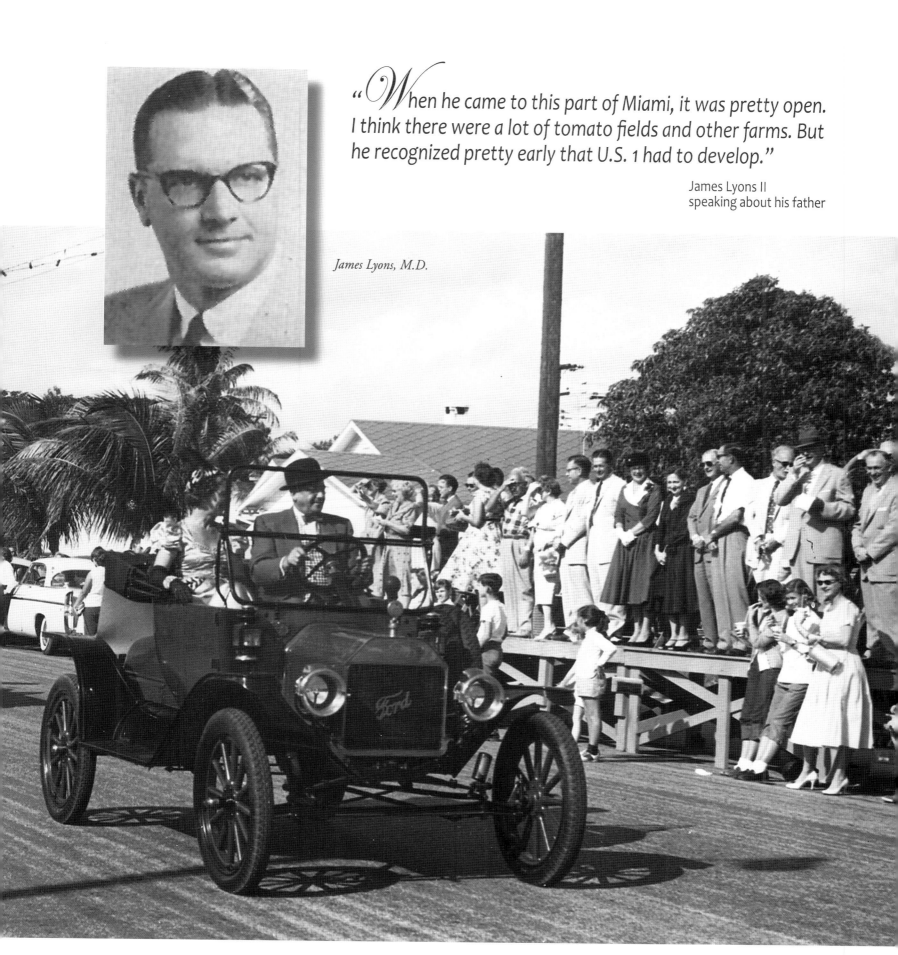

"*When he came to this part of Miami, it was pretty open. I think there were a lot of tomato fields and other farms. But he recognized pretty early that U.S. 1 had to develop.*"

James Lyons II
speaking about his father

James Lyons, M.D.

By the 1950s, South Miami was a thriving community. Residents enjoyed community events, such as this parade.

A Building and a Vision

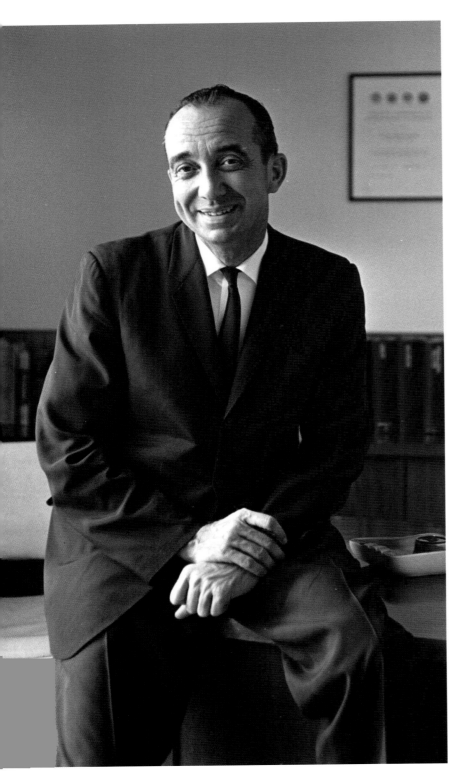

Raymond Poore was South Miami Hospital's first administrator.

For about 20 local doctors, the skeleton building on South Dixie Highway and 62nd Avenue provided an opportunity. The doctors, many of whom had moved to South Florida after World War II, were launching their practices. Some were not on staff at nearby Doctors' Hospital in Coral Gables or Mercy Hospital in Coconut Grove, and the process to join was lengthy and difficult. The physicians often had to navigate the roads into downtown Miami's Jackson Memorial Hospital to admit patients. The doctors needed a place of their own — a hospital with easy access to the southern part of Dade County.

On May 14, 1959, the group held its first organizational meeting at Dr. Lyons' Coral Gables office on Biltmore Way. Their goal was to lease the far-from-completed building and transform it into a hospital.

The group met almost weekly and sketched out a rough organizational structure. James Vaughn, M.D., a young doctor who had moved to South Florida in 1950 after a stint in the U.S. Army, was elected chief of the medical staff. Helen Hudnall, a West Virginian who had been in Miami for a decade and had worked at Doctors' Hospital in Coral Gables, came aboard as director of nursing. Banker Omar Stang, president of First National Bank of South Miami and a patient of Dr. Vaughn, chaired the first Board of Directors.

To handle the job of opening and managing the hospital, the group hired Raymond Poore, who had worked as a business manager and assistant administrator at Mercy Hospital. Poore brought his experience and a strong work ethic to South Miami. "For Ray Poore, building the hospital was really a labor of love," Dr. Vaughn said. "He worked so hard to get things off the ground. His only agenda was to get the best hospital up and running."

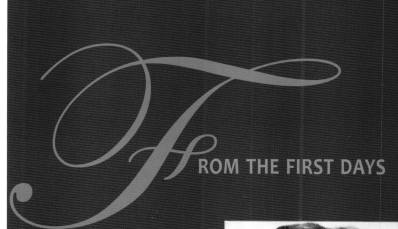

After several months of negotiations, the lease for the building was signed on August 17, 1959. The group had the option to purchase the building for $1.08 million after three years. The leaders set out to build a hospital from scratch — designing rooms, ordering supplies and even picking paint colors. "I remember that I had some of the responsibility for the nursing station," Ms. Hudnall said. "I bought everything. I would walk through the building with all the construction going on. It was very exciting to see something from the beginning."

One of the biggest challenges was raising money. To complete the interior of the building and cover pre-opening expenses, the group launched a campaign to sell $1 million in bonds. In order to join the medical staff, each doctor was required to purchase a $10,000 bond. Other bonds were sold to patients, local businessmen and friends. "Finances occupied a great preponderance of our time since we didn't have any money," Dr. Hallstrand remembered. "We did whatever we could to raise money." Hospital leaders conducted tours of the building and held barbecues at some of the medical staff members' houses to generate interest and support.

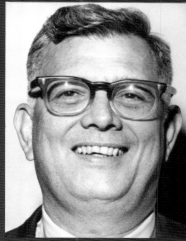

James Vaughn, M.D.

James Vaughn, M.D.

James Vaughn, M.D., knows intimately the history of South Miami Hospital. He was there every step of the way. The Georgia native arrived in Miami in 1950, a few years out of the University of Maryland Medical School and fresh from Army service. Dr. Vaughn came south because he knew an established doctor in the area and recognized the community's potential for growth. He joined a cadre of young physicians setting down roots.

Dr. Vaughn built a presence as a family doctor and also worked as an anesthesiologist at Mercy and Doctors' Hospitals. Like other community doctors, he wanted a hospital close to his practice and helped spearhead the campaign to build South Miami Hospital. He was the hospital's first chief of staff, served many years on the Board of Directors and remained a vocal hospital leader for more than four decades.

"I worked on the hospital day and night," he said. "It really was my mission. I was always doing things for the hospital — going to meetings, talking to people in the community about it and trying to help it be successful."

Joining him side-by-side was his wife, Phyllis Vaughn, M.D., a fellow physician whom he met in medical school. The two doctors became the public face of the young hospital and, along with other pioneers, nurtured its growth.

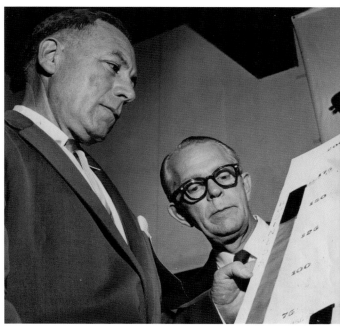

Omar Stang (left) with Val Stieglitz, president of the South Miami Chamber of Commerce

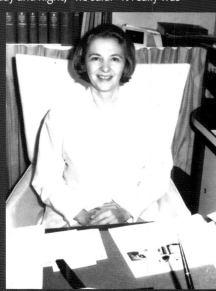

Phyllis Vaughn, M.D.

A South Miami Spirit

Beyond finances, the logistics of converting an office building into a hospital proved daunting. "Construction, planning, drawing and organization all went forth simultaneously on a wartime crash program as detailed drawings were handed to the contractor by the page," Poore said at the time. "Haste makes hair-raising problems and we had more than our share." Because much of the structure was already complete, the leaders had to compromise and adapt. The office elevators could not hold hospital beds, so with some inventive design, workers removed the elevators' interior rails and bumpers on the beds.

On February 22, 1960, nearly 10 months after the first organizational meeting, South Miami Hospital opened its doors to 15 patients. Room rates were $29 for a private room, $19 for a semi-private room and $15 for a ward bed.

Considering the quick pace of construction, the hospital was impressive. The first floor included the pharmacy, emergency room, kitchen and cafeteria. The second floor housed eight suites of private offices for physicians and dentists. The third floor remained an unfinished shell with a future capacity of 44 beds. The laboratory, X-ray department, and one 23-bed nursing unit were located on the fourth floor. Four 22-bed nursing units made up the fifth and sixth floors. The seventh floor housed the surgical suite, central supply and maternity, including the delivery and labor rooms, nurseries and a 12-bed postpartum unit. On the rooftop sat a 200-ton air conditioner to cool the entire building, a boiler room and living quarters for the engineer. It was affectionately dubbed the penthouse suite.

When the first patient, the wife of hospital Board member Jack Davis, was admitted, the pioneers felt an enormous accomplishment. "What we did in such a short period of time was really amazing," Dr. Vaughn said. "I am sure many doubted that we would actually open. We built a hospital for our community, our patients."

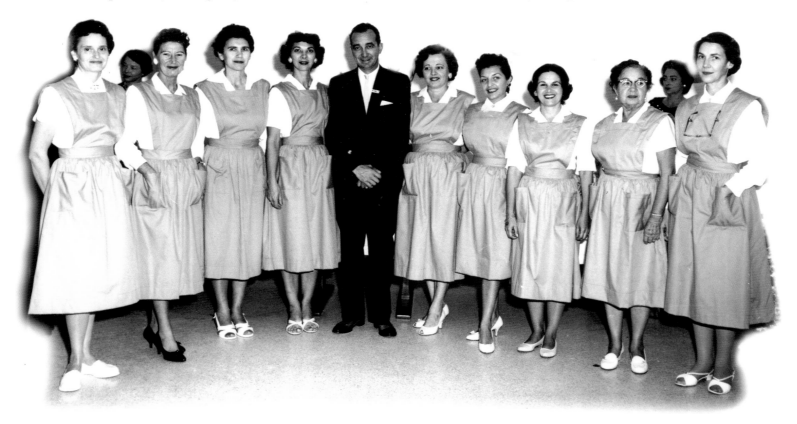

The Pink Ladies volunteered at the hospital, helping with daily tasks and raising funds. Here, they pose with Ray Poore.

On February 22, 1960, nearly 10 months after the first organizational meeting, South Miami Hospital opened its doors to 15 patients. Room rates were $29 for a private room, $19 for a semi-private room and $15 for a ward bed.

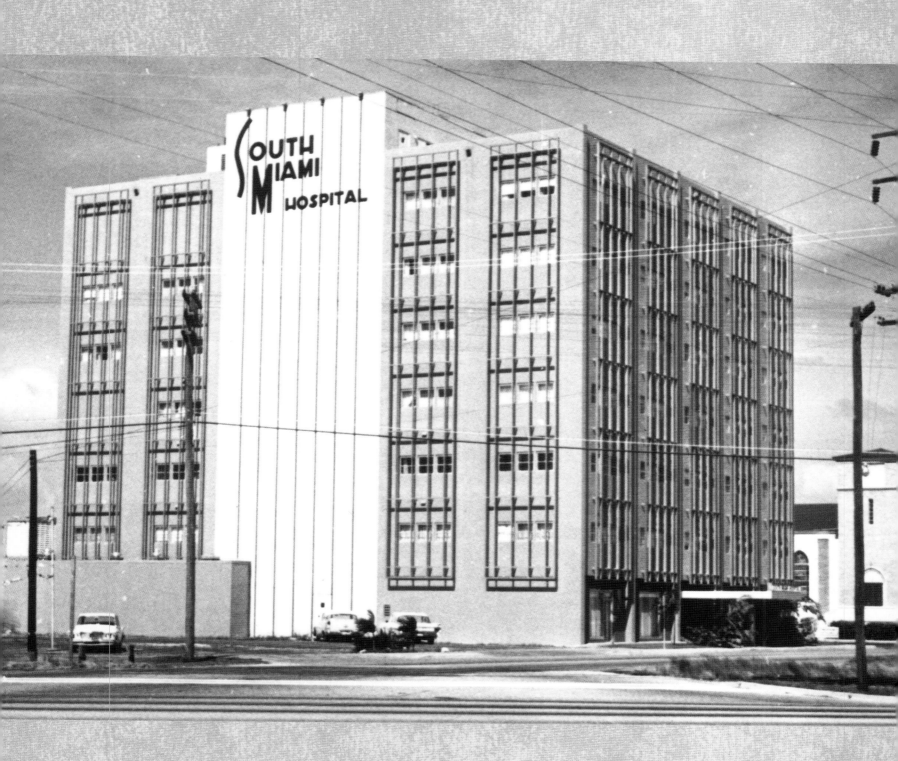

A HOME BY CHANCE

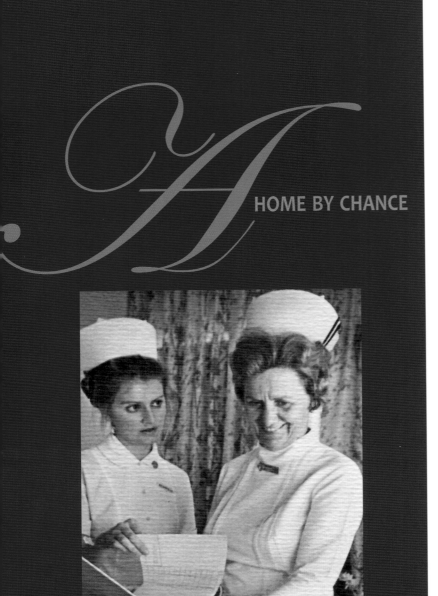

Helen Hudnall, R.N., (right) and Carol Klimchak, R.N.

Helen Hudnall, R.N.

Helen Hudnall, South Miami Hospital's first director of nursing, arrived in South Florida in 1949 by chance — literally. After a cold winter day in her native West Virginia and a fall on some ice, Ms. Hudnall craved a place where the sun always shined. A flip of a coin picked Miami over southern California. The young nurse moved and quickly settled into a job at Doctors' Hospital in Coral Gables. Over time, she got to know James Lyons, M.D., and some of the other founders of nearby South Miami Hospital.

As the Lyons building began to turn into a hospital, Ms. Hudnall joined the South Miami group to create a nursing department. She often donned a hard hat and walked amid the construction. Like so many early employees, Ms. Hudnall was a jack-of-all-trades — manning the hospital's only nursing station, dispensing medications and even maintaining equipment. With Raymond Poore by her side, she helped develop South Miami Hospital's philosophy of pampered patient care.

"The challenges of the early years were amazing — opening the hospital and watching it grow," Ms. Hudnall remembered. "It was really one of the highlights of my life."

A certain spirit emerged at South Miami Hospital. It had a personal feel. The doctors saw themselves not simply as physicians but as builders of a community hospital. "Our charter made us different," said Bernard Silverstein, M.D., a cardiologist. "The bylaws dictated that a majority of the members of the Board of Directors had to be doctors. This meant that the doctors could really shape the hospital and make decisions. We really had a sense of being a part of its growth and development."

The employees shared that personal connection as well. Ray Poore developed a reputation as an active and accessible leader. "He was not sitting in his office," remembered Trudy Armstrong, R.N., who joined the hospital right after it opened. "He made rounds with the nurses and visited patients. He really set the tone for all of us to be involved and to really care."

With personal care at its foundation, the hospital thrived. By the end of the first year of operation, it had admitted more than 6,100 patients and employed more than 200 people. Despite that success, money — or a lack of it — was a constant problem. The hospital operated at a loss, and vendors and suppliers waited months for payment. Personal notes from physicians were used as collateral until funds could be found to cover expenses. At one point, auditors representing the Methodist Church evaluated the hospital for possible acquisition. After reviewing the finances, they declined to get involved, concluding that South Miami Hospital was going bankrupt.

The leaders turned to community members to find funds. The hospital's Ladies Auxiliary organized a fair in the parking lot off 62nd Avenue. The group solicited donations of jewelry and valuables from grateful patients and, in turn, sold them to benefit the hospital. In 1961, the hospital raffled off a new Rambler. Sometimes, the fundraising was more formal. "As president of a bank, Omar Stang really helped us," Dr. Vaughn remembered. "He loaned us money to make payroll and, through his connections in the community, got others to be involved in the hospital." Even with all the support, South Miami ran on a shoestring budget. "Often it felt as though we got through by love and a prayer," Dr. Vaughn said.

*T*he leaders turned to community members to find funds. The hospital's Ladies Auxiliary organized a fair in the parking lot off 62nd Avenue. The group solicited donations of jewelry and valuables from grateful patients and, in turn, sold them to benefit the hospital. In 1961, the hospital raffled off a new Rambler.

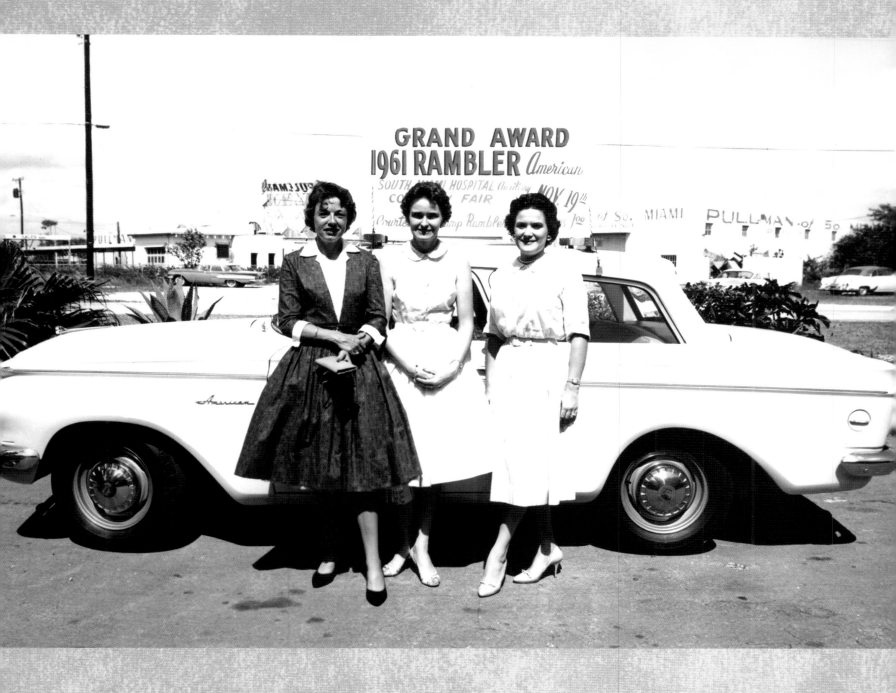

Pampered Patient Care

With community support and the hospital running at more than 90 percent capacity, South Miami kept growing. In January 1962, it opened a cardiac unit with 24 beds on the third floor. A year later, the hospital reached an important milestone.

On February 14, 1963, the Joint Commission on Accreditation of Hospitals awarded it a full three-year accreditation. Plans also took shape for a seven-story service building adjacent to the main hospital. To offset the cost of the additions, the hospital found a benefactor in the form of an unassuming retired executive. William Calhoun had been a steady supporter of the hospital and joined the Board of Directors in early 1962. He had a long and successful career at Sears Roebuck and Company, where he rose to vice president of personnel and sales and led the company's efforts to develop a profit-sharing plan.

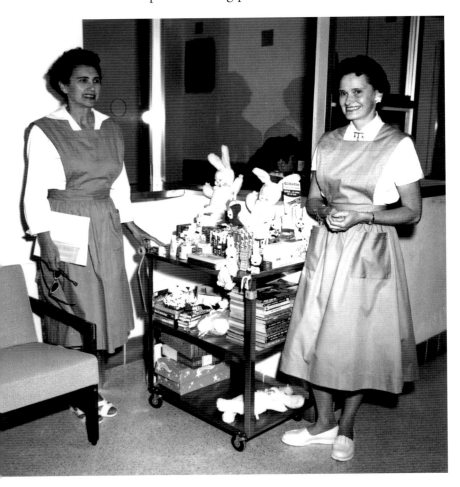

Calhoun brought his everyman persona to South Miami. "There was no bravado with him," remembered Dr. Silverstein. "He was not an obvious millionaire." In the summer of 1963, the quiet, dignified Calhoun made his most significant donation to South Miami. He walked into Ray Poore's office on the ground floor and waited outside so as not to disturb the busy administrator. When a secretary finally ushered him in, he gave a surprised Poore shares of Sears stock worth more than $100,000. The donation represented the largest gift yet to the hospital and allowed the expansion to move forward. Calhoun did not want any attention or input on how the money was used. "You're the one who knows how to run a hospital, not me," he told Poore. "Now if you want some advice on merchandising, I can help you."

The service building, dubbed the Calhoun annex, opened on February 22, 1964, the hospital's fourth anniversary. Calhoun's donation, along with a government grant, paid for the building. The 18,000 square feet included administrative offices, storage areas, a carpenter shop, a print shop, two laboratories, a new recovery room, a doctors' lounge, and physical and oxygen therapy rooms. At the Calhouns' request, the building was dedicated to the Ladies Auxiliary and the Candy Stripers (the youth volunteer group).

The annex relieved some space pressures in the main hospital. Much of what was located on the third floor moved to the new facility. In the newly open space, the hospital added beds and a nursing station to the west side of the floor. The construction was the final step in the original plans, giving South Miami a total of 170 beds.

The Pink Ladies sold magazines and trinkets from a portable gift cart.

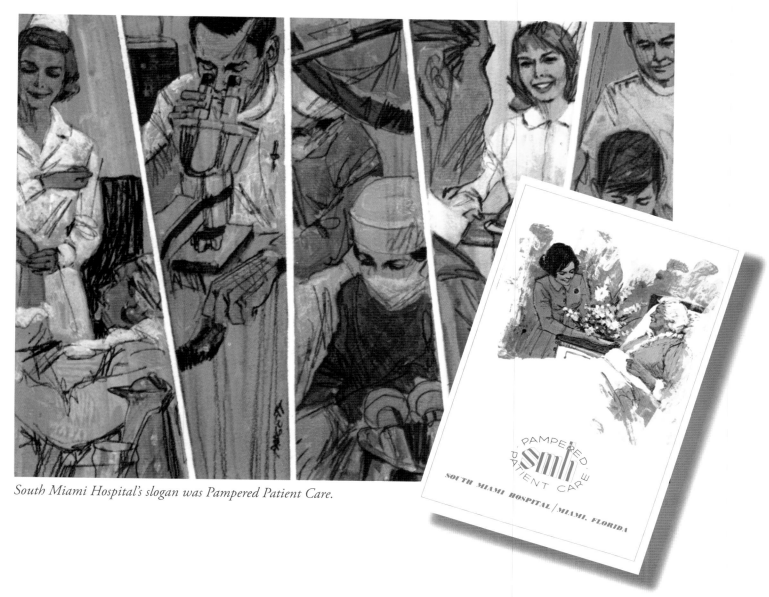

South Miami Hospital's slogan was Pampered Patient Care.

The successful expansion validated the original group's vision. "Imagine the euphoria when every room, every bed was filled and the founders were proven right: the community needed this hospital," reflected Joseph George, M.D., years later. Yet the progress brought a hint of what would be the hospital's biggest problem — space. Located in the center of a burgeoning community that included a downtown business district on Sunset Drive and a population of more than 10,000, its footprint was limited. Land for expansion was scarce. Hospital leaders recognized that they had to concentrate on the core mission inside the building: offering the highest quality care for patients.

This philosophy, called Pampered Patient Care, was embraced by employees and became the hospital's calling. "It is a service rendered our patients far beyond the call of duty," Director of Nursing Helen Hudnall said at the time. "It is an affectionate type of service, an attempt to do anything possible, and sometimes impossible, to please our patients for any reasonable or unreasonable request. Frequently, their desires are anticipated and are fulfilled without request." This included not just the immediate physical needs but extra things, such as assistance in using the phone, a cup of coffee, a back rub, a pillow and a compassionate ear.

The hospital built its reputation on the personal attention it gave patients. Administrator Raymond Poore focused on the details — from the noise level in the hallways, even posting signs to "Join Our Quiet Please Club — Help Stamp Out Noise," to the food served in the cafeteria. He referred to the patients as customers and made their satisfaction a high priority. Local newspaper columnist Herb Rau even labeled South Miami as the "Fontainebleau of hospitals" — after Miami Beach's famed hotel.

The Next Step

South Miami ended its fifth year of operation entrenched in the community. Employees numbered more than 400 and the annual payroll exceeded $2 million. Despite its success, the 1964 expansion proved inadequate and leaders once again confronted the issue of space.

"At South Miami we have about 30 patients a day discharged and as fast as they leave, the beds are filled with new patients," Ray Poore told the newspaper. Often the census reached more than 100 percent. Patients slept in the halls and on some days all but the most critically ill were turned away.

Part of the problem was South Florida's changing demographics. Miami was now a full-fledged metropolis with thousands of new residents flocking to the area. In February 1962, Dade County's population reached one million. Between 1960 and 1970, the county would grow by 35 percent. Most of the settlement centered around the outlying areas, and South Miami's population nearly doubled to almost 20,000. Neighboring communities of Coral Gables, Kendall, Homestead, Perrine and Richmond Heights experienced their own population booms. The development came with a price — a strained infrastructure. Population "growth has been exceeded by the growth of only two things — the need for more hospital beds and roads," noted a local newspaper.

South Miami's leadership responded. "As the area around South Miami grows, as more and more beds are needed for the sick in this area, it becomes obvious that South Miami Hospital must expand. It cannot stand still — it cannot remain the same size," G. Thomas Samartino, M.D., wrote in an employee newsletter in 1966.

With a clear impetus for expansion, the Board approved for the first time a master plan that would address, among other things, how and where to add beds. The financial picture also stabilized. In 1966, the hospital finalized the purchase of the building and the property under it. Negotiations also began to buy some of the surrounding land, including nearly five acres of the Huskamp Motors property to the south and

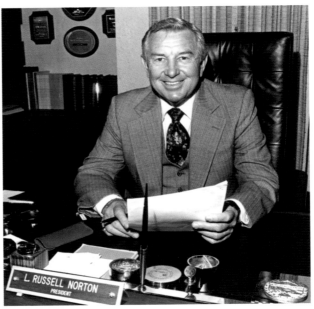

L. Russell Norton

neighboring tracts belonging to local residents. In total, South Miami had 11 acres on its site. For those who had been in the trenches carving out a hospital in makeshift circumstances, it was a rewarding time. "We finally had the opportunity to look more positively into the future," Dr. Hallstrand said.

To finance the next stage, South Miami formalized its fundraising efforts. Another bond drive began, and the hospital established a development office. A community group, the Associates, also organized to support the hospital. Business and social leaders paid annual dues of $25 and enjoyed programs such as tours of the hospital, guest speakers and "minute-men" talks about the hospital's future. Among the charter members was banker Russell Norton, who would become a Board member and longtime South Miami supporter.

The ambitious plans inspired optimism. Yet the leaders never lost sight of the hospital's original mission. "We are growing," Ray Poore said at the time, "but we are not going to lose our individual concern for the personnel or the patient."

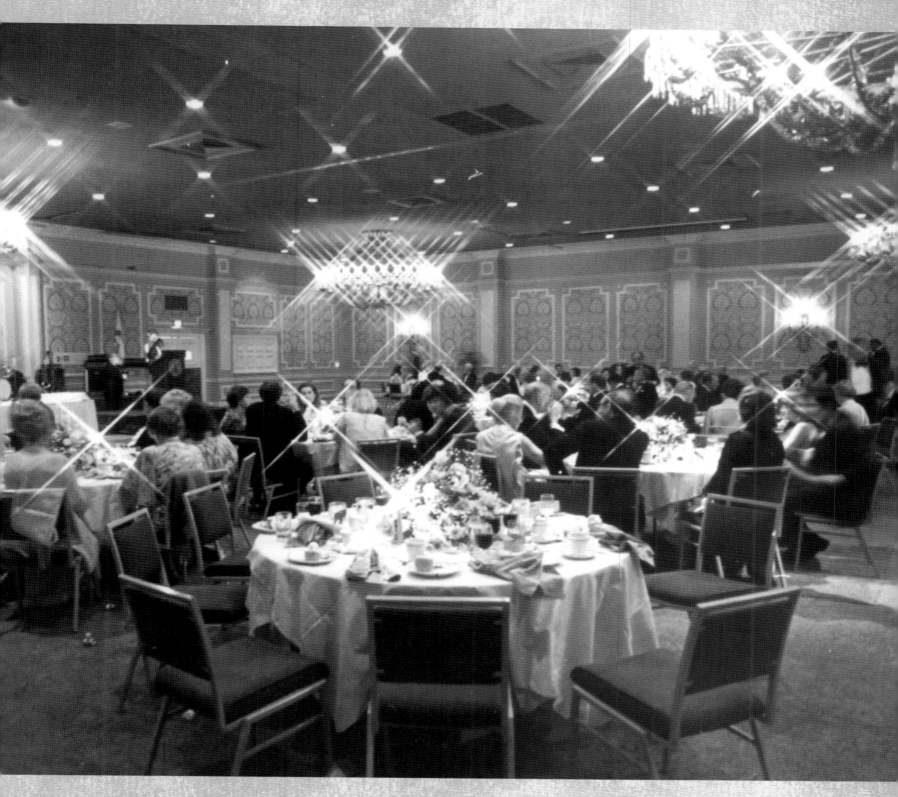

The Associates, a group of business leaders who wanted to raise money for the hospital, sponsored the annual Mercury Ball. The ball took its name from Mercury, the Greek god of culture and tradesmen, and giver of good things. Each year, the gala raised money for a specific hospital need, including diagnostic equipment and special services. The tradition continues today with a signature event planned by the Associates and South Miami Hospital Foundation.

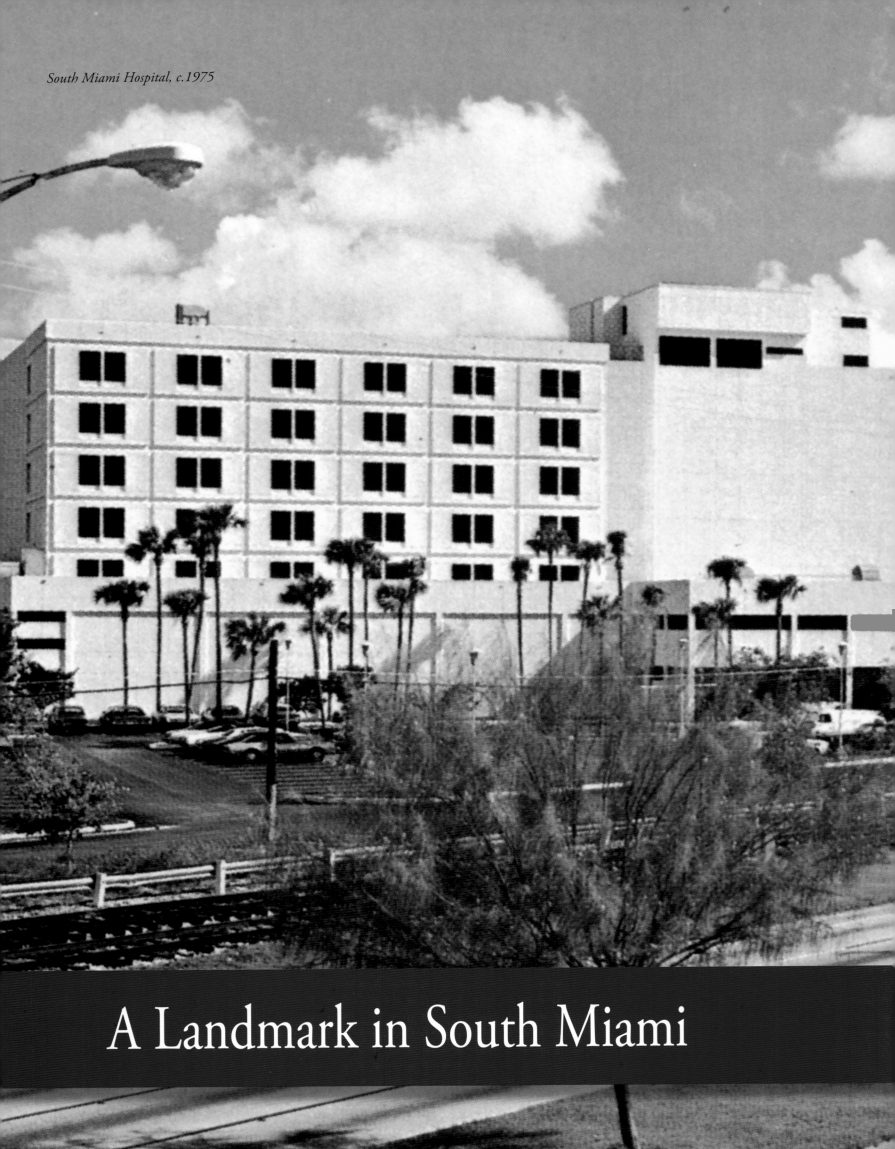

South Miami Hospital, c.1975

A Landmark in South Miami

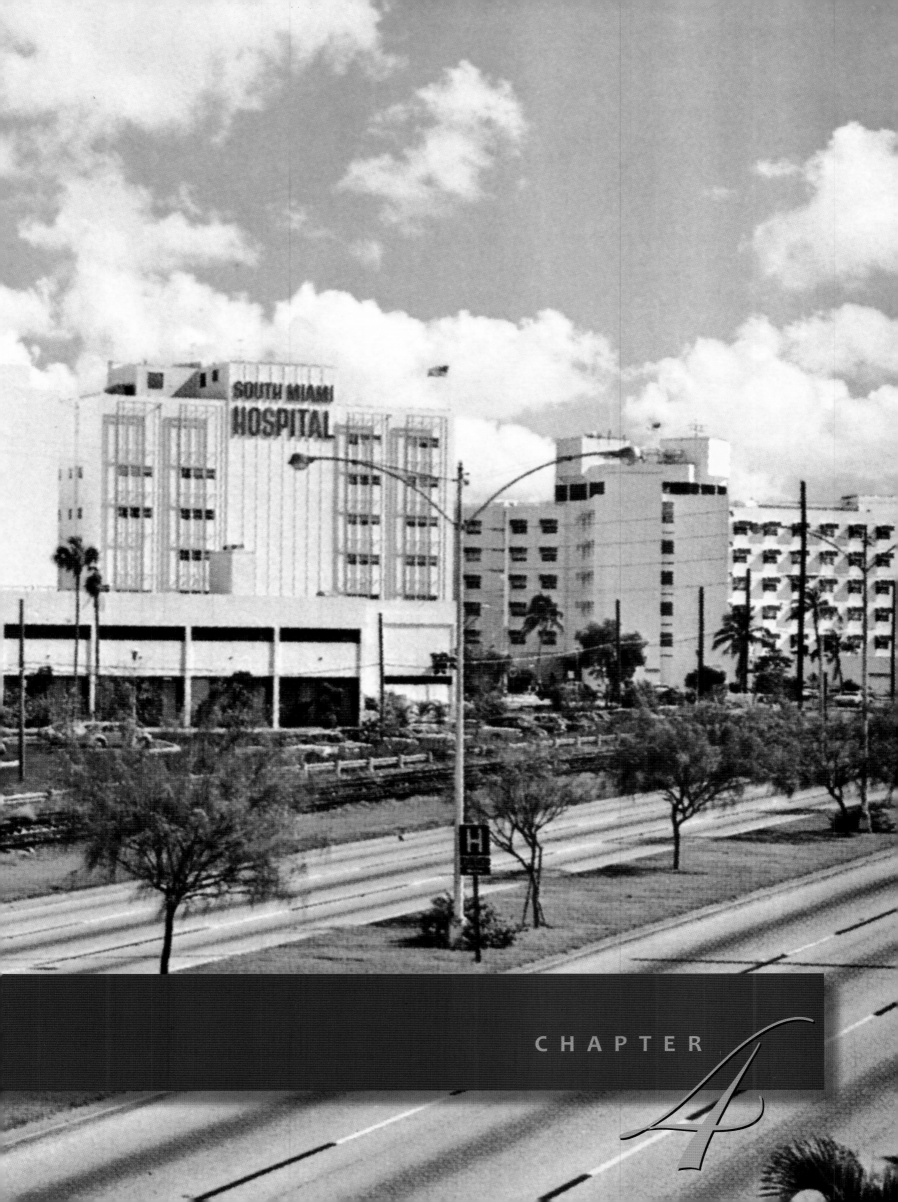

"This institution is and will always be a community hospital. It will not belong to one doctor, to a group of doctors, to one lay person, to a group of lay people, or to any combination of factions or cliques. It will remain universal in scope, will absorb within its boundaries all shades of ethical practices, and will always strive for excellence in patient care."

Victor Dabby, M.D.
President, South Miami Hospital Board
1978

The leaders of South Miami had ambitious plans for the hospital's future. From the beginning, the hospital operated at near capacity, and by 1968 patients filled 98 percent of South Miami's beds each day. A local newspaper even reported that a sign proclaiming, "We need beds, please," adorned a wall on the first floor.

The impetus for expansion was clear. With the purchases of surrounding acres, the hospital now had more land and fundraising had begun. The leaders would just have to decide what to build, what services to offer and how to pay for it all.

The administration and Board of Directors developed a phase one expansion plan that would transform the hospital. It included a new building with 137 patient beds, an expanded emergency department, a 12-bed intensive care unit, a new main entrance, and ancillary services such as a pharmacy and respiratory therapy. While the overhaul was still in the planning stages, however, hospital leaders had an unexpected opportunity.

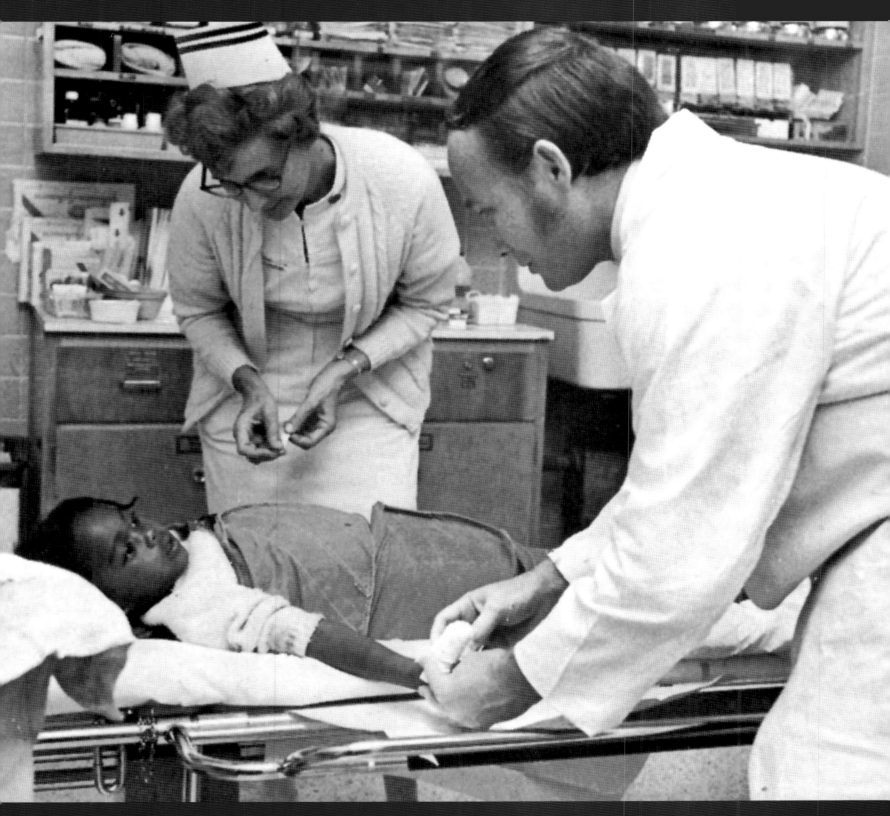

*The expanded Emergency Room offered
a complete range of medical care.*

An Unexpected Opportunity

A building across S.W. 62nd Avenue from the hospital was under construction and slated to become a recuperative center. In the summer of 1970, the owners of the building offered it to the hospital. Realizing that the structure would provide almost immediate beds, the Board agreed to the $850,000 purchase. It invested more than $1 million to convert the building into what was dubbed South Miami Hospital East — complete with 160 patient beds.

On February 21, 1971, the new building opened. It did not replace the planned expansion but simply solved an immediate need. "For some time there had been an unmet demand for general hospital beds in the area. South Miami Hospital had a serious bed shortage and in our long-range expansion program, the situation would not have improved in less than three years," said Board member Claude Holmes, M.D., at the time. "East provided immediate bed relief, particularly private rooms, of which we always had shortages; enabled us to expand our medical staff; and provided space flexibility during the construction of phase one. It has helped us to maintain our 'Pampered Patient Care' philosophy during a critical period of growth."

With the new building, South Miami Hospital was now divided by a main thoroughfare, 62nd Avenue. Employees transported patients from one building to another, often using a green-flowered van known as Daisy. The added beds achieved their goal. In 1971, the hospital admitted more than 10,400 patients, up from 8,600 the previous year.

The hospital also broke ground on phase one of the expansion project. With a two-year construction timeline, South Miami unveiled the new areas in 1973. The emergency department opened in March, two months ahead of the rest of the project. The expansion, dedicated on May 20, 1973, featured a cardiac unit within the new intensive care unit, a new surgical area measuring 10,000 square feet and major upgrades throughout the hospital. It was akin to the delivery of a long-awaited baby, Ray Poore noted.

Facing page: Raymond Poore (middle) oversaw the hospital's expansion.

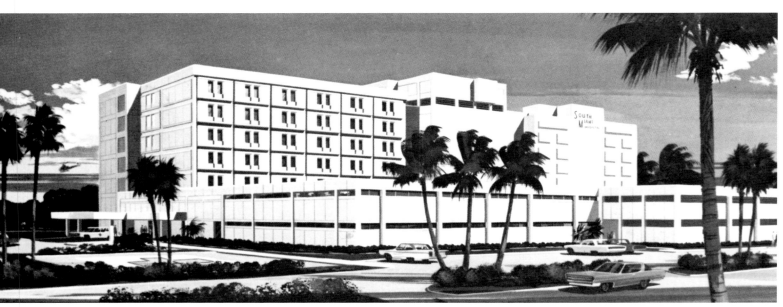

Rendering of phase one, the Pavilion project, 1976

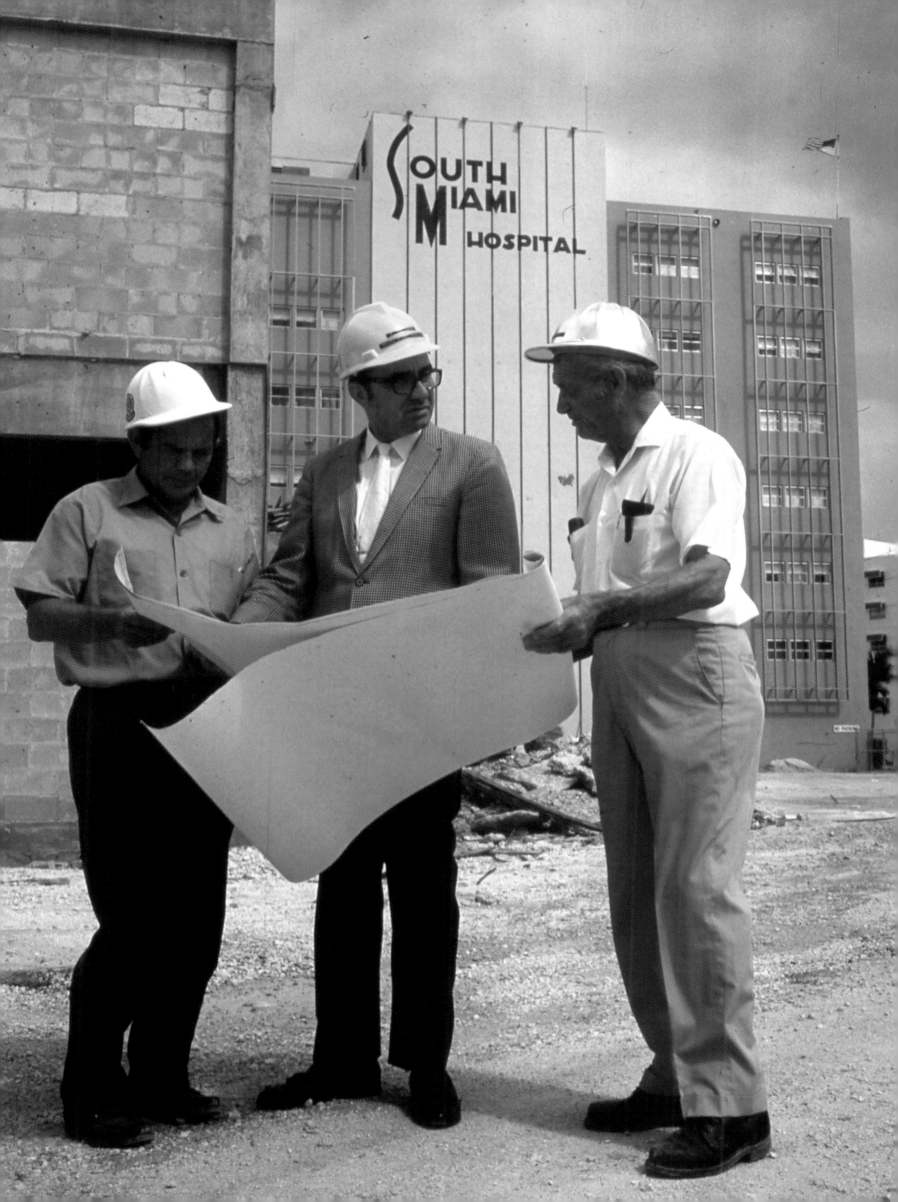

Challenges and Changes

By the end of 1973, with the expansion and East Building, the hospital had 373 beds. Admissions for the year neared 14,000. Yet the growth brought challenges. Managing the renovated hospital was a much more complicated proposition. "We are no longer the little hospital on the corner of U.S. 1 and 62nd Avenue," Ray Poore observed in 1973. "We must now acknowledge that we are 'big business' and must take a long, hard look at ourselves and determine our future course of action."

With the larger hospital's increased financial demands, coupled with a national economic crisis, boom time did not last. The nation was experiencing an oil crisis, rapidly declining stock market and rising inflation. That left people with less money to spend and industries across the board — including healthcare — felt the impact. South Miami Hospital's daily patient census declined to an average 75 percent, and the hospital finished the year with a financial loss.

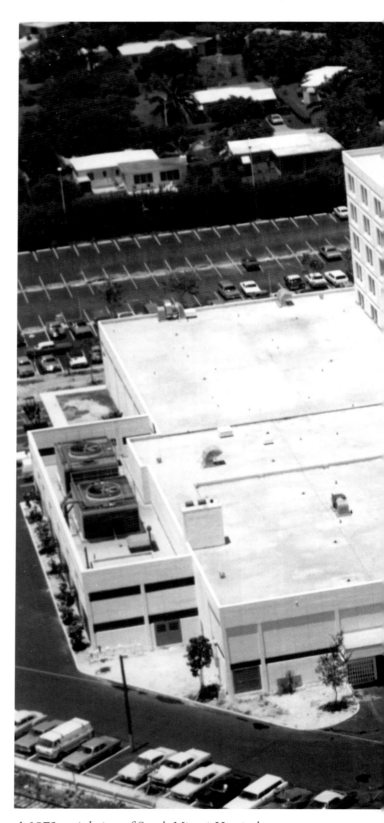

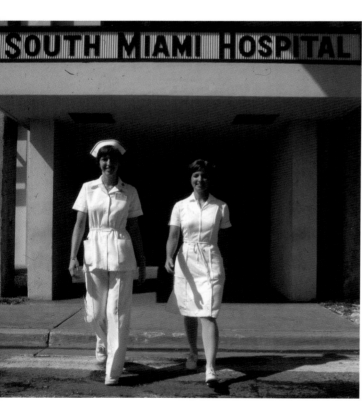

Hospital personnel crossed SW 62nd Avenue to care for patients in South Miami East.

A 1973 aerial view of South Miami Hospital

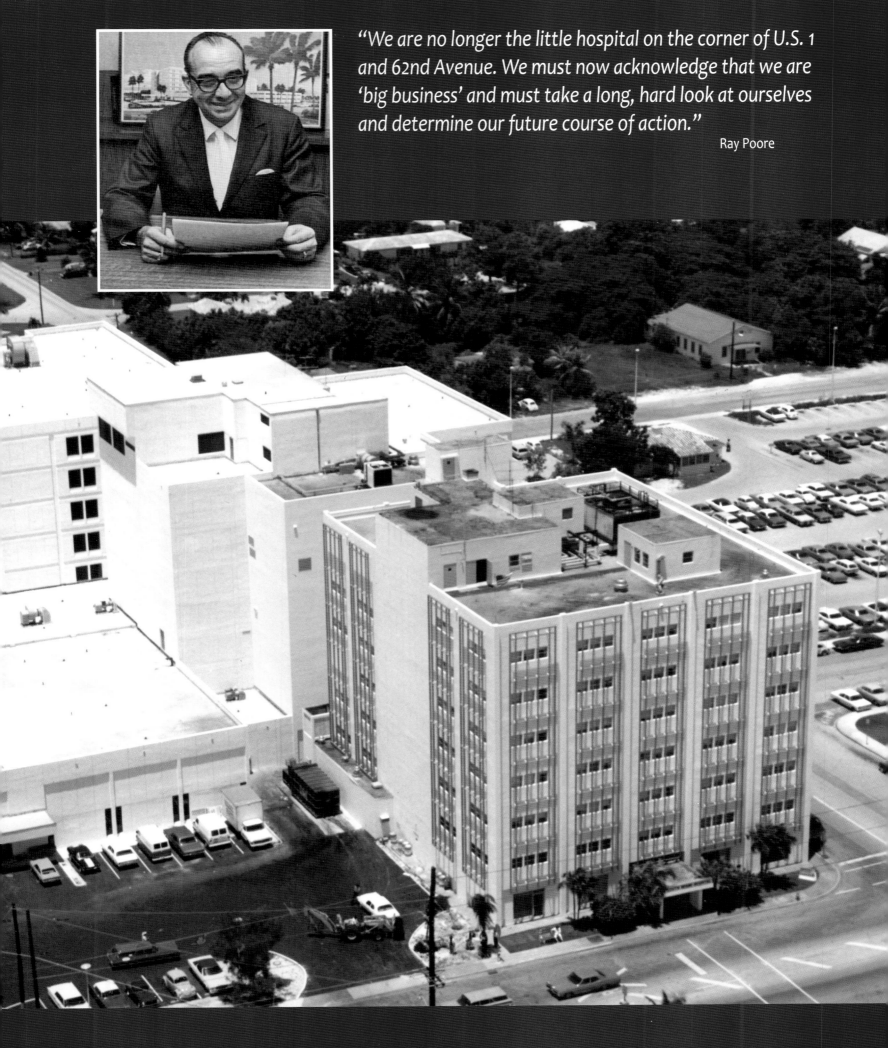

"We are no longer the little hospital on the corner of U.S. 1 and 62nd Avenue. We must now acknowledge that we are 'big business' and must take a long, hard look at ourselves and determine our future course of action."

Ray Poore

The difficult economic climate led leaders to take a step back and evaluate. With the help of consultants Booz, Allen & Hamilton, who had spearheaded the expansion plans, the Board refocused its efforts. In one significant change, Ray Poore resigned in March 1974. For those who worked beside him since the hospital's opening, Poore's departure was a personal loss. "It was a very painful day," said nursing chief Helen Hudnall. "He had given his heart to the hospital." While there was no denying that Ray Poore was a major reason why the hospital got off the ground, some on the Board believed it was time for new blood. South Miami was transitioning from a small community hospital to a large medical center.

Dr. Holmes took over as acting administrator until a new leader was found. In November 1974, Donald Cook, who had been with Booz, Allen & Hamilton, assumed the post. Cook was a familiar face at the hospital. As a South Miami consultant, he knew the hospital's personnel and problems and identified growth areas. With a national economic recession and rising medical costs, Cook believed that the best way to increase revenue was to increase programs. "A shortage of services exists," he said at the time. "If met, they would alleviate the bed surplus."

With this in mind, in 1975 the hospital expanded and renovated its obstetrics department to reflect emerging trends in prenatal care, family rooming and natural childbirth. By the next year, the hospital opened an inpatient and outpatient alcohol rehabilitation program housed in the East Building. The comprehensive program was unique in Dade County. It offered family counseling, group therapy and follow-up care. The hospital also opened its cardiovascular laboratory, developed cancer services, built a new full-service laboratory and created a diabetes treatment center. The breadth of services allowed South Miami to meet the community's demand and harness advancing technology.

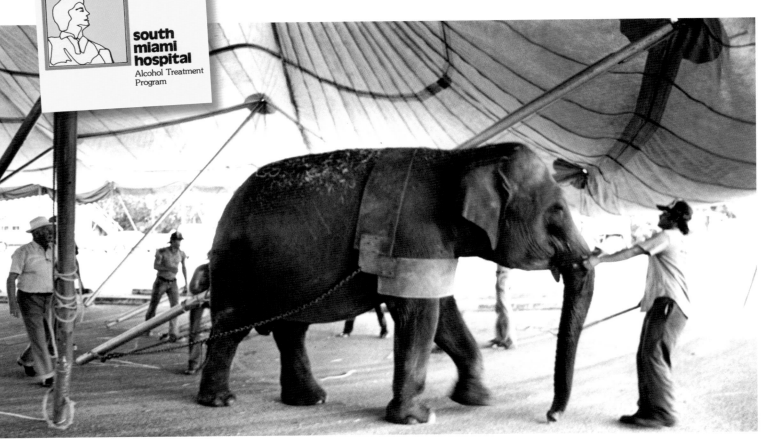

Dolores Morgan, M.D., believed that recovery and sobriety needed to be a continuous journey. At this homecoming luncheon for the Addiction Treatment Program's alumni, Jessie the elephant helped erect a tent. The luncheon was one of many programs that kept alumni connected to South Miami long after their hospital stay.

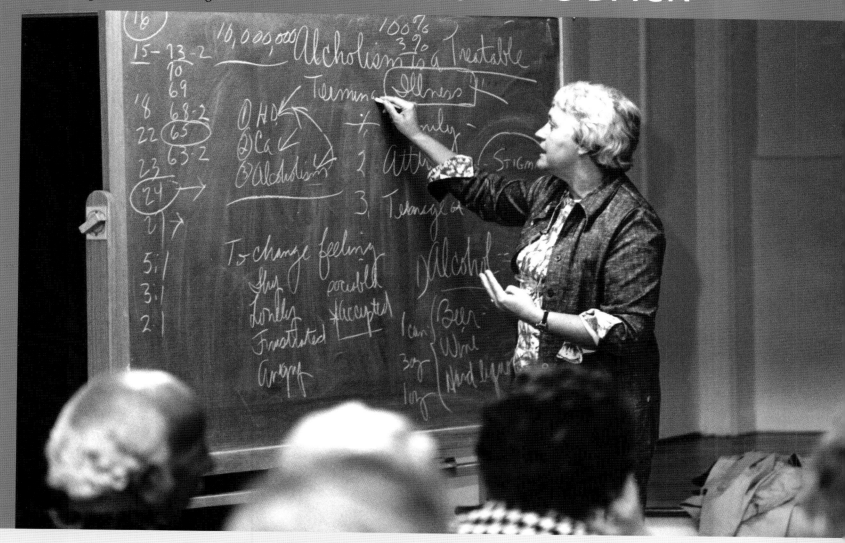

Dolores Morgan, M.D., instructing class

South Miami Hospital Alcohol Treatment Program

In 1976, South Miami Hospital opened the Alcohol Treatment Program, the only hospital-based addiction care in South Florida. The brainchild of Dolores Morgan, M.D., and Administrator Donald Cook, the program approached addiction treatment as a continuing journey. Patients stayed at South Miami Hospital for 28 days of detoxification and intensive counseling, then partici-pated in two years of outpatient therapy, support groups and family counseling. "We offer a broad-scoped, comprehensive plan," Dr. Morgan said at the time. "We are here to help those alcoholics for whom there has previously been little or no help."

The philosophy was groundbreaking. Dr. Morgan had studied other successful programs and brought the best practices to South Miami. "Dr. Morgan had a one-track mission — recovery," said Rick Wolfson, who started working at the program in 1983 and served as its director from 1993 to 2008. "Her philosophy that patients did not have to suffer alone was the program's hallmark. She gave addicts hope and a path to recovery."

Today, South Miami Hospital's Addiction Treatment Program treats patients from all over the world. Since its founding, it has helped more than 25,000 people lead more sober lives.

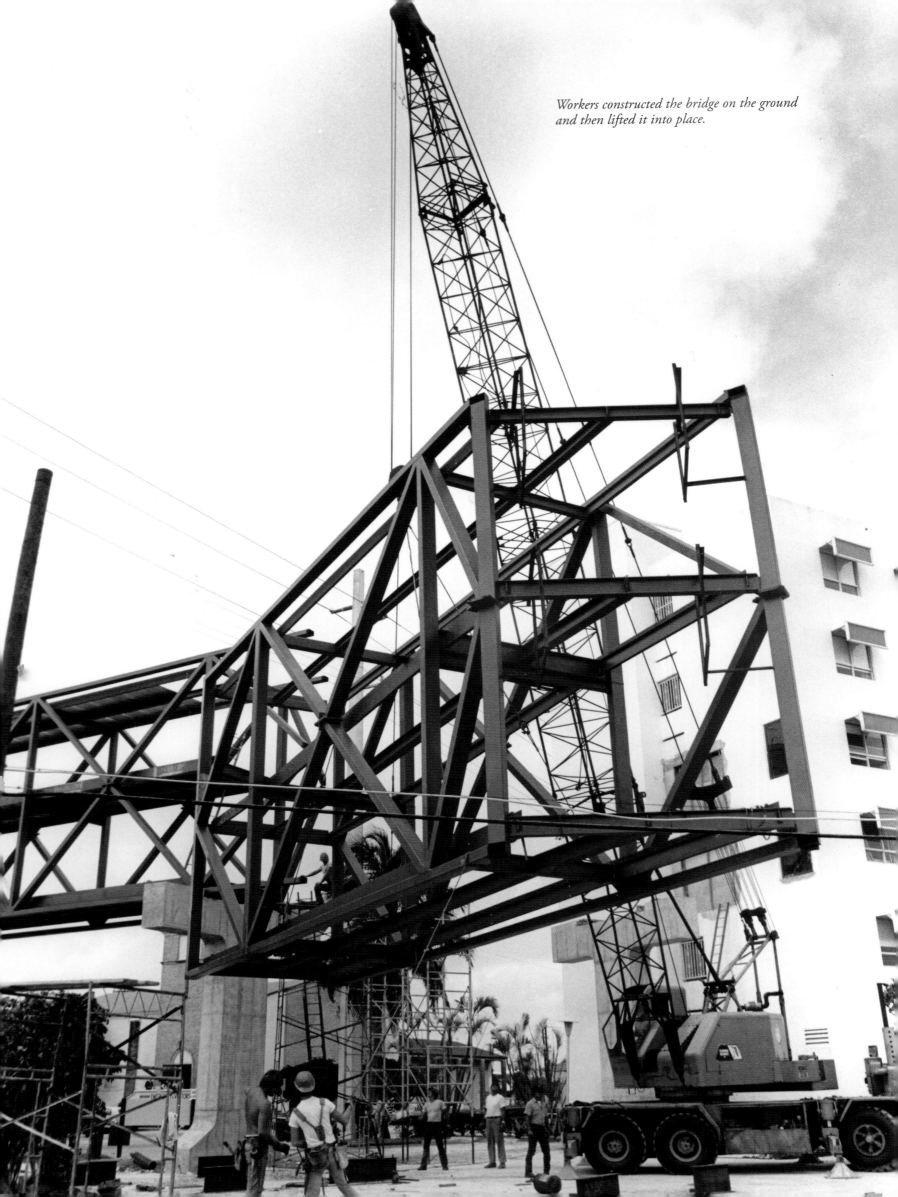

Workers constructed the bridge on the ground and then lifted it into place.

In 1977, Cook and the Board came up with an innovative solution to South Miami's unique setup across a major street. As the hospital grew, transporting patients across 62nd Avenue was becoming increasingly problematic. Data indicated that employees crossed the street more than 1,400 times a day and transported between 30 and 50 patients. The trips were time-consuming and even dangerous, as the staff had to navigate traffic in all weather conditions. Leaders planned for a double-decker pedestrian bridge to link the East Building with the main building between the third and fourth floors. The bridge would make South Miami the first hospital in South Florida to use air rights for patient travel. Employees embraced the idea, donating more than $153,000 to the $600,000 project.

Construction began in September 1978. The task — how to get this massive structure in the air — proved daunting. Engineers designed the bridge much like a child's erector set. Workers, using more than 40 tons of steel, constructed its pieces on the ground and planned to lift it in place. In what was dubbed the Valentine's Miracle of 1979, with onlookers cheering, two large cranes lifted and positioned the basic structure between the buildings. Eight months later the 175-foot bridge opened, complete with four-foot-high windows, air conditioning, carpeting and phone service. The impressive structure solved the traffic issue and finally unified South Miami Hospital.

In April 1979, in the midst of the bridge project, Donald Cook resigned to take a similar position in Los Angeles. Cook's tenure had brought targeted growth and new services. Yet amid the progress was a wave of unrest. Inflation, spiraling costs and the first steps of managed care left the hospital on shaky financial ground. Some on the Board questioned the management and what was perceived as unchecked spending.

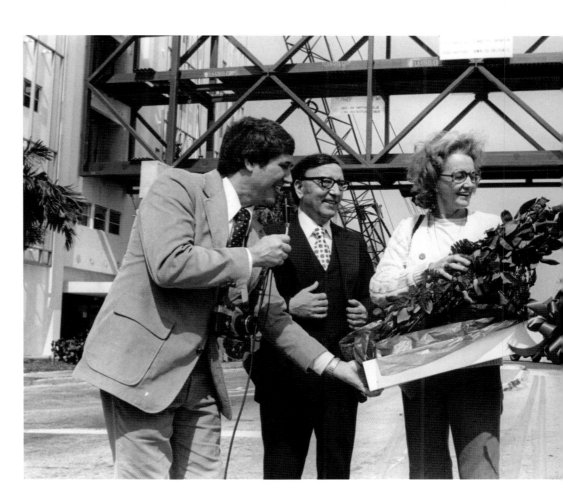

Donald Cook (left), Victor Dabby, M.D., and Roseanne Kelley, R.N., celebrated the opening of the bridge, which connected the East Building to the main hospital.

To succeed Mr. Cook, the Board looked to Merrill Crews, the administrator at neighboring Larkin Hospital. As an experienced hospital manager, Crews knew that the healthcare industry was in the midst of change. With insurance issues and proposed Medicare limits, hospitals were generating less revenue. So he initially focused his attention on containing costs and tightening the hospital's spending. South Miami began to share purchasing of some supplies with other hospitals, as the increased volume produced cost savings. In addition, the hospital concentrated on energy management that included eliminating unnecessary lighting and using task lighting when possible.

But growth was still a necessity. This meant investing in services to draw more patients to South Miami, which was typically 67 percent full. The hospital renovated the obstetrics department, and it became one of South Florida's busiest. It also improved cardiac care, adding the latest diagnostic equipment and centralizing services on the fourth floor of the main building. Under the guidance of James Margolis, M.D., South Miami became a leader in the newest treatment for heart disease — coronary angioplasty. With this minimally invasive procedure, doctors threaded a tiny balloon catheter through the groin into the heart's artery and inflated it so blood could flow freely. When Dr. Margolis brought the technique to South Miami in December 1978, he was one of a handful of pioneers doing angioplasties in the United States. By 1983, nearly 250 procedures were performed annually at the hospital.

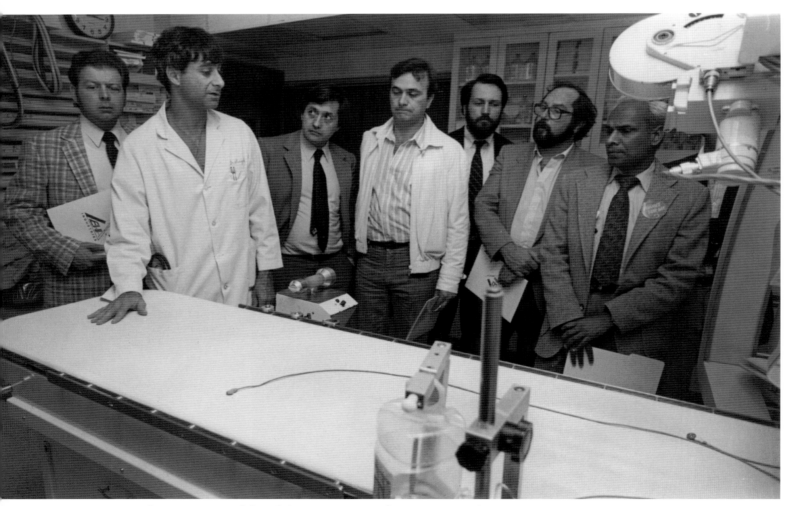

James Margolis, M.D., (second from left) was a pioneer of coronary angioplasty.

PTCA: How it Works...

CLOGGED CORONARY ARTERY

PCTA cases involve arteries that are constricted by fatty deposits which jeopardize critical blood flow.

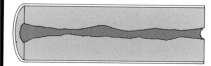

CATHETER INTRODUCTION

Inserted through a minimal incision, typically in the groin, the balloon catheter is directed through the artery system until reaching the affected area.

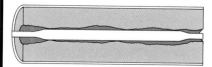

ONCE SITUATED

A series of brief inflations are initiated about the blockage.

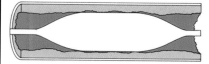

BLOOD FLOW RESTORED

Normally several inflations are all that is required to compress placque and slightly enlarge the interior artery walls creating improved blood flow.

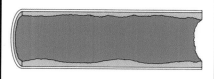

South Miami Hospital broadened its cardiac services to include coronary angioplasties, the latest techniques in cardiac rehabilitation and support groups for patients suffering from heart disease.

South Miami Hospital Wants *YOU* to Have a Healthy Heart!

That's why we created the HEART TO HEART CLUB for you or someone you know who has experienced a heart attack or other form of heart disease.

The HEART TO HEART CLUB is for people who are interested in cardiac rehabilitation. It's a forum for learning and group support. Physicians and other professionals offer programs and answer questions in all areas of concern to recovering patients and their families.

Membership is free. Meetings are held at 7:30 p.m. on the fourth Tuesday of every month at South Miami Hospital, U.S. 1 and S.W. 62nd Avenue, in the Penthouse, located on the 7th floor of the Tower Building.

The HEART TO HEART CLUB is another Community Health Education Program of South Miami Hospital. For more information call Community Relations, 622-8105.

Come join us. After all, who couldn't benefit from a good "HEART TO HEART?"

HEART TO HEART CLUB
south miami hospital

1981

South Miami Hospital...
LOOKING BACK

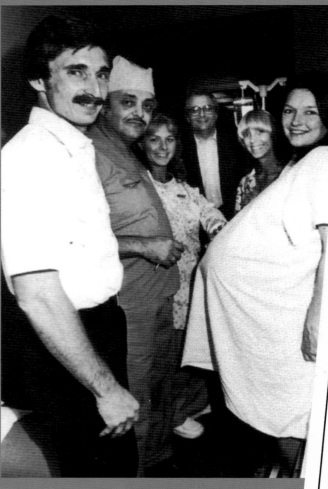

Patty Adams keeps her spirits up, with the support of husband Kent, Dr. Donald Hanft, nurses Debbie Sears and Gerry Myers and Manuel Suarez-Mendizabal, M.D.

PACE SETTER MAGAZINE

SOUTH MIAMI HOSPITAL • FALL 1981 • VOLUME FIFTEEN • NUMBER THREE

Quadruplets — A Florida First!

EENY MEANY

MINEY MO.

Family-Centered Maternity Care

On September 16, 1981, South Miami Hospital's maternity team, led by Donald Hanft, M.D., delivered Florida's first surviving quadruplets — Douglas, Brooke, Paul and Lindsay Adams. The delivery was planned with military precision and went off without a glitch. As one obstetrician reached for a child, another cut the cord, then handed the baby to a pediatrician, who carried the newborn to an adjoining room for the neonatologist to examine. The small army had practiced well in advance of the main event. The babies, born by cesarean section at 36 weeks, were strong and healthy. "It was an amazing experience to share," Dr. Hanft said just after the delivery. "I am on cloud nine."

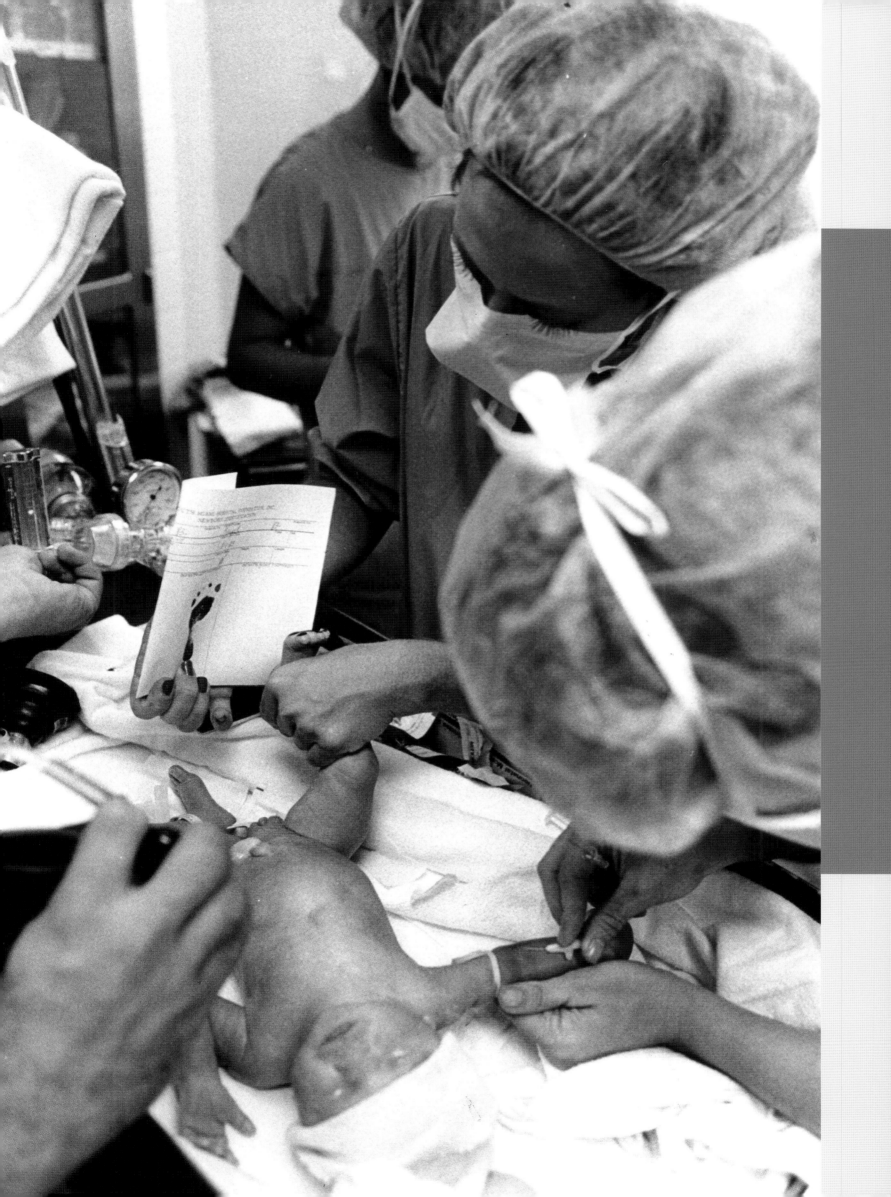

As South Miami celebrated its 25th anniversary in 1985, plans emerged to guide the hospital's future and guard against some of healthcare's downtrends. "In the ever-changing healthcare industry, it is impossible to stay ahead while standing still. We evolve not only to survive, but to improve upon the already excellent level of care we deliver and, yes, even to prosper. And so, we advance," Merrill Crews wrote in a newsletter. "South Miami Hospital is moving. We're moving like never before. And as our long-range plan unfolds, we will be an active participant in some of the most exciting — and effective — developments in Miami healthcare."

The long-range plan called for more hospital beds in high-demand services, bringing the total to 567. It also outlined construction that included a six- to eight-story parking garage, medical office building, North Tower building with 29 obstetric suites, an outpatient center and a larger emergency room. When completed, the hospital's footprint would nearly double, increasing from 439,620 to 714,000 square feet.

The leaders' vision put resources in growth areas — outpatient and emergency services, physician offices and obstetrics.

The ambitious building program brought questions and protests from a surrounding neighborhood whose residents felt threatened by encroaching development. They looked warily at the prospect of a major medical center in their backyard. To answer the neighbors' concerns, hospital executives held 34 public meetings and workshops. They listened and compromised by adding more landscaping and surface parking and limiting the size of the new buildings. "A required element of our future development is that South Miami Hospital now and always plays a positive and responsive role toward the communities it serves. That is especially essential regarding the city whose name our facility bears," Crews said. "Great pains have been taken to fulfill rather than inhibit the needs of South Miami's citizens while providing an upgraded physical plant."

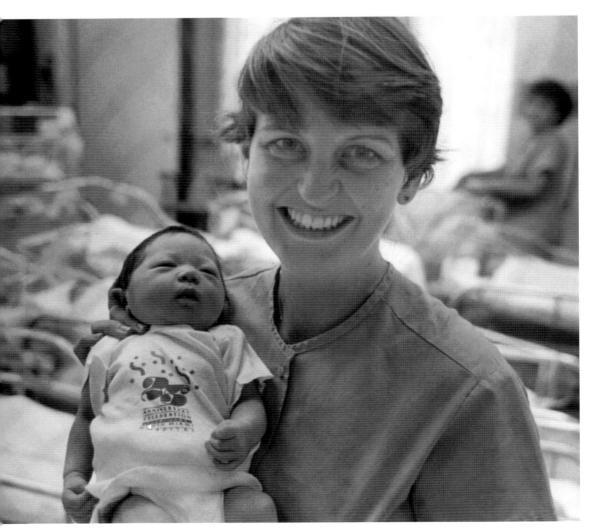

Newborns received special T-shirts marking South Miami Hospital's 25th anniversary.

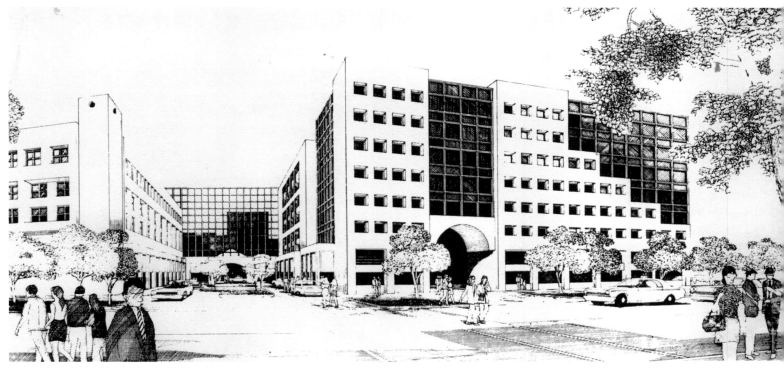

The expansion included a new entrance, garage and medical office building.

The open communication and concessions worked. Within the next few years, South Miami Hospital began renovations. It also added a free-standing diagnostic center, a freestanding ambulatory center, expanded cancer and radiation therapy, and home healthcare. The specialized services helped cushion the hospital against the tide of financial pressures. "It was an exciting time at South Miami," said Wayne Brackin, who joined the hosptial in 1985 as an administrative resident. "We were at the center of all this new technology and our physicians were driving the clinical innovation."

Yet South Miami's leaders felt that it was not enough. To be financially stable, South Miami needed to serve more patients. Hospitals could not afford to run operations as they had, and Merrill Crews and the Board looked beyond the traditional community for growth. They found a surprising opportunity for expansion in deep South Dade. Homestead's James Archer Smith Hospital was in financial trouble and South Miami Hospital could offer a solution. If all went well, a partnership between the two would bring financial security to a struggling community centerpiece and financial strength to a full-service medical center.

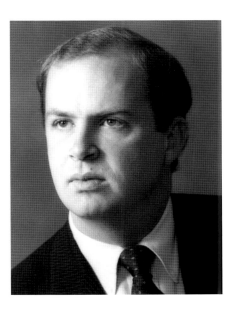

"It was an exciting time at South Miami. We were at the center of all this new technology and our physicians were driving the clinical innovation."

Wayne Brackin
administrative resident

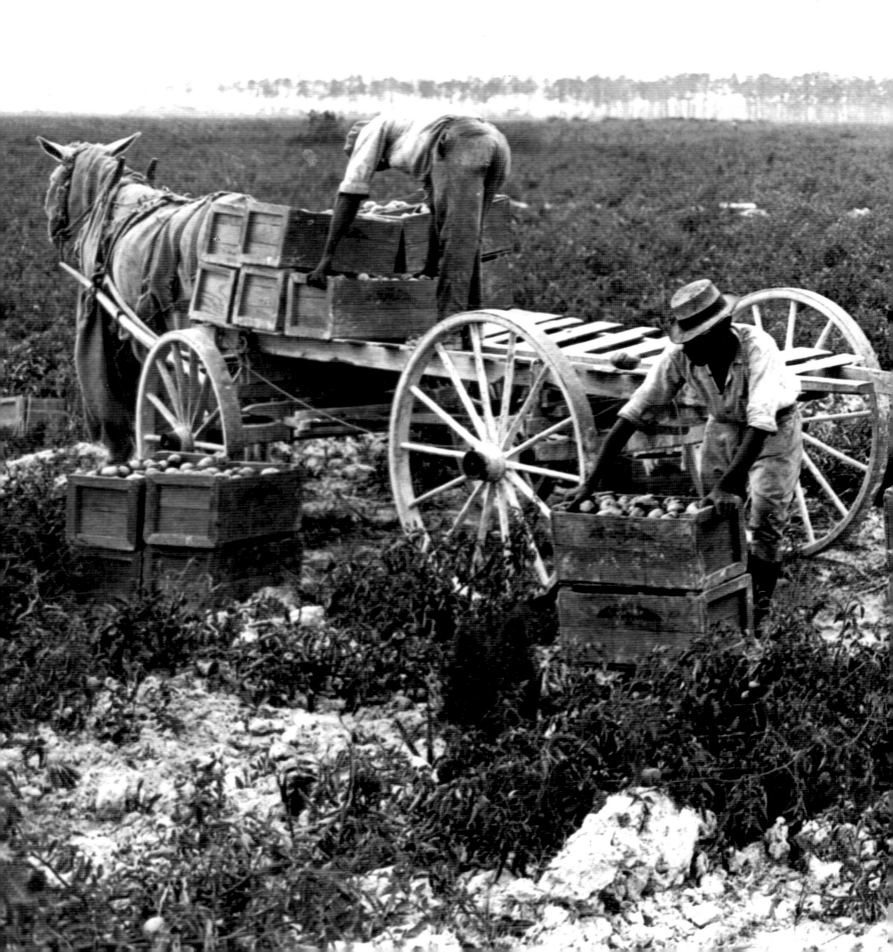

Tomato field in East Glade, c.1909

At the Center of Homestead

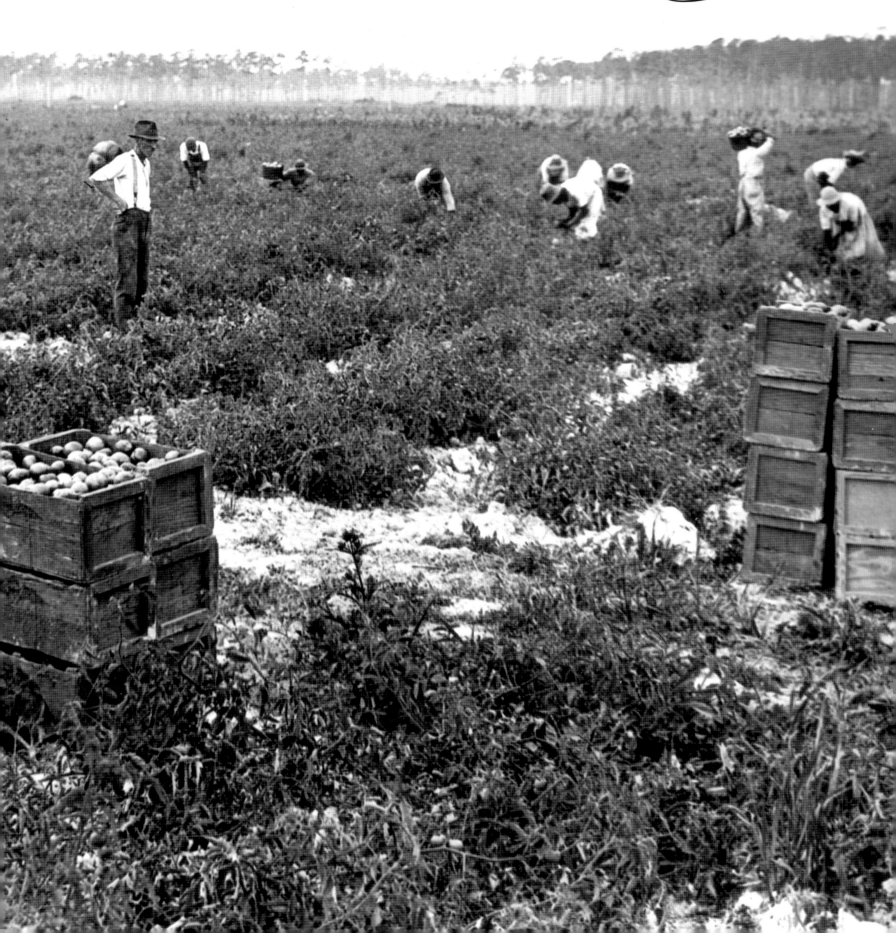

"It is a human institution... We have tried to run a hospital that makes every patient feel upon entering that every person cares as to whether or not he recovers, and concern is given 24 hours of the day, all year long, to every detail of welfare and comfort extended to the patient."

Report from the Board of Directors
James Archer Smith Hospital
1949

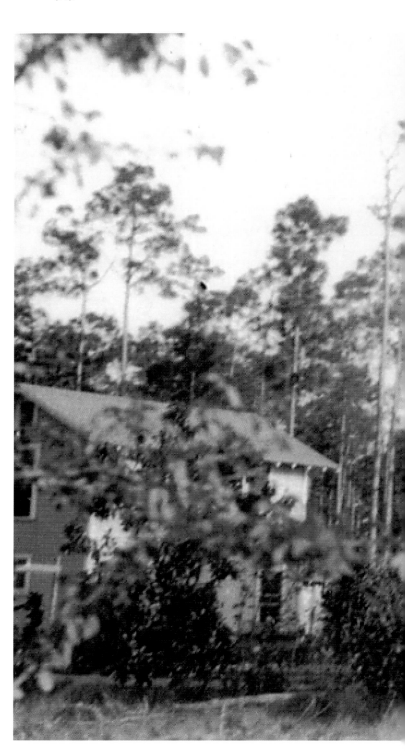

*I*n 1919, a young doctor named James Archer Smith settled in Homestead, a town about 20 miles south of Miami. He came looking for unspoiled land, game to hunt and people to heal. Dr. Smith grew up on a spit of land near the Florida-Georgia border — and his heart never left the backwoods. After some time in North Florida and a stint in World War I, the doctor came to Miami in 1917. But he found the city of nearly 30,000 too big and too developed.

Dr. Smith was at home in Homestead. The community was still in its infancy, incorporated just six years earlier. The rural area was hospitable, with a small-town feel. It included a school, drug store, three churches, a women's club and a library. The 1,200 residents lived off the land and clung proudly to their agricultural heritage.

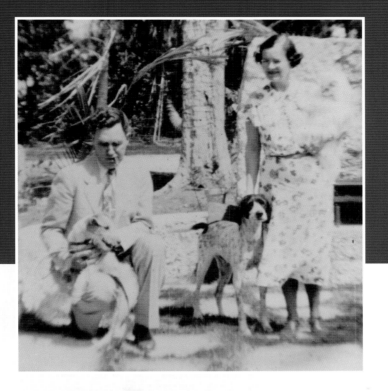

Left: Dr. Smith and his wife, Ada, with their dogs on the patio of their home.

Bottom: Dr. James Archer Smith's house was located on N.E. Sixth Street and Krome Avenue, c.1925.

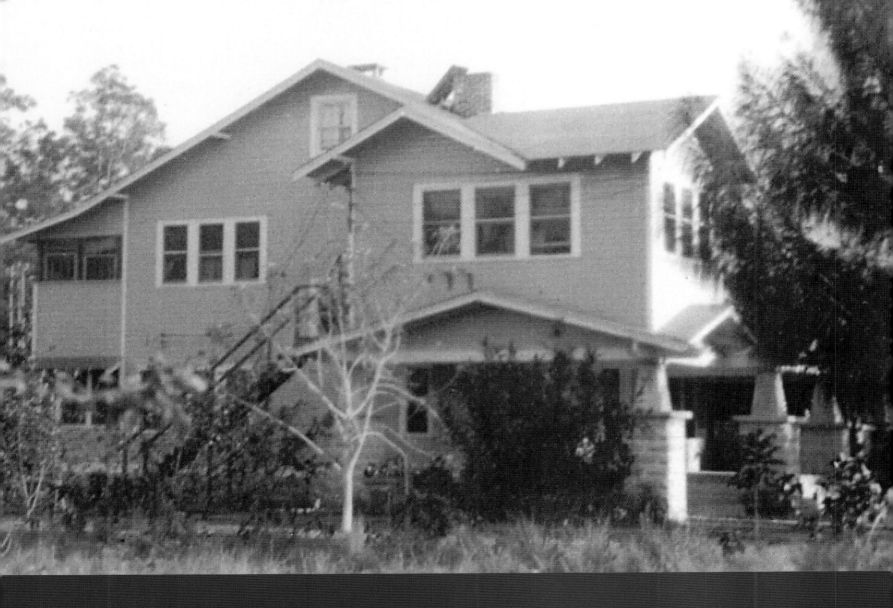

A Wilderness Becomes a Town

Just a few years before Dr. Smith arrived, Homestead was a wilderness. It was not until 1903, when surveyors for Henry Flagler's Florida East Coast Railway began readying the area for a railroad extension south from Miami, that a few pioneers discovered the location. William Alfred King, the section foreman, built the first permanent buildings in the community — a depot, offices, a tool shed and several homes for the railroad workers. The camp was made of portable structures. As soon as a section of the railroad was completed, workers tore the camp down and reassembled it to follow the tracks' progress. Its only inhabitants were associated with Flagler's project. Despite the isolation, the fertility of the land and the impending transportation brought optimism. A November 27, 1903, *Miami Metropolis* newspaper article described the promise that James Ingraham, a railroad vice president, saw in the location. "Mr. Ingraham is delighted with the terminal site," it read. "He says that it overlooks an immense prairie, over which the sails of craft on the bay can be seen toward the east while toward the south can be seen the mangrove swamps …"

The nascent community had not yet received an official name. Initially it had been called homestead country — simply a description of the homesteaders who gathered there. Some proposed calling the place Ingraham, in honor of the railroad man. But Ingraham would not hear of it. "It would hardly be fair to take all the glory of it to myself," he wrote in response to the idea. "…I therefore suggest that the place be named 'Homestead.' It is the homestead country, and the name has an attractive sort of a sound that may help bring people to it and establish it as a center."

By the summer of 1904, the railroad reached the now formally named Homestead, and with it more land opened up and settlers followed. William Horne, who owned a bicycle and grocery store in Miami, approached Flagler's men about opening a store for the workers and a boarding house for the occasional visitor, and got the support he needed. After Horne secured land, the railway's trains transported his building materials. He opened his store and living quarters and, with his wife, Ida, planted some tomato crops.

Others joined them and, by 1907, Homestead counted enough children in its population to open a school. The residents still grappled with the difficulties of pioneer life, including summer flooding, disease-carrying mosquitoes and an abundance of horse and deer flies that left their livestock soaked in blood.

The challenges, however, produced action. On January 27, 1913, 28 registered voters gathered to discuss the incorporation of Homestead. Their primary motivation was organizing to combat pollution from outhouses and shallow drinking wells. After enthusiastic discussion, 23 voted to incorporate and elect R.F. Tatum as mayor, and J.D. Redd, John Calkins, J.U. Free and G.D. Budd as councilmen. One of the group's first moves was to buy an acre of land outside Homestead's limits for a town dump.

The council also arranged to pave two main streets, buy a fire engine and build a city hall. The railroad chugged to and from Miami with regularity, bringing visitors and goods. Progress was starting to make the wilderness look more like a town.

"I therefore suggest that the place be named 'Homestead.' It is the homestead country, and the name has an attractive sort of a sound that may help bring people to it and establish it as a center."

James Ingraham
Vice President
Florida East Coast Railway

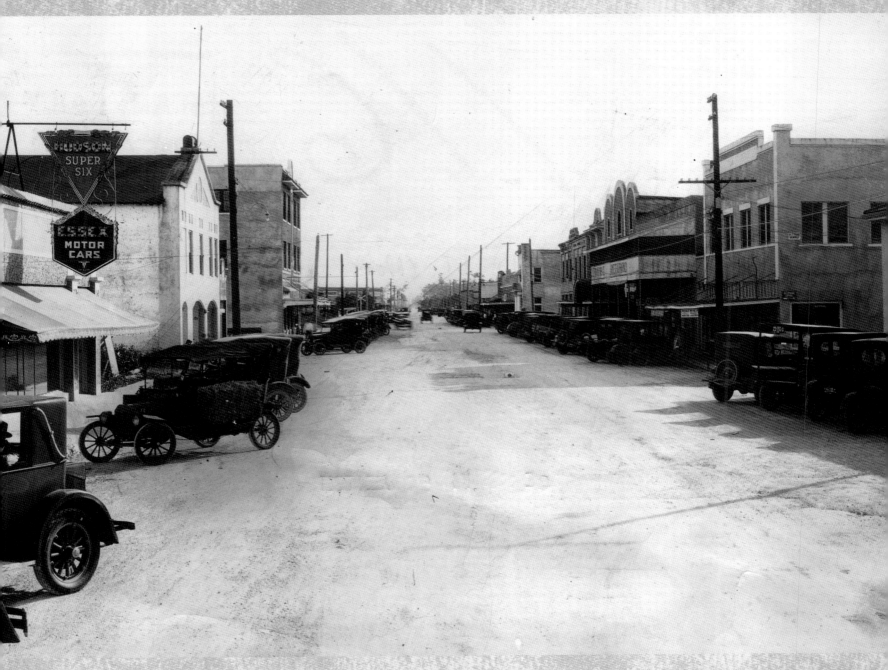

Looking south on Krome Avenue, c. 1920

In 1917, Florence Hunt added another piece to this developing community — a hospital. Ms. Hunt first began caring for South Dade residents as a nurse in private homes, seeing patients one at a time. The demand grew and she rented a two-story house in neighboring Florida City at First Street and N.W. First Avenue and named it the Florida City Hospital.

After two years, the area's local doctor, John Tower, M.D., convinced Ms. Hunt to move to Homestead. Dr. Tower had arrived in Homestead in 1910, an accomplished doctor hoping the warm climate would improve his ailing respiratory sys-tem. A 1901 graduate of Northwestern University Medical School, Dr. Tower had worked in Illinois, Minnesota and Kansas. When he came to South Dade, he cared for residents regardless of their race or ability to pay.

In September 1919, Hunt opened a six-room bungalow on Palmetto (Fourth) Street, which was called both Hunt Hospital and Homestead Hospital. She later added an oper-ating room and her practice flourished, espe-cially with women delivering babies. When she got too busy, she called a Miami nurse, Genevieve Fisk, to help.

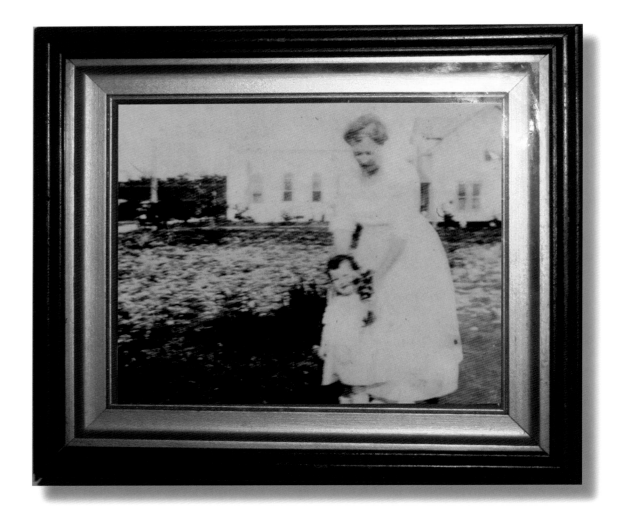

Florence Hunt is pictured with her daughter, Maude. Ms. Hunt ran hospitals in Florida City and Homestead.

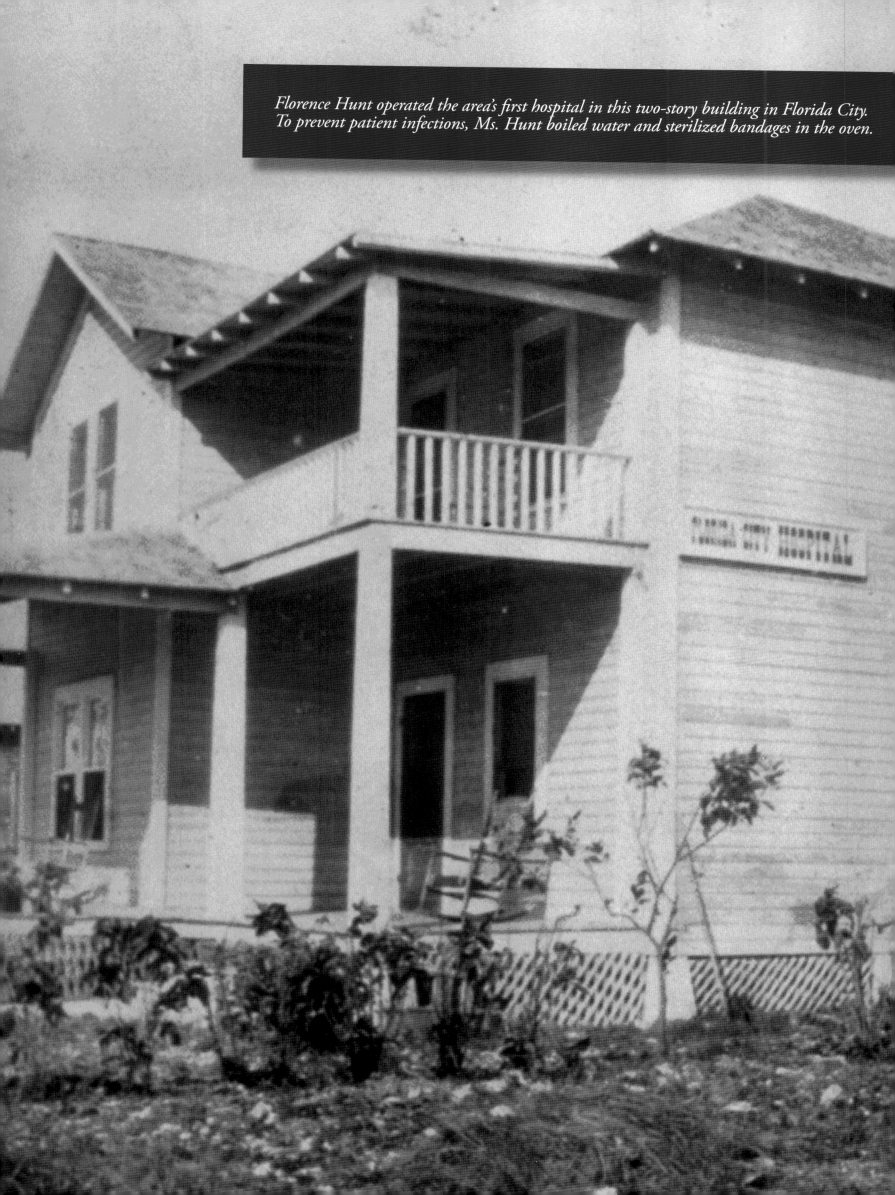

Florence Hunt operated the area's first hospital in this two-story building in Florida City. To prevent patient infections, Ms. Hunt boiled water and sterilized bandages in the oven.

To handle the community's growing medical needs, Ms. Fisk opened her own hospital in 1922 at N.W. Pine (First) Avenue and Campbell Drive (Eighth Street). The setup was modest — just a handful of beds in a simple-framed house. The staff included Fisk, a second nurse named Lena Cavender and the newly arrived Dr. Smith. They were later joined by another local doctor, A.M. Logan, M.D. Fisk's hospital was the center of medical care in the community.

Homestead relied on the makeshift establishment — what Dr. Smith called a "five-room house made over into a hospital." At first, it may have been adequate. The city's population was a little more than 1,300 and Dr. Smith and the others were indefatigable caregivers, part of the residents' extended family. But like the rest of South Florida, the community grew during the 1920s.

The great real estate boom brought people and development to the agricultural enclave. Krome Avenue property sold and resold at a frenetic pace. A downtown tract of land that cost $200 at the start of the decade sold for $1,500 in 1924 and nearly $100,000 a year later. During the height of the boom, developers announced plans for three large hotels, a 1,000-seat theater with a ballroom, four stores and a gasoline station.

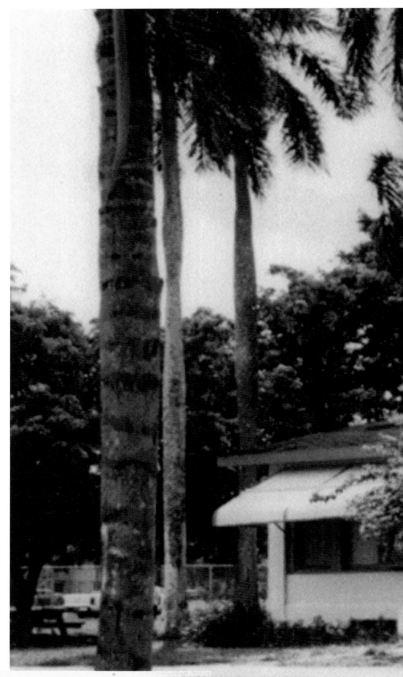

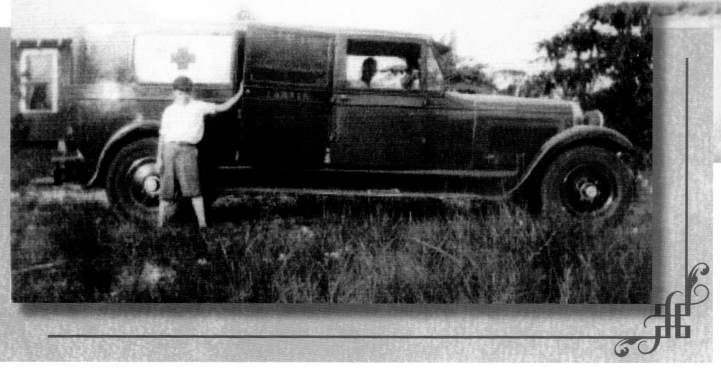

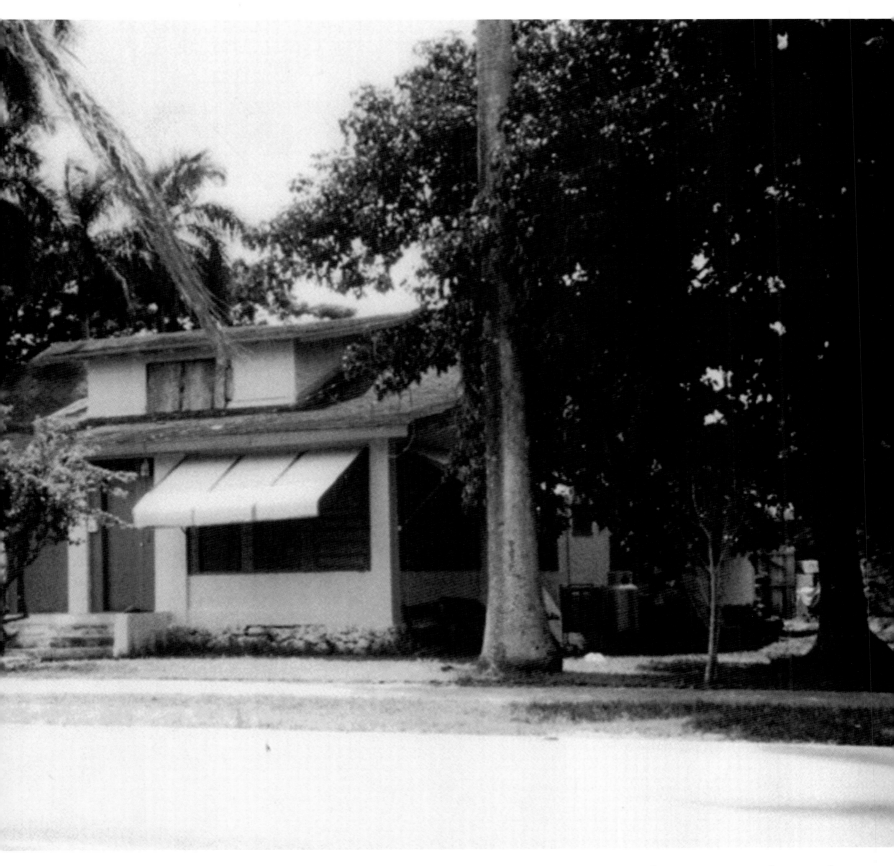

Above: Genevieve Fisk established the Post Graduate Hospital in 1922. It remained open until James Archer Smith was built.

Facing page: The Turner Funeral Home car served as the rural community's ambulance, transporting patients to Homestead's makeshift hospitals or to Miami for care.

A Need and a Hospital

The ambitious ideas were never realized. The 1926 hurricane destroyed much of South Florida, ending the real estate boom. The economic hardship of the Great Depression left many in the area struggling to make ends meet. For Homestead, agriculture remained the mainstay. Farmers cultivated crops including tomatoes, mangoes, potatoes, broccoli and corn. Most of the now more than 2,300 residents worked in the fields or packing houses.

With the trying times and growing population, providing healthcare to the community was a problem. Dr. Smith and his colleagues lacked adequate resources. While South Dade was connected to Miami by railroad and the now-completed South Dixie Highway, it remained isolated. Dade County Hospital opened in 1927 and offered care, but its location at 8500 S.W. 107th Avenue was still too far from deep South Dade. In fact, Dr. Smith, who was chief surgeon of the hospital, traveled approximately 50,000 miles a year to and from his office at the old Bank of Florida building at Krome Avenue and the Kendall facility. The unpaved roads made the trek arduous.

As early as 1926, Smith, who was then part of the City Council, began pushing for a larger, modern hospital in the area. After a few missteps, the effort gained footing, due in part to the merging of need and politics.

President Franklin Roosevelt answered the suffering of the Great Depression with an alphabet soup of government programs that hoped to stimulate the economy by creating jobs. Labeled the New Deal, these efforts included the Civilian Conservation Corps (CCC), which employed men to preserve and develop natural resources, and the largest employment program, the Works Progress Administration (WPA). Among its many features, the WPA hired the unemployed to build roads, public buildings and airport landing fields.

The WPA's mission fit perfectly with Homestead's goal of building a hospital to serve South Dade. In July 1938, the city's newspaper made its first mention of a $65,000 community hospital to be built as a WPA project. Community leader and Dr. Smith's longtime friend J.D. Redd donated the site — a 2.5-acre tract on N.W. First Avenue and 12th Street. Redd was a pioneer in Homestead and one of its most prominent citizens. He operated a general store and then the area's first department store. He served on the City Council from its incorporation until 1935, and the Dade County Commission from 1921 to 1935 and again from 1937 to 1942.

In November 1938, the federal government and local officials approved a $46,000 hospital with construction set to begin the next year. The WPA already had a presence in Homestead. WPA workers were building the library at 212 N.W. First Avenue and a municipal park. They resurveyed and remapped the city. J.E. Gossman, who supervised the library construction, was in charge of building the hospital.

While the hospital had its roots as a federal project, it was a decidedly community affair, with Dr. Smith as the driver. The WPA required the City of Homestead to share the hospital's cost — nearly one-third of the estimated budget. Dr. Smith almost single-handedly ensured that Homestead would not have to dip into its municipal accounts. He helped organize fundraisers, including themed dinner dances, picnics, raffles and fish fries. He used the force of his personality to convince, cajole and beseech friends, family and grateful patients to donate to the hospital. "He was a persuasive con man," said his son affectionately, years later, "and he usually got his way."

With the trying times and growing population, providing healthcare to the community was a problem. Dr. Smith and his colleagues lacked adequate resources.

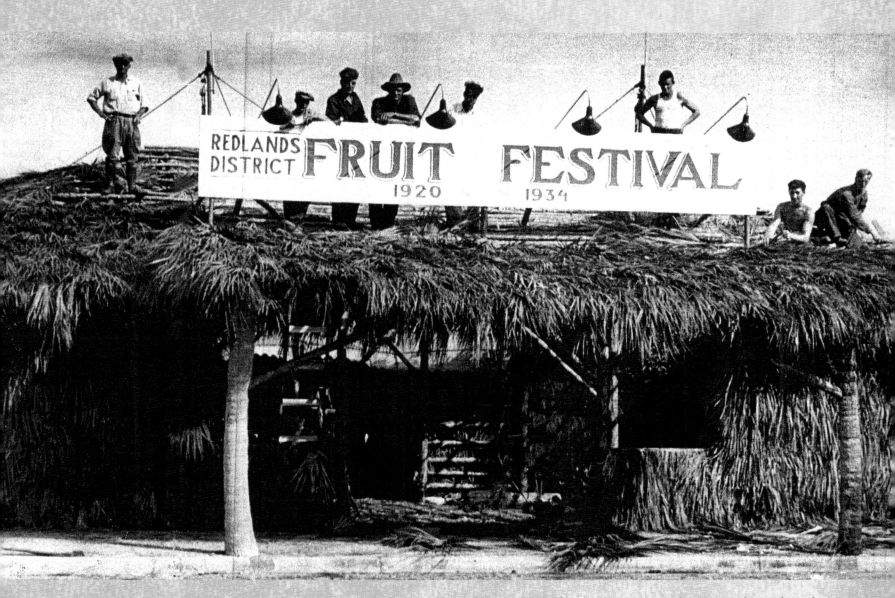

Agriculture was the main industry in early South Dade.

A Name and a Start

By 1940, the hospital was well under way. It was a grassroots effort, with the community pitching in to help. Until the building was ready, a stretcher, oxygen tent, baby incubator and operating table sat in storage at the First National Bank of Homestead. In May, about 150 community leaders and residents gathered at a picnic dinner on Dr. Smith's front lawn. During the event, the mayor proposed naming the hospital after the beloved physician. Although Dr. Smith protested, preferring that the name reflect the Homestead area, every guest voted to name the building after its "father." James Archer Smith Hospital was officially created. The first Board members equally represented the surrounding communities of Homestead, Redland, Silver Palm, Princeton, Goulds, Florida City and Perrine. In a prophetic comment that foreshadowed future conflicts, Mayor Tom Harris pledged that the Board would have complete charge of the hospital's management. "The city will keep out of it," he said.

James Archer Smith Hospital admitted its first patient, W.M. Brodie, on August 9, 1940. The building included 10 patient rooms, one operating room, one delivery room, a kitchen and X-ray facilities with equipment from Ms. Fisk's defunct hospital. Dr. Smith and Dr. Logan staffed the hospital. Room rates were $5 a day for a semi-private room, $6 a day for a private room and $7 a day for a corner room. The superintendent, as the administrator was called, was Elinor Robertson, who had spent five years at Dade County Hospital in Kendall at S.W. 107th Avenue.

With its opening, the community found its cause. "You are getting the best hospital building and equipment that money can buy and I know that you all are as proud of it as I am," Dr. Smith said at the time. "Everyone I have contacted for donations has given me money willingly and generously, and I can't thank them enough."

Residents and organizations sponsored individual rooms. The doors read like a Who's Who of Homestead's elite. Dr. Smith and his wife sponsored one, as did Mr. and Mrs. Charlie Fuchs of the famed Fuchs Bakery. The Rotary Club's room honored Dr. Tower, who had died a year earlier.

By the end of the first month, hospital personnel had treated 29 patients. The closing of both Hunt Hospital (1936) and the Fisk Hospital (1940) made JAS, as locals affectionately called it, the sole hospital in the area. In a sad twist, Ms. Hunt died just a month after James Archer Smith opened.

While James Archer Smith had a modern feel, leaders prided themselves on the intimacy of "their" hospital. The spirit that drove this rural community — its population hovered around 3,000 in 1940 — shaped the hospital as well. The community was like a family who took care of each other.

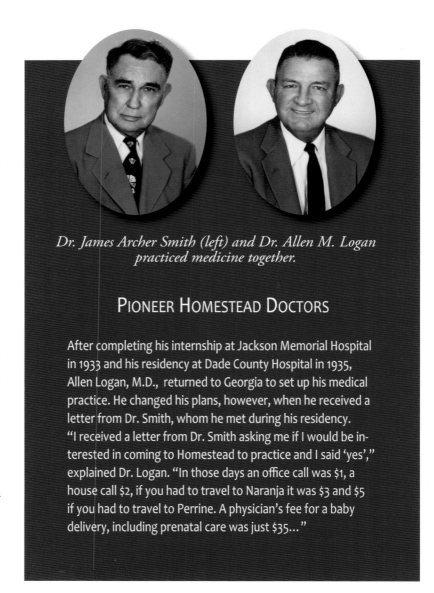

Dr. James Archer Smith (left) and Dr. Allen M. Logan practiced medicine together.

PIONEER HOMESTEAD DOCTORS

After completing his internship at Jackson Memorial Hospital in 1933 and his residency at Dade County Hospital in 1935, Allen Logan, M.D., returned to Georgia to set up his medical practice. He changed his plans, however, when he received a letter from Dr. Smith, whom he met during his residency. "I received a letter from Dr. Smith asking me if I would be interested in coming to Homestead to practice and I said 'yes'," explained Dr. Logan. "In those days an office call was $1, a house call $2, if you had to travel to Naranja it was $3 and $5 if you had to travel to Perrine. A physician's fee for a baby delivery, including prenatal care was just $35..."

"It was really a godsend.... If it wasn't for the hospital we would have had to travel to Kendall or Miami for care."

Charlotte Schmunk
Hospital volunteer

"It was really a godsend," remembered Charlotte Schmunk, who was born at Fisk Hospital in 1925 and became involved with James Archer Smith and served as president of its Ladies Auxiliary. "If it wasn't for the hospital we would have had to travel to Kendall or Miami for care." Perhaps out of necessity, the hospital and its doctors became the glue that tied Homestead residents together.

"We were like a family," Ms. Schmunk said. With his gregarious personality, Dr. Smith would walk the halls, telling jokes and greeting everyone he encountered with the familiarity of an old friend. The more formal Dr. Logan carried himself with a bit more reserve. Patients were more likely to swoon over his sophisticated style than slap his back. Still, both shared an unwavering dedication to the patients, hospital and community. They made house calls, often traveling throughout deep South Dade day or night. As true family physicians, they cared for parents, children and grandchildren. In the case of the Schmunks, Dr. Smith delivered both Charlotte and her son.

James Archer Smith Hospital opened August 9, 1940. Drs. Smith and Logan staffed the 10-bed hospital.

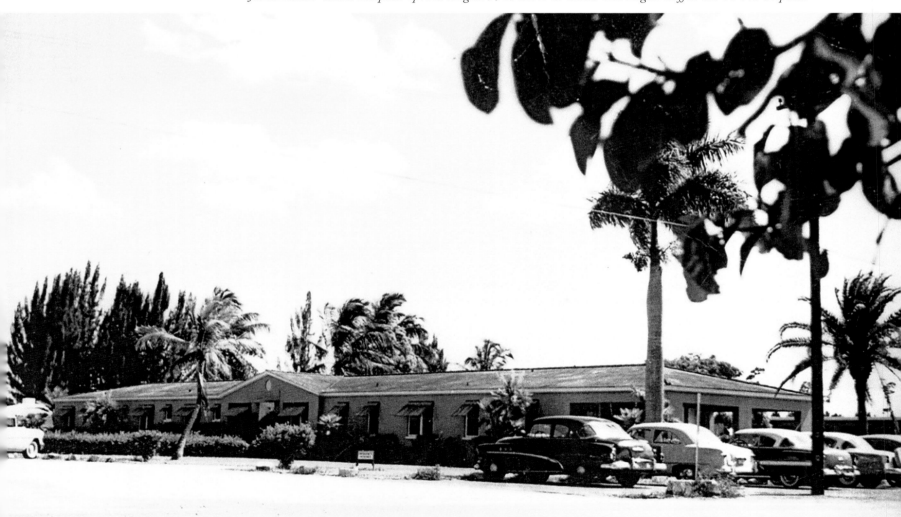

Additions and Expansions

Four years after admitting its first patient, James Archer Smith was ready for growth. The hospital added eight rooms and new kitchen facilities in an $18,000 renovation. As it had done in the past, the community rallied around the hospital to raise funds for the improvements. Activities included baseball games, dances and a chicken dinner at Dr. Smith's house, where items such as a birdcage and nylon stockings were auctioned.

In 1949, the hospital grew yet again. By converting some of the private rooms into semi-private ones, James Archer Smith became a 25-bed hospital. The project also expanded the emergency room and laboratory. Still, the expansions were small and the hospital remained the homey, friendly place of its founding.

The new decade did little to disrupt the tranquil lifestyle of Homestead. The population in the city limits grew to 4,500, but daily life was still about the land. While Miami was taking its first steps toward becoming a metropolis, South Dade was very much country. Residents farmed and rode horses; children played undisturbed in the yard or helped their parents tend crops.

Nonetheless, James Archer Smith needed to adapt to the community. By 1953, the hospital had doubled in size with a new 30-bed wing, a new operating room, and a delivery room and nursery. For the next decade, the hospital's footprint remained the same. A small renovation in the early 1960s brought new offices, an enlarged kitchen with a dining room and more beds. James Archer Smith became a 75-bed institution.

The era was also one of charter changes and ownership questions — an issue that would plague the hospital for years to come. The city had initially leased the hospital to a nonprofit corporation, James Archer Smith Hospital, Inc., and its Board of Directors helped manage the hospital. After some question about the terms of the lease, the city amended the charter — and the change gave local government strong influence over hospital operations.

Part of this was due to the timing and technicality of the law. By the mid-1960s, community leaders and hospital officials realized that the nearly 30-year-old building was outdated. Hospital leaders wanted a replacement and hoped to get federal aid to finance a new building. To qualify for both U.S. Department of Housing and Urban Development loans and grant money from the Hill-Burton Act (which provided government money to build and improve hospitals), the city needed to have budgetary control over James Archer Smith.

The legal changes allowed the hospital to qualify for federal funds. Residents of Homestead and community groups helped as well. In a 1966 election, taxpayers approved the sale of revenue bonds for the new hospital building. The Ladies Auxiliary began organizing an annual dinner dance — the Champagne Ball — that raised money and awareness for the hospital.

In March 1969, a 75-bed building replaced the original James Archer Smith. The $2.5 million, three-story hospital had the latest technologies, including an intensive care unit, a coronary care unit, physical therapy suites and a respiratory therapy department. Room rates reached $37 for a semi-private room and $48 for a private room. Each came equipped with a telephone and television.

Five years later, the hospital tapped into more federal money to support another expansion. In May 1974, it added a 48-bed wing that included a critical care unit, pediatric ward and prayer room. More than 175 employees now worked at James Archer Smith.

"We had most everything at the hospital. People did not have to go up the road for their healthcare," remembered Barbara Dempsey, who worked in food services at the time. "Patients could stay in the neighborhood and that was comforting. Our patients were people we knew — who we went to church with or saw at the grocery store."

Yet the congeniality belied a brewing conflict. With city officials now having authority over hospital operations, the mix of politics and healthcare proved explosive. The next decade at James Archer Smith would have a soap-opera quality with infighting, a revolving door of leadership and a fight for survival.

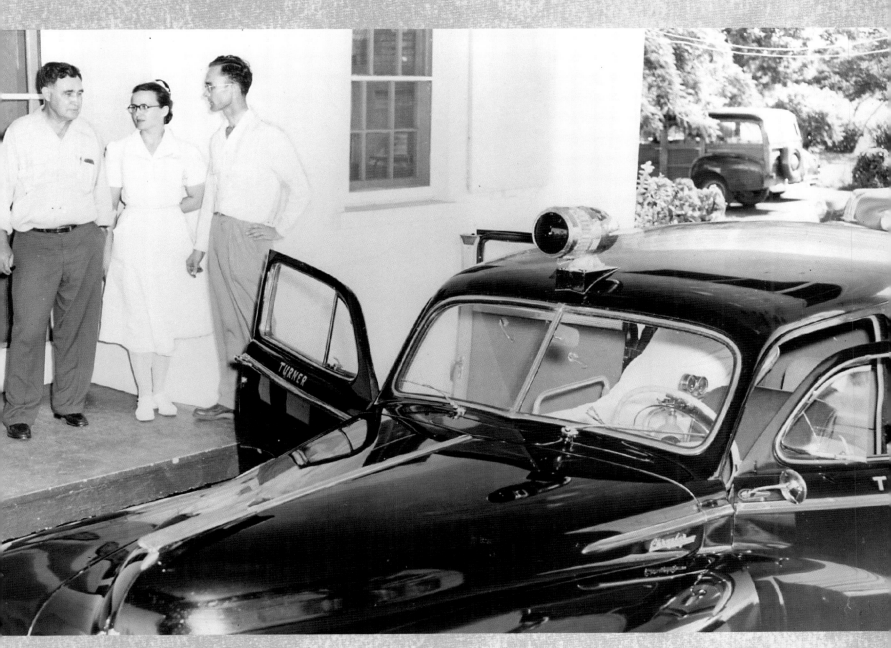

Dr. James Archer Smith (left), an unidentified nurse and Ed Branam of the Turner Ambulance Service stand at the front door of James Archer Smith Hospital on July 28, 1950.

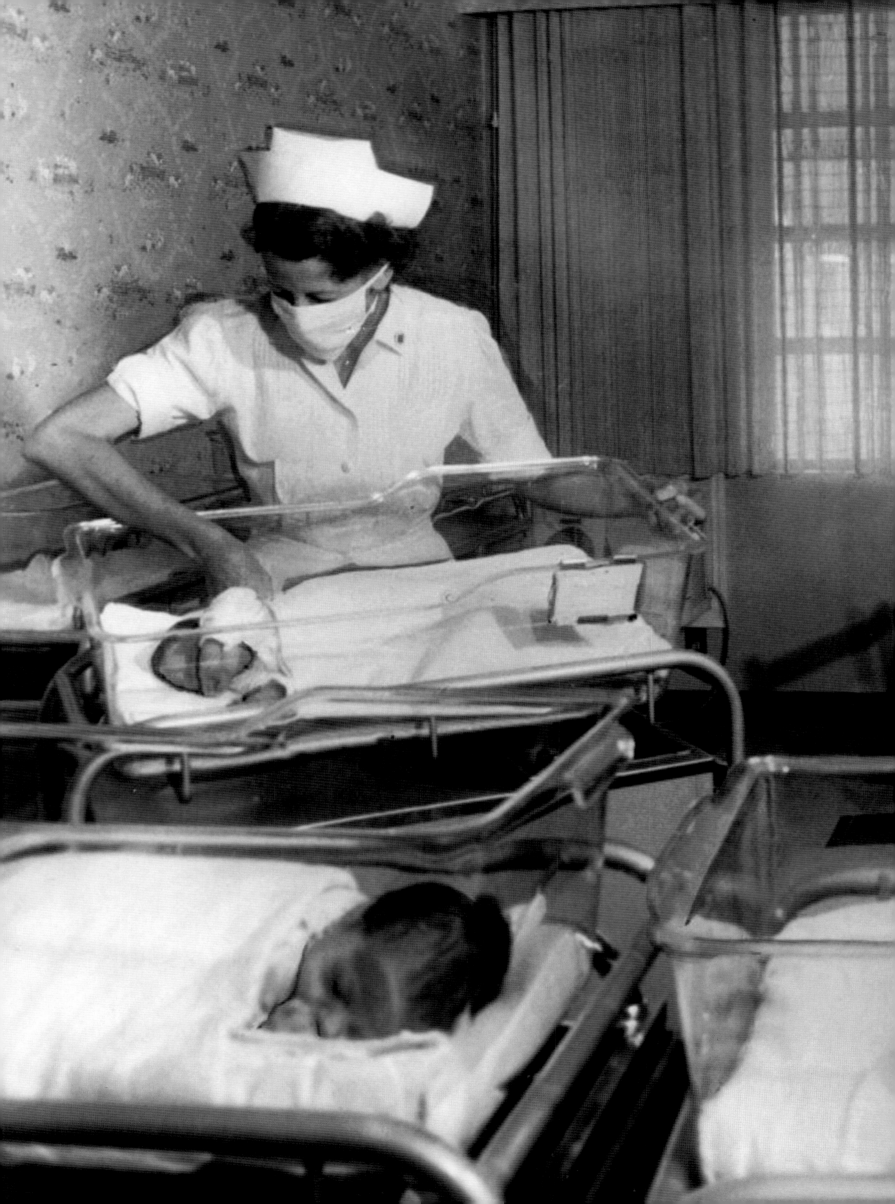

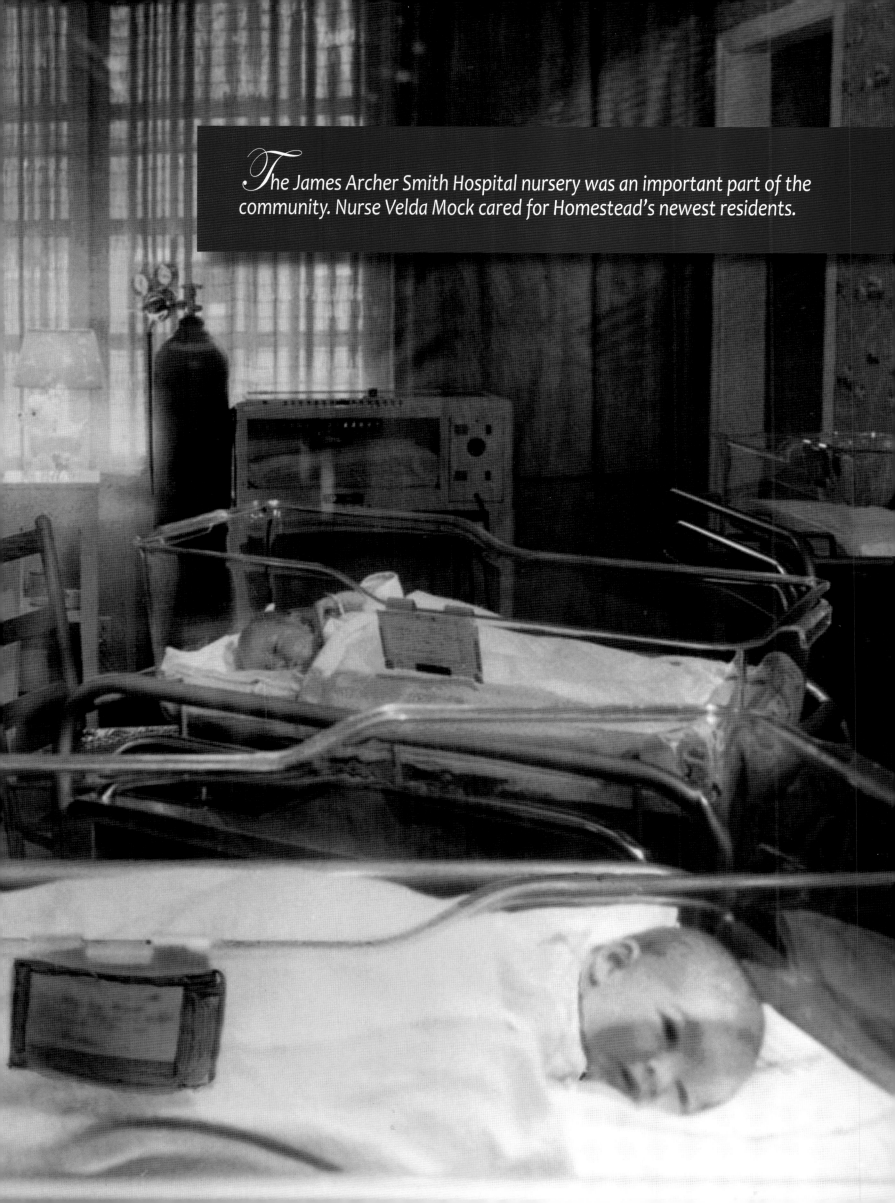

The James Archer Smith Hospital nursery was an important part of the community. Nurse Velda Mock cared for Homestead's newest residents.

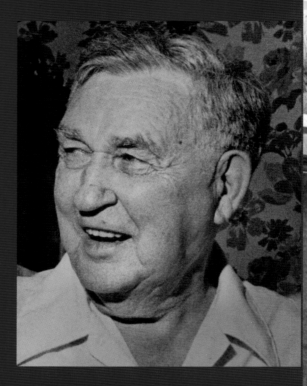

James Archer Smith, M.D.

He was called Homestead's uncrowned king, benevolent dictator and unofficial mayor. Whatever the title, James Archer Smith, M.D., was the city's leading citizen. Dr. Smith was born in 1891 near Madison, Florida, about 20 miles from the Georgia border. His father cultivated cotton and tobacco on the family's plantation and the boy learned early to love the land. He enjoyed a Huck Finn kind of childhood, fishing and hunting in the surrounding woods and streams.

Dr. Smith attended the University of Florida and then Atlanta Medical School (later Emory University). He married a local girl, Ada Palmer, and practiced in North Florida before serving in France during World War I. After the war, he came to Miami and in 1919 settled in Homestead, where he lived and cared for patients until his death at age 91 in 1982.

Dr. Smith was a beloved country doctor with big-city smarts. He could quote Shakespeare, fish for his dinner and hunt big game. In fact, he proudly displayed his prize catches throughout his house. He was also a practical joker. Legend had it, for example, that one Christmas he asked the police chief for the jail keys because he wanted to see a patient. Later at bed check, all 20 prisoners were gone. Dr. Smith had released them, with a wink and Christmas wishes.

In Homestead, there was little he did not do. He was elected to the City Council in 1923 and held office for eight years before resigning — too opinionated for the delicacies of politics. He served on the volunteer fire department, played baseball for the local team and for a time had a nursery just outside of town. He even donated royal palms to beautify Krome Avenue.

Most of all, he was the neighborhood doctor. He tended to the young and old, delivered babies and, in an era of deep segregation, cared for residents regardless of race. When making a house call, he might ask what was for dinner and sit right down to eat. Dr. Smith never kept track of payments. He would take vegetables or fruit in place of money — whatever a family had — and was known to leave a few dollars on the table if the situation warranted.

It was fitting that the community's hospital bear his name. He was the city's caretaker and pushed hard for its creation. Nevertheless, it was a formal honor for a man without formality. A longtime hospital volunteer, Charlotte Schmunk, said Dr. Smith was "like an old shoe that you loved and never got tired of wearing."

Facing page: Dr. James Archer Smith and his wife, Ada Elisabeth Palmer Smith, in their house on N. Krome Avenue

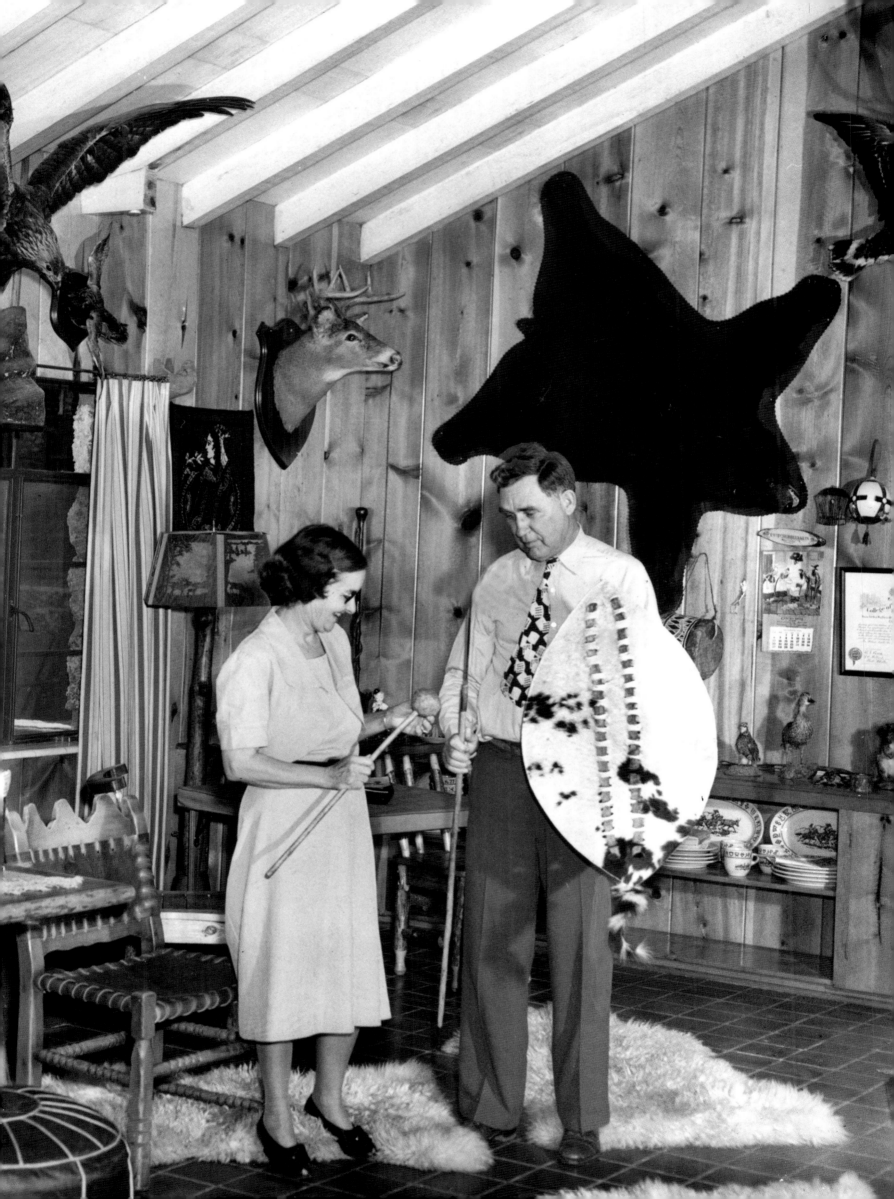

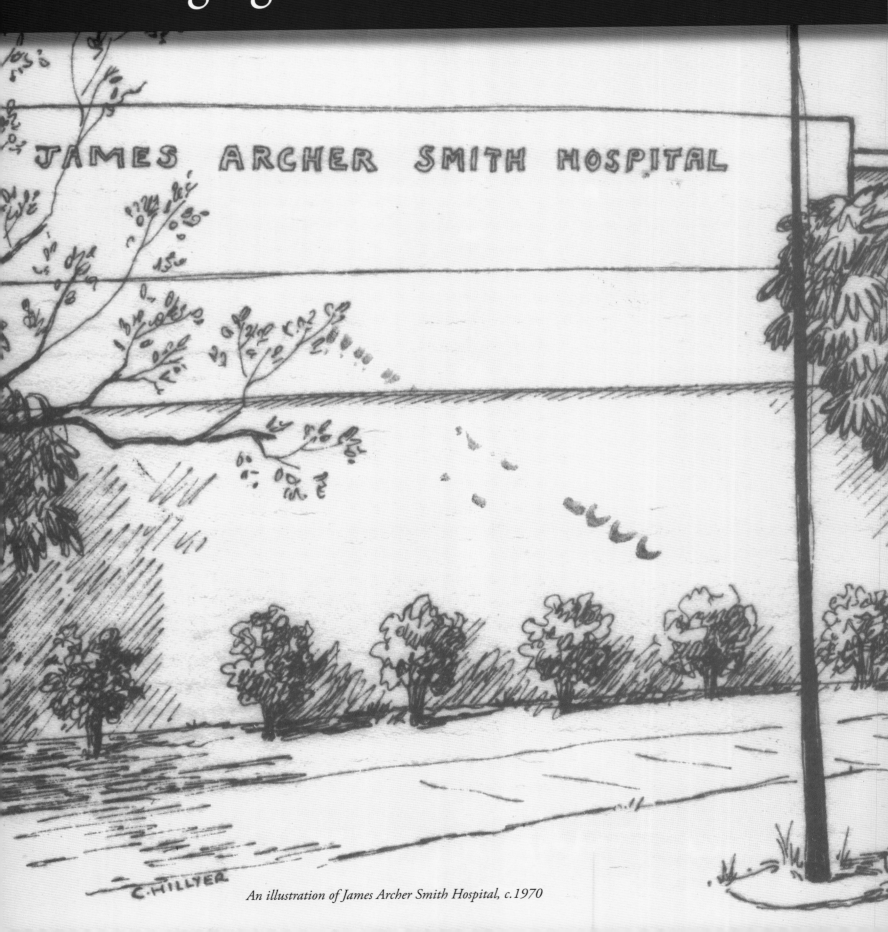

Merging Interests

An illustration of James Archer Smith Hospital, c.1970

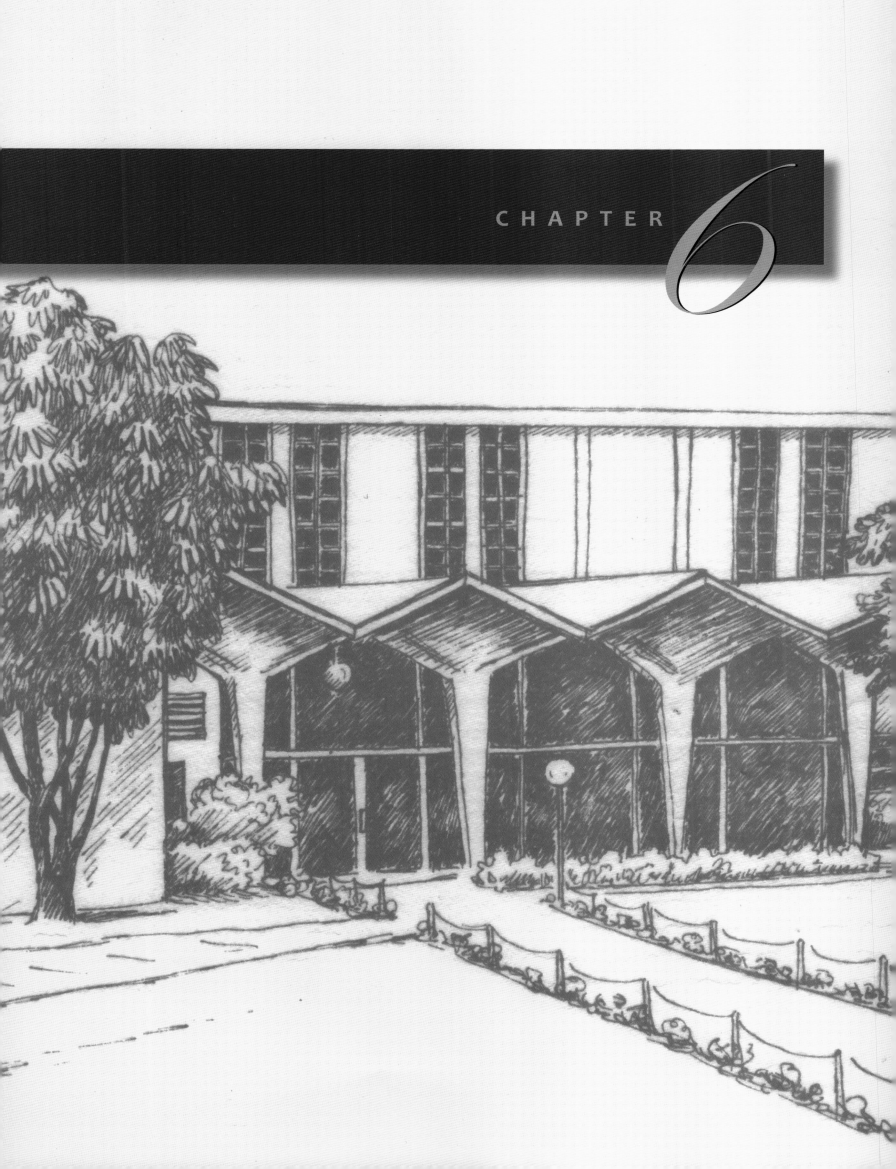

CHAPTER *6*

"Throughout its history, James Archer Smith Hospital has faced many challenges. But every one of them has made the hospital stronger in the community of Homestead. And the strengths of this institution have been the foundation for the future — a future which promises more challenges, progress and a lot of excitement."

Vincent B. McKee
CEO, James Archer Smith Hospital
1970

James Archer Smith Hospital began its 35th year in 1975 with an improved facility and more services. The hospital served a tight-knit Homestead community, whose population would double from about 13,000 at the decade's start to more than 26,000 by 1980. While the area still was a prospering agricultural region, the community was broadening beyond farming. An urban core developed around Krome Avenue. Homestead built a new City Hall and opened a regional library and new high school.

The hospital remained a source of pride, but its mission to serve the community's healthcare needs became muddled by challenging circumstances. Even with the hospital's new wing, its facilities were lacking, especially in comparison to the fast-growing hospitals to the north, Baptist and South Miami. The 1973 addition of Miami Dade General Hospital at 9333 S.W. 152nd Street (later called Coral Reef Hospital) added competition in the southern part of Dade County. As a small rural hospital, it was becoming harder and harder for James Archer Smith to offer patients the latest technologies.

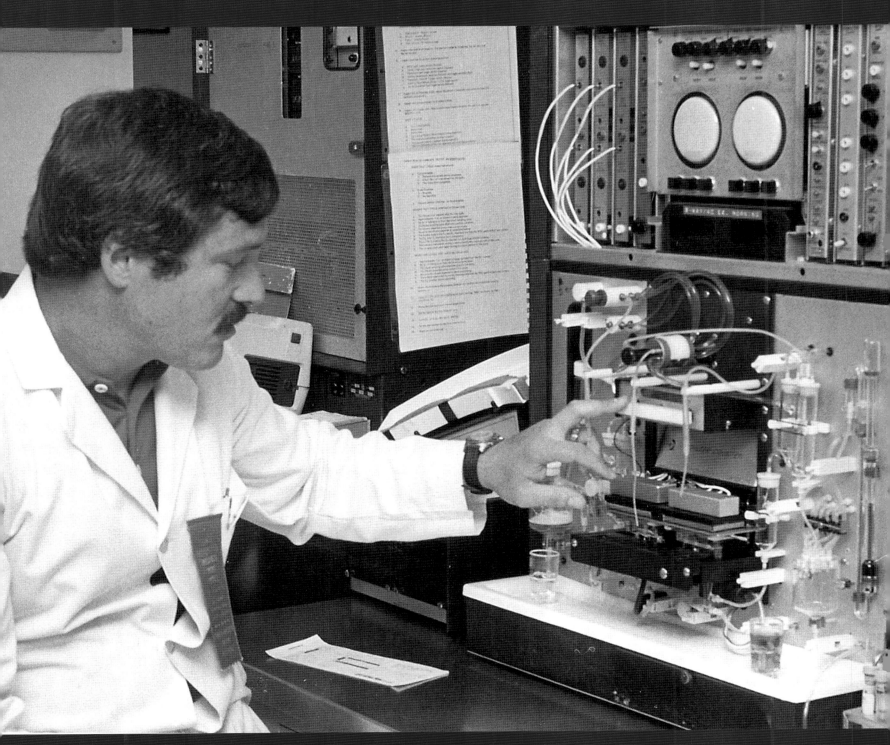

By 1975, James Archer Smith Hospital included a new building with cardiac services, a laboratory, physical and respiratory therapy and pediatric care. Despite the range of services, the hospital faced financial problems.

A Push to Sell

As the 1970s ended, a storm of criticism swirled around James Archer Smith. Outside auditors questioned the hospital's financial foundation, citing delays in patient billing, inconsistent operating procedures and unneeded expenditures. They pointed to important hospital equipment that was not purchased and roof and air-conditioning repairs that were left undone.

James Archer Smith's unique management structure compounded the problem. The City of Homestead had overarching control over the hospital. While City Council members appointed a supervisory Board to help James Archer Smith's leaders, the situation remained highly charged. Local politicians could, and often did, interfere with hospital business. Meetings about hospital policy were open to the public and often deteriorated into shouting matches. Local newspapers ran accounts of the spectacle and controversy.

Some issues were clear. The hospital needed updated equipment, capital improvements and tighter management controls. Some residents believed that the change could not happen with local government involved. They argued that politicians brought their own ideas to the hospital, creating turmoil and a lack of clear leadership.

In 1981, Homestead voters faced a referendum question — whether to sell James Archer Smith Hospital. The idea was that the city could rid itself of a financial burden and a new owner could improve the hospital and run it efficiently. The faction in favor of the sale even outlined where the city's proceeds could go — to renovate the senior citizens center, improve parks and streets, and hire more police officers.

Despite the hype, the question was far more complicated. The hospital had symbolic meaning to a community with a strong sense of pride. Equally important was the hospital's mission to care for all residents, regardless of their ability to pay. A new owner could limit services for the poor. With passionate feelings on both sides, the election grew emotionally charged.

About a week before the vote, the City of Homestead heard from James Archer Smith himself, an aging medical and community leader who weighed in on the controversy with a letter to the local newspaper. Dr. Smith acknowledged the problems with the hospital, and had even expressed embarrassment about the situation, but still believed that it belonged to the Homestead community. The citizens built it, paid for it and used it. "How can the City of Homestead sell something that morally does not belong to it?" he wrote. He urged citizens to vote no on the sale and "with more effort make the hospital an institution we can all be proud of and which can give the best medical care...which was the original intention anyway."

> "*How* can the City of Homestead sell something that morally does not belong to it? With more effort we can make the hospital an institution we can all be proud of and which can give the best medical care...which was the original intention anyway."
>
> Dr. James Archer Smith

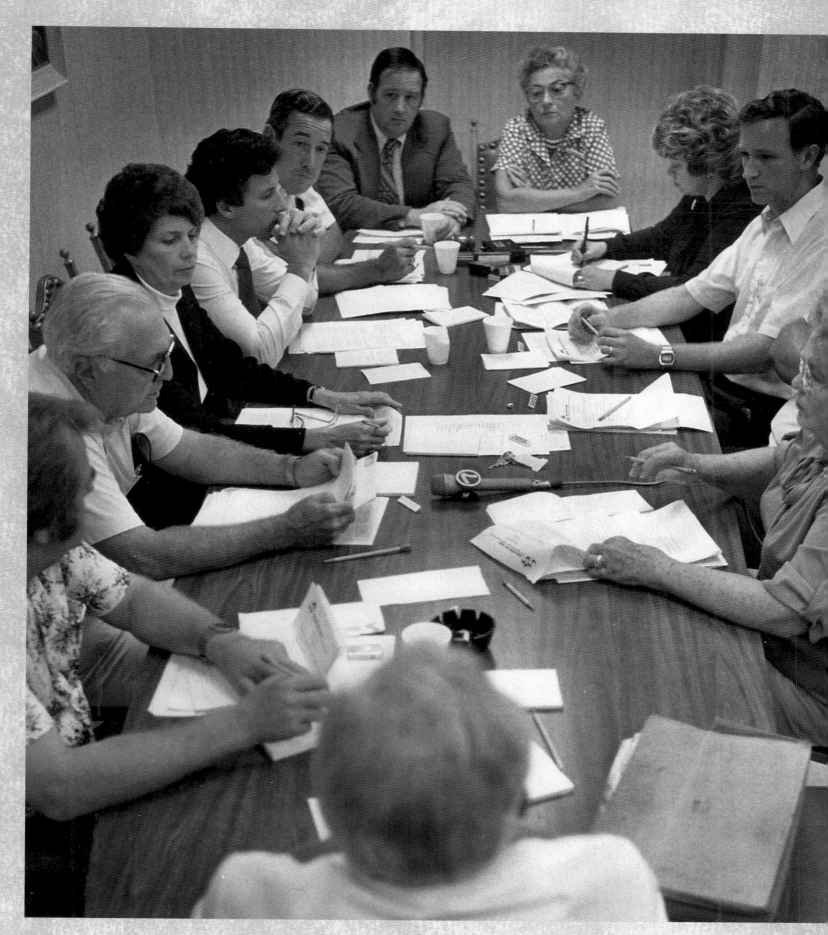

Board members of James Archer Smith Hospital in November 1980

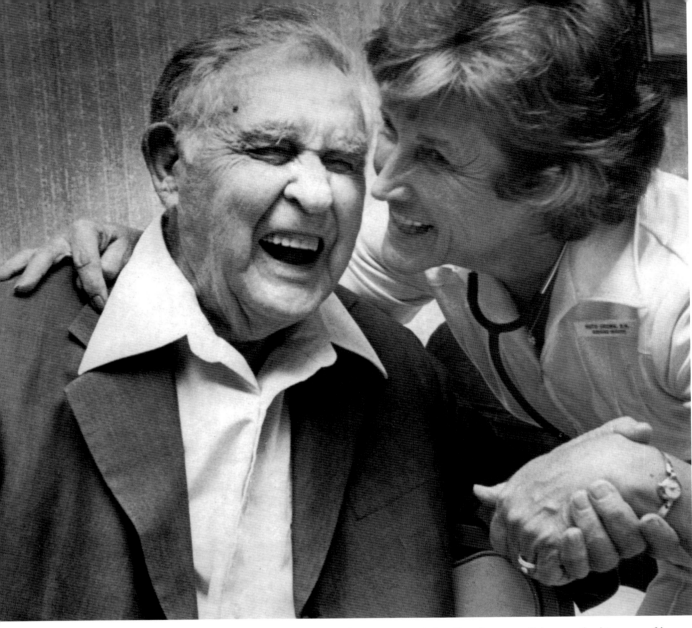

James Archer Smith, M.D., shared a laugh with Ruth Brown, R.N. Dr. Smith was well-known for his sense of humor. "If you can't see the funny side of life, you might as well quit," he said often.

The referendum on the sale of the hospital failed by a three-to-one margin. James Archer Smith remained in the city's hands. Nine months after residents voted to keep his namesake hospital, Dr. Smith died at 91. He had seen patients up until about two years before his death.

The vote certainly reflected a commitment to the hospital's founding mission but did little to solve the problems. James Archer Smith still faced local politics and lacked resources. The City Council and the hospital's leadership looked for answers with outside management. They hired Nashville-based Hospital Corporation of America (HCA), the nation's largest hospital management firm, to run James Archer Smith. For a fee of about $250,000 annually, the company handled the day-to-day affairs of what was the largest business in Homestead, with 340 employees and a payroll of $6 million a year.

HCA did not solve the problems. The City Council, hospital Board and HCA leadership clashed. At one point, four of the 11 hospital Board members resigned in frustration. The executive director position became a now-you-see-him-now-you-don't job with one HCA executive after another trying to straighten out the mess.

Publicly, HCA touted its strengths. In 1983, just as the management contract was up for review, the company presented a progress report. HCA pointed to streamlined operations that had saved more than $1 million, increased patient revenue and improved employee morale. Some building repairs also were made. "In other words," the report concluded, "the City of Homestead and James Archer Smith Hospital have realized a more than threefold return on their original investment of the HCA management fee."

The reported successes notwithstanding, the City Council and hospital leaders paused when it came time to extend HCA's contract. Some questioned the management fee and others pointed to the turnover of HCA officials and a lack of communication between the hospital and its "distant" headquarters in Nashville.

A Change in Management

In the midst of the negotiations, another player emerged — South Miami Hospital. In the summer of 1983, Executive Director Merrill Crews presented a proposal to manage James Archer Smith. Crews stressed what he termed South Miami's strengths — financial stability, strong management and a local presence. He pledged that South Miami would straighten out James Archer Smith within two years. Crews also distanced himself from controversy. "Politics belongs in one place — government," he said. "We don't play politics at South Miami."

For South Miami Hospital, the management of James Archer Smith would expand its service area south. This was especially important with Baptist Hospital's growth and the heightened competition for patients. South Miami leaders were looking to find new sources of revenue.

Many in Homestead welcomed South Miami's interest. The hospital had an established presence and promised a certain degree of professionalism. "HCA's [management years] haven't been the smoothest for the city-owned hospital. What primarily gives South Miami Hospital the edge over HCA is that SMH is local," an editorial in the city's newspaper declared. "The hospital's managers are aware of local problems and needs which would prove to be beneficial… If the South Miami Hospital management team can operate James Archer Smith in the same fashion it does its own hospital, the Homestead community will have an excellent facility in its backyard."

Regardless of the support, the City Council and hospital Board had a mind of their own. After heated deliberations and more discussions about selling James Archer Smith, the Board did not renew the HCA contract and did not hire South Miami. Instead, it hired Joseph Jacobs, a hospital administrator from Maryland, to run James Archer Smith, without a larger organization behind him. It was akin, one employee noted, to being in the ocean without a vessel.

Jacobs approached the job with high hopes. "I understand they have some challenges down there," he said, "but I am confident that I will be able to work well with the employees." Jacobs recognized that foremost among the challenges was the aging physical plant. Within his first month on the job, he identified the greatest needs as replacing furniture for patients and acquiring new X-ray and other diagnostic and lab equipment. He also proposed an ambitious $9 million renovation. It would include a new 50,000-square-foot building with an emergency department, operating rooms, outpatient center and critical care beds. The expansion would add services and better serve Homestead's 25,000-plus residents.

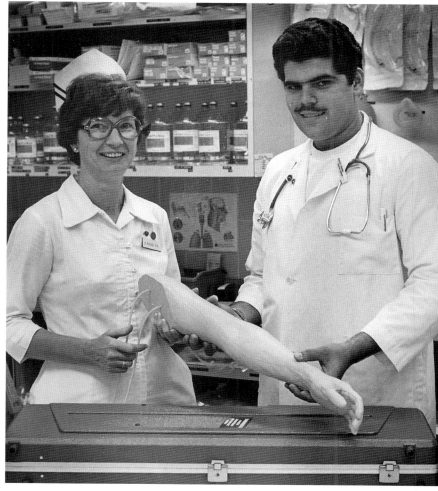

Coordinator of Nursing Services Ms. Keesee, R.N., and Ernest Triana prepare for emergency medical training.

The renovations were much needed. Medical technology was changing dramatically and the hospital needed to keep pace. "The facility is a hospital for the '60s," then Homestead Mayor Irving Peskoe said. "It is not a hospital for the '90s." Jacobs and hospital leaders pushed ahead. In what must have felt like "here we go again" for those familiar with the hospital, the financial realities were daunting. After more than $200,000 and a year's planning, the hospital halted the expansion in January 1987. An independent audit showed that the hospital had lost almost $500,000 in the last year. Occupancy rates averaged under 58 percent — not enough for the hospital to break even. It simply could not absorb the cost of expansion. Less than two months later, Jacobs resigned in the sixth leadership change in seven years. Once again, the question returned, just who was running James Archer Smith Hospital?

In May 1987, a committee appointed by the mayor recommended that the city should no longer be involved with James Archer Smith. For nearly two decades, politics had influenced hospital policy and decisions. Major personnel decisions and budget requests had to clear the City Council, an elected body with members who had little expertise in hospital matters. In addition, each election ushered in new leaders who appointed their own members to the hospital Board.

The report concluded that it was time to end the conflict and instability. "Cities ought not to own hospitals," it read. "They are community service organizations, not government agencies." For an area that cherished its independence and way of life, this was difficult to accept. "I really think the day is going to come when the hospital will have to go another way," said Vice Mayor Paul Brookshire. "Residents have held onto it out of nostalgia. When reality hits the pocketbook, things change."

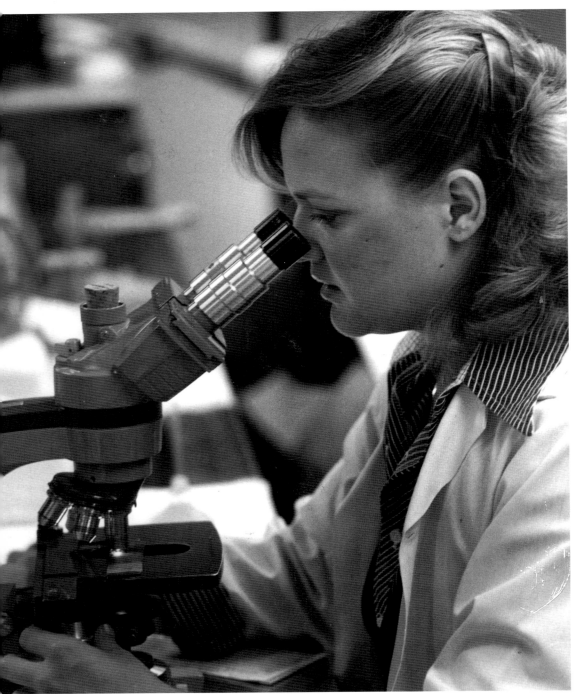

The 1980s were a difficult time for James Archer Smith Hospital. As staff cared for patients and performed medical tests, politicians debated the hospital's future.

James Archer Smith Hospital...
LOOKING BACK

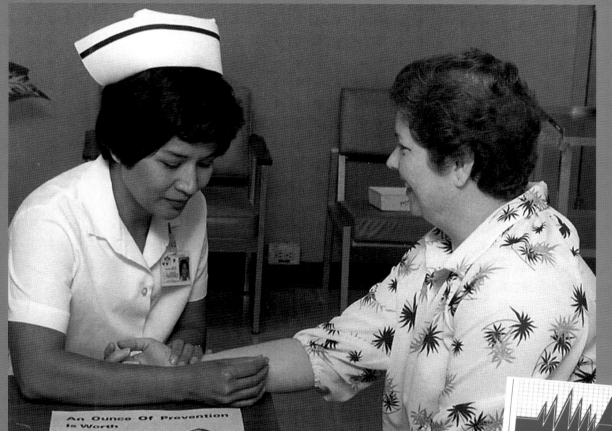

Elisa Kellawlan, R.N., performs a tuberculosis test.

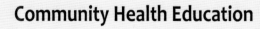

Community Health Education

James Archer Smith had a long tradition of offering community programs to Homestead residents on topics such as quitting smoking, diabetes, infertility and childbirth. Health fairs, blood pressure screenings, cancer screenings and tuberculosis testing emphasized wellness and prevention. Today, Homestead Hospital continues its community focus. In 2009, more than 1,500 people came to Homestead Hospital for programs ranging from parenting tips to information about joint replacement surgery.

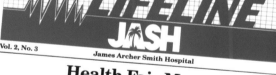

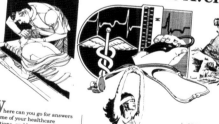

LIFELINE
JASH

Vol. 2, No. 3   James Archer Smith Hospital

Health Fair Mania Comes To Krome Avenue

Where can you go for answers to some of your healthcare questions, and have health screenings or minor tests conducted? And where you can feast on the finest health care foods, get a nutrition work-up, learn about exercise, and safety tips for children? And while you're doing these things, where else can you be entertained by high school jazz bands, clowns, cartoon characters, and celebrities? Give up?

All these things are happening on one action-packed day on Saturday, March 5th when the second annual James Archer Smith Hospital/Homestead Chamber of Commerce Health and Safety Fair lights up the town.

The fair, which takes place from

10:00 a.m. to 4:00 p.m., will be held on Krome Avenue from Fourth Street to Second Street.

"Having a health fair gives everyone a chance to learn about good health care and to see how their daily habits affect their total health picture," said Paula Yudenfriend, health fair coordinator. "And having the fair on Krome Avenue will give the entire community a chance to get together and reacquaint themselves with the revitalized downtown area.

"The theme of this year's fair is education," said Yudenfriend. "We want to educate the public both about preventive health care and the importance of child safety."

While the fair will feature an array of health screenings and

(Con't on page 2)

A Familiar Face

It was clear that James Archer Smith could no longer stand alone. The 120-bed hospital needed management expertise and an infusion of capital for improvements. After prolonged discussions about keeping the hospital's current structure, selling it or collaborating with a larger institution, the City Council reached agreement. In March 1988, the city signed a three-year management contract with South Miami Hospital. James Archer Smith leaders gave South Miami full authority to manage the hospital's day-to-day operations. "After all of its bumbling and Machiavellian intrigues, the Homestead City Council appears to have hit upon a sound interim solution to James Archer Smith Hospital's seemingly interminable problems," an editorial in *The Miami Herald* concluded.

South Miami sent Vice President Dennis Blay to Homestead to run the hospital. His team confronted bad news. A closer look at the financial situation noted a $330,000 shortfall for the first three months of 1988. The group evaluated departments, streamlined operations and focused on improved billing. The efforts worked. An audit in September pointed to a dramatic improvement in the hospital's bottom line. "There have been significant changes in management since South Miami took over," the independent audit said.

In July 1989, Dennis Blay left and South Miami sent its assistant administrator, Wayne Brackin, to Homestead. In his four years at South Miami, Mr. Brackin had earned a reputation as a focused manager with a personable and approachable nature. At age 30, he was one of the youngest hospital administrators in Florida, bringing high energy and a willingness to engage with the community. "I knew right away that we needed to have a peaceful relationship with city officials — from council members to the manager," Mr. Brackin remembered. "I spent a lot of time talking with them. I worked on building fundamentals and having people know that I was around."

For a hospital accustomed to a stream of new faces and turmoil, Brackin fit the bill. Jerry Case, a

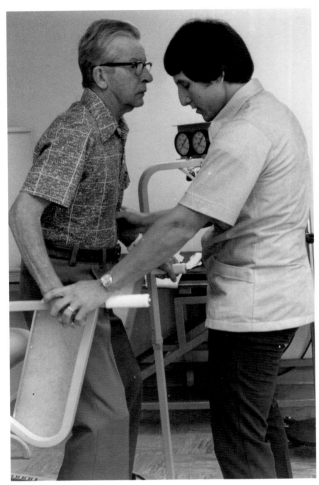

The hospital provided a range of services including physical therapy.

longtime Homestead resident and hospital Board member, remembered that the community embraced the affable executive. "He was a listener and that was something we didn't always have," Case said. "He got all the facts and then made decisions." Still, the larger issue of the facilities and needed renovations persisted. "As far as turning it around, South Miami has done a good job," then City Manager Alex Muxo said. "The problem is the hospital critically needs capital improvements." The hospital needed a complete overhaul, including a new emergency room, operating rooms, intensive care unit and updated equipment such as CT scanners. South Miami could not afford to invest what was estimated to be more than $7 million for a temporary management contract.

Within a few months of South Miami's arrival, the City Council put the hospital up for sale. After inquiries from several prospective buyers, South Miami emerged as the only viable candidate. Baptist Hospital declined to bid, citing the cost.

> "*As* far as turning it around, South Miami has done a good job. The problem is the hospital critically needs capital improvements."
>
> Alex Muxo
> Homestead City Manager

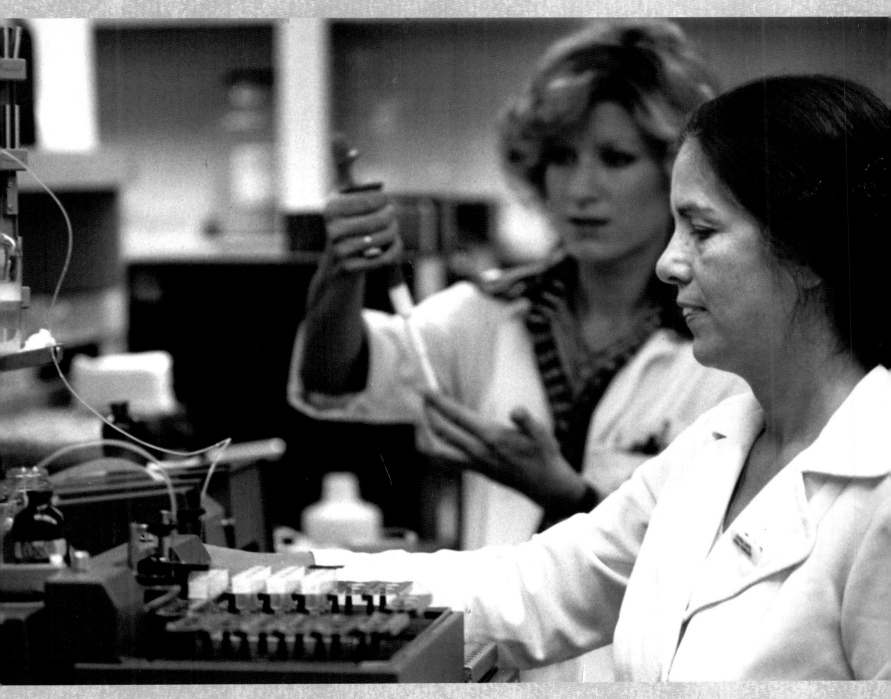

South Miami Hospital brought stability to James Archer Smith.

Booming in Kendall

At the time, Baptist Hospital, with more than 2,300 full-time employees, was a formidable presence in the community. Under the guidance of Administrator Brian Keeley and Board Chairman Robert Cole, the hospital had recently expanded. The shovel donated by Arthur Vining Davis for groundbreakings was busy as the hospital embarked on a series of construction projects that transformed its verdant campus. It 1986, Baptist broke ground on the Lake Pavilion on the site of the Davis Building. When completed in 1989, the three-story building would house inpatient rooms, a new rehabilitation center and a new maternity center. In a historic twist, while demolishing the Davis Building, construction workers found a time capsule full of faded photographs of the 91-year-old Arthur Vining Davis wielding the official groundbreaking shovel and helping cement the building's cornerstone in 1959. Similarly, hospital leaders placed a copper time capsule with current and historical documents and photos in a column outside the entrance to the new building.

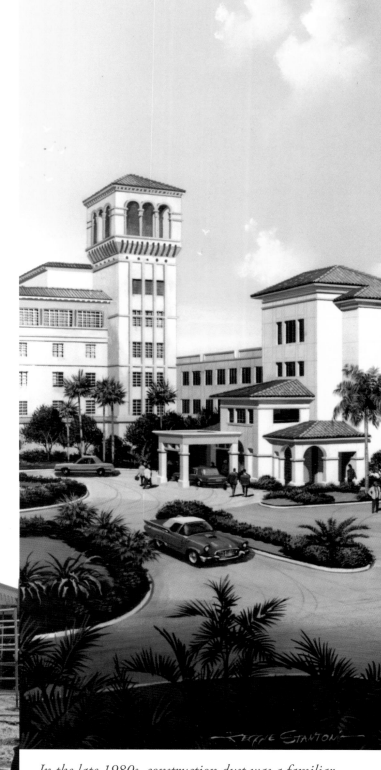

In the late 1980s, construction dust was a familiar sight at Baptist Hospital. New buildings included the Lake Pavilion and Medical Arts Building.

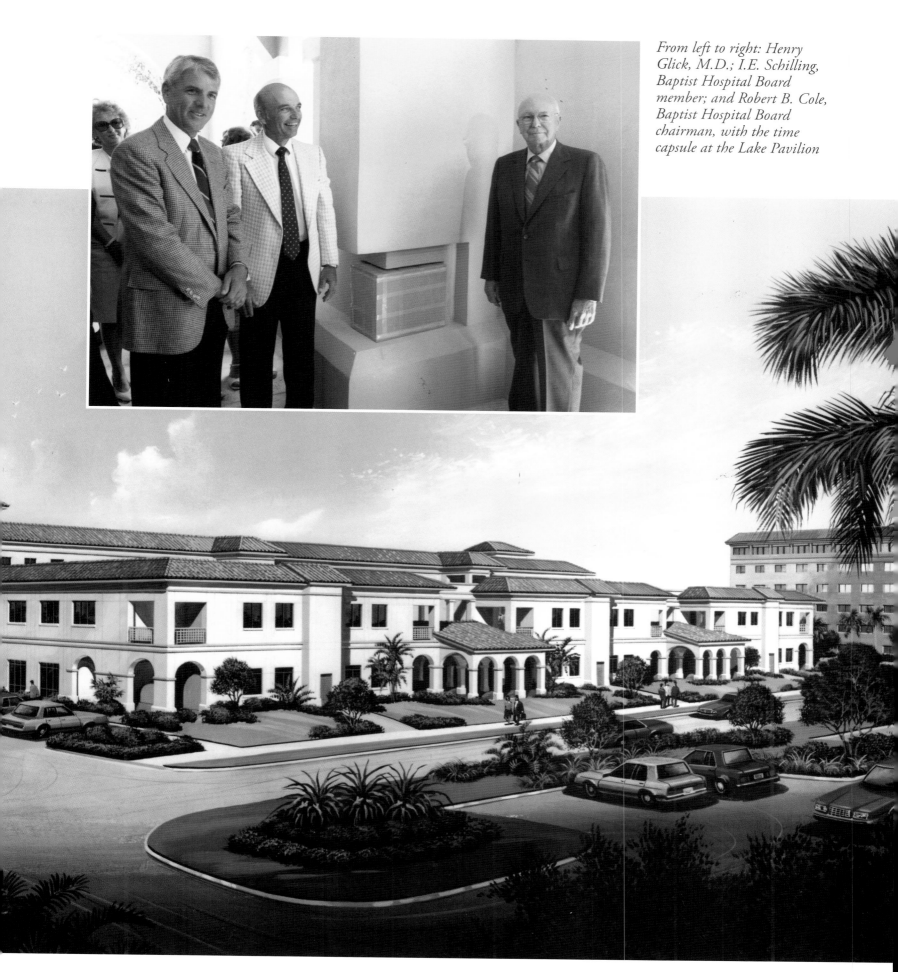

From left to right: Henry Glick, M.D.; I.E. Schilling, Baptist Hospital Board member; and Robert B. Cole, Baptist Hospital Board chairman, with the time capsule at the Lake Pavilion

A rendering of the Family Birth Place and Davis Center for Rehabilitation

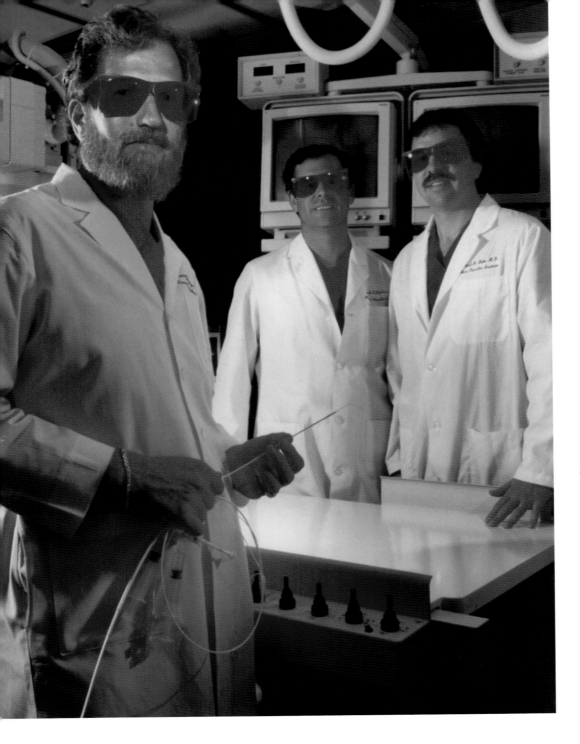

Left to right: Drs. Barry Katzen, Jack Kaplan and Michael Dake were the Institute's first interventional radiologists. They performed various procedures, including using lasers to pulverize plaque in the arteries of the leg.

In 1986, the hospital also broke ground on a six-story Medical Arts Building to house outpatient diagnostic and laboratory services and doctors' offices. Designed to be inviting and state-of-the-art, the building would look more like a downtown office than a hospital.

That same year, Baptist Hospital began planning for a new innovative service, what became known as Miami Vascular Institute (today's Baptist Cardiac & Vascular Institute). Barry Katzen, M.D., a charismatic Miami native who had built a reputation in Virginia as a leader in the developing field of interventional radiology, came to Baptist Hospital in late 1986. His goal was to redefine how doctors treated patients and to expand the hospital's radiology program.

To support the Institute, the hospital invested $2.5 million to build a dedicated area with two in-

terventional suites and the latest imaging technology. When it opened in November 1987, it began what would grow to become one of Baptist Hospital's busiest and most celebrated services. "We got up and running with our fingers crossed," Mr. Keeley said, "but we immediately saw the potential and success. We realized that the Institute worked and would keep growing, so it made sense to move forward."

In 1987, Baptist also broke ground on a $12.5 million Surgery Center. The 60,000-square-foot center would increase the number of operating rooms from 10 to 18, giving Baptist the second largest surgical facility in Dade County, behind Jackson Memorial Hospital. In addition to incorporating the latest equipment, the new Surgery Center would allow the hospital to increase its surgical caseload by more than 30 percent.

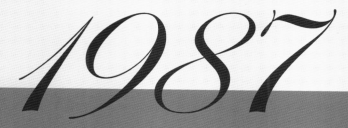

1987

Baptist Hospital...
LOOKING BACK

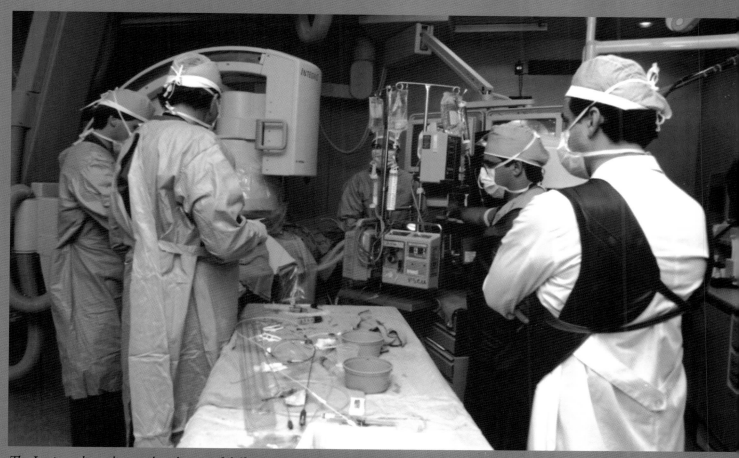

The Institute brought together doctors of different specialties.

Baptist Cardiac & Vascular Institute

In 1987, Miami Vascular Institute (today's Baptist Cardiac & Vascular Institute) opened. With support from a forward-thinking medical staff and hospital leaders such as Brian Keeley and then Vice President Lee Huntley, interventional radiologist Barry Katzen, M.D., the Institute's founding medical director, proposed a multidisciplinary approach to treating the cardiovascular system. Under the collaborative model, doctors of different specialties would work side by side in consultation to determine the best course of treatment. Patients with blocked arteries could consult with specialists who together would determine the best approach — whether it was open surgery or a less invasive method. Today the Institute is one of the most successful in the United States. Its doctors pioneer the latest treatments, participate in research trials and lecture around the world.

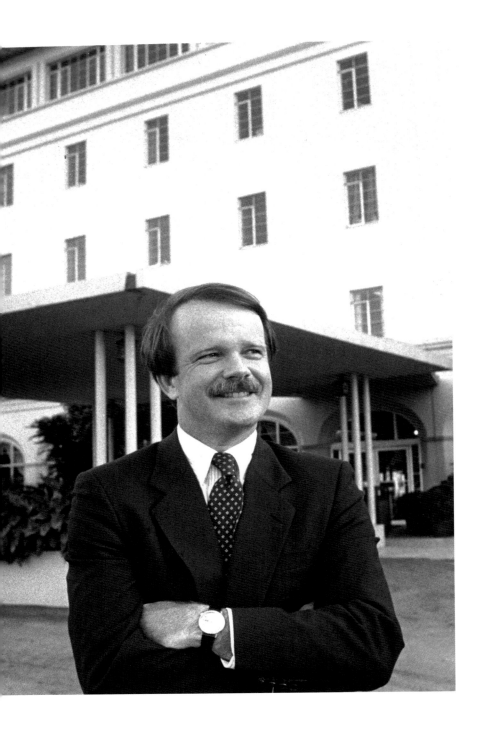

Taken together — the Lake Pavilion, the Medical Arts Building, Miami Vascular Institute and the new Surgery Center — the projects constituted Baptist Hospital's most ambitious construction program to date. When many hospitals were struggling financially, Baptist developed specialized and profitable services. "It was a time of bricks and mortar growth," said Ana Lopez-Blazquez, who was hired in 1987 as assistant director of planning and within two years became the department's director. "We were like a sleeping giant with tremendous opportunities. We saw a need for a service or building, justified its development, planned it and then turned it over for construction."

But Ms. Lopez-Blazquez, Brian Keeley, Robert Cole and other hospital leaders focused on more than bricks and mortar. Nationwide, hospitals were affiliating with other hospitals with the idea that a larger group could benefit from economies of scale, the consolidating of business services, and, most importantly, negotiating better managed care contracts. Those that did not affiliate often sold out to for-profit companies that were gobbling up hospitals and trying to turn them into money-makers. "We were not sure how it was all going to settle, but there was a massive consolidation in the industry," Keeley said. "As strong as we were, we were not strong enough to be successful over time. It seemed to be: either merge or be taken over. Eat or be eaten, so to speak."

It seemed appropriate, then, that Baptist would vie for James Archer Smith Hospital. However, Baptist Hospital had charted its success with a culture of fiscal responsibility. The Board made decisions after careful study, asking questions such as "Can the hospital afford this?" and "Does the hospital really need this?"

"For the hospital it was really about being financially sound and having strong fundamentals. The Board really stressed that," said Chief Financial Officer Ralph Lawson, who joined Baptist Hospital in 1989 after working with Baptist for the two previous years as a partner at the national accounting firm of Deloitte Haskins & Sells.

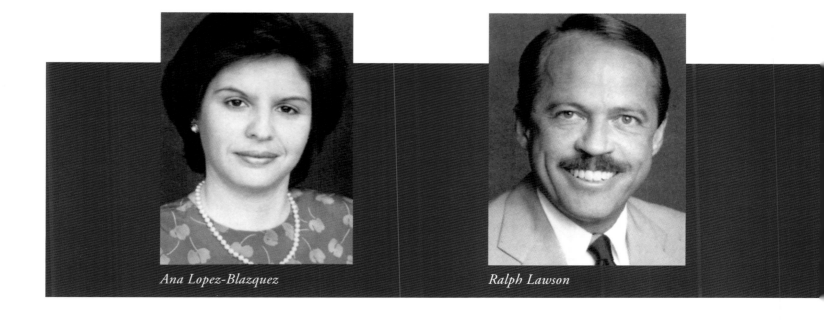

Ana Lopez-Blazquez

Ralph Lawson

The City of Homestead and hospital officials estimated that James Archer Smith needed $7 million in capital improvements, but Baptist's appraisal nearly doubled the figure, making it too costly. "The bottom line is we are not able, financially, to put up the kind of money we feel it needs for it to be the kind of hospital we want it to be," said a Baptist spokeswoman at the time.

It was also a case of poor timing. Hospital leaders wanted to broaden Baptist's direction, but they were still defining their goals. "We evaluated James Archer Smith and the numbers did not work," Ms. Lopez-Blazquez said. "We were also still refining our growth strategy and understanding the managed care market. It did not seem like it was the right time."

With Baptist Hospital out of the picture, South Miami moved ahead to purchase James Archer Smith and expand to a high-growth area. The arrangement included a price of about $9 million with the caveat that most of the money would be reinvested in the hospital for the much-needed improvements. Even though some believed the City of Homestead was selling the hospital too cheaply, there also was a groundswell of support. Many of the community leaders and businessmen, as well as those associated with the hospital, believed that this solution gave the hospital what it needed — management and capital for renovations. The Greater Homestead/Florida City Chamber of Commerce publicly advocated for the move. Newspaper editorials extolled the stability and record of success that South Miami brought to the hospital.

The City Council put the question of James Archer Smith's future to the voters in a referendum. Although technically the results were nonbinding, the Council agreed to honor them. On November 7, 1989, 70 percent of the residents who cast ballots voted in favor of the sale and its financial terms. The community had spoken.

With the residents of Homestead firmly behind the sale of James Archer Smith, the city and South Miami Hospital began negotiating the details. A few stumbling blocks remained. The issue involved South Miami's reinvestment in the hospital and a schedule for the renovations. The City of Homestead wanted assurances that South Miami would show its commitment to the community right away by making improvements in a timely manner. By November 1990, the principals agreed. South Miami promised to spend more than $7 million upgrading the hospital over the next three years.

One month later, on December 21, 1990, South Miami Hospital took ownership of James Archer Smith. The two hospitals would merge — becoming South Miami HealthSystem. Those who had worked hard to save the hospital were satisfied. "Who's the real winner in this? It's the community," said City Manager Alex Muxo. "These improvements have been needed for a long time."

A Turnaround

South Miami Hospital began transforming James Archer Smith. It purchased more than $650,000 in equipment, including the latest radiologic technology, began remodeling the interior of the aging building and planning for the emergency room expansion. To complete the new look, Wayne Brackin and his team made a symbolic decision — to change the hospital's name. In October 1991, James Archer Smith became Homestead Hospital. It was a move to both distance the hospital from its controversial past and link its identity to the community. Mr. Brackin recognized that residents were connected emotionally to James Archer Smith and the hospital's beloved namesake. He surveyed leaders in the community and spoke to Dr. Smith's widow. "We

wanted to be sensitive to the hospital's history," Brackin said, "but also set the course for its future."

While the situation and morale at the newly christened Homestead Hospital were improving, things at South Miami Hospital were problematic. The hospital struggled to cope with the financial impact of managed care and the change in traditional insurance payments. Revenues and reimbursements dipped. Money, or the lack of it, became a critical issue. "It was a difficult time for the hospital," said James Stewart, M.D., who joined the medical staff in 1972. "We were physician-run and proud of our culture of personalized patient care. Unfortunately, we were not equally prepared or successful in dealing with managed care."

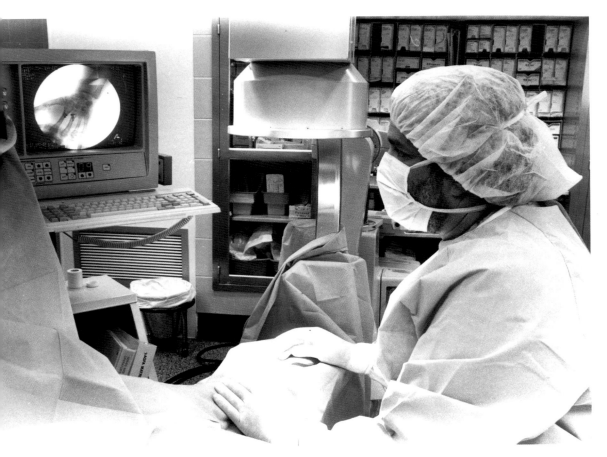

South Miami Hospital updated James Archer Smith Hospital with new equipment. Here, Ronald Chassner, M.D., performs surgery with a C-Arm Image Intensifier.

Facing page: With the change in ownership, Homestead Hospital received a facelift. At the renovation's groundbreaking were (left to right) Sandra Schwemmer, M.D., City Manager Alex Muxo, Homestead Mayor Tad DeMilly, Wayne Brackin, City Councilwoman Eliza Perry, South Miami HealthSystem CEO John Geanes and Homestead Hospital Board Chairman Rev. William Chambers III.

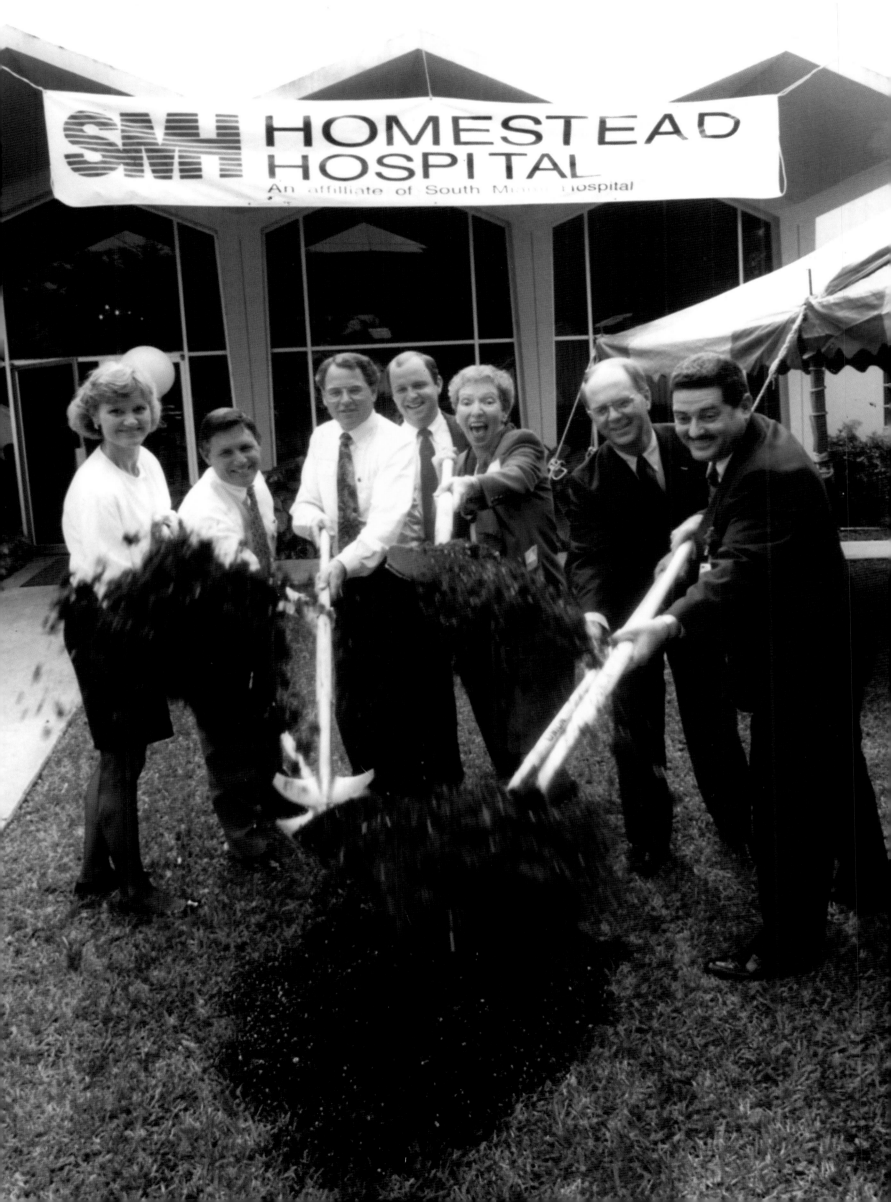

In 1991, Merrill Crews resigned and John Geanes, a vice president for North Broward Hospital District, took over. Geanes' background was in marketing. While he had an understanding of how to bring patients to South Miami, the hospital was still grappling with serious financial problems. Medical costs soared; new technologies demanded significant investments and the hospital's revenues could not keep up. The hospital laid off 30 employees from maintenance and dietary services and rumors swirled that it was for sale. For-profit companies already were making inroads in South Florida. Columbia Hospital Corporation, a Texas-based company, had recently purchased Victoria Hospital in downtown Miami and Coral Reef Hospital in South Dade (renaming it Deering Hospital), and was negotiating for Kendall Regional Hospital.

HealthSouth Corporation, located in Birmingham, Alabama, purchased Doctors' Hospital in Coral Gables in February 1992.

In a time of uncertainty, the South Miami administration worked to reassure nervous employees. "There seems to have been an endless supply of rumors," a June 1992 employee newsletter read. "To put a major rumor to rest — this hospital is not for sale."

Neighboring Baptist Hospital was more stable. The hospital was earning accolades for its working environment. Organizations such as the Florida Nurses Association and magazines such as *Working Mother* and *Good Housekeeping* recognized the hospital for its employee benefits and progressive policies, especially toward women in the workplace. The hospital's culture valued employees and this led to a loyal and satisfied workforce.

Baptist Hospital had a long tradition of a supportive workplace environment. Its daycare center for employees' children dates back to April 1964.

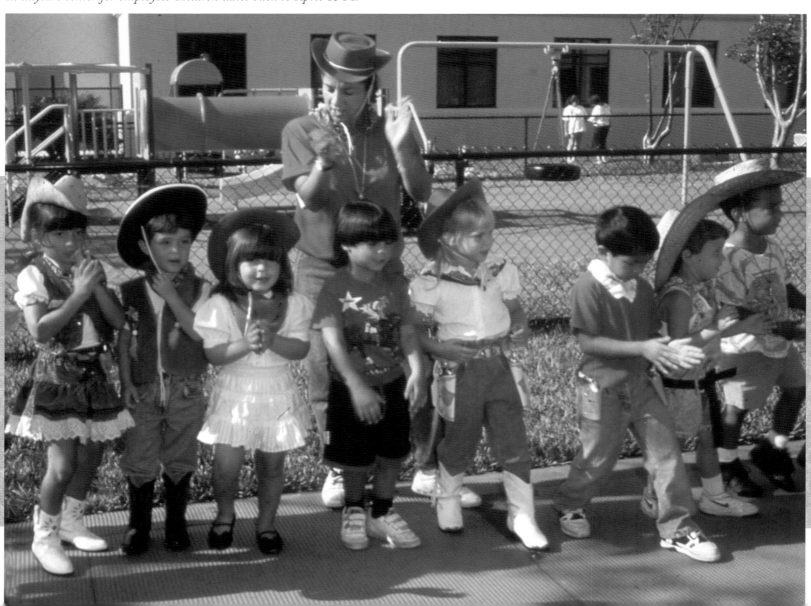

The leadership team also was beginning to build a strategy to expand beyond the traditional hospital. In 1990, it opened an outpatient health center at the Beacon Center at 8301 N.W. 12th Street to provide walk-in medical care, occupational health services and physical therapy. The satellite facility joined the West Kendall Family Center at 9000 S.W. 137th Avenue. West Kendall opened in 1986 as a small center for educational programs. In 1992, it expanded to include physical therapy. The idea was to bring health services into neighborhoods and expand Baptist's patient base. "Baptist Hospital is not going to be a hospital anymore," Keeley said in 1992. "We're going to be a medical center that delivers a lot more than hospital care. We'll be a wellness center, an outpatient center, provide more home healthcare than ever and, coincidentally, we'll be a hospital that has inpatients."

The expansion did not mean that Baptist was moving away from its core mission. The conservative philosophy that guided the hospital required growth that was thoughtful and purposeful. The approach paid off, as the hospital remained financially sound in a challenging era. "We're not going to get too big. We aren't out there buying up hospitals outside our service area or getting into business ventures we know nothing about," Mr. Keeley said at the time. "Some hospitals get involved in some pretty esoteric things. They lose a lot of money because they are inexperienced in these areas. We're going to stay in our area — provide superior healthcare services to our community."

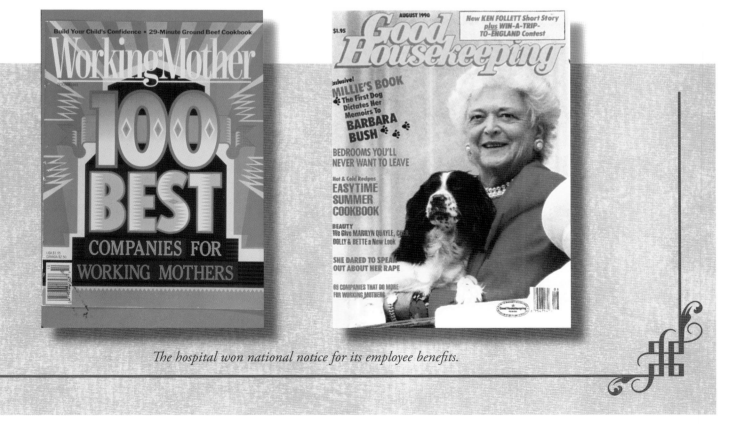

The hospital won national notice for its employee benefits.

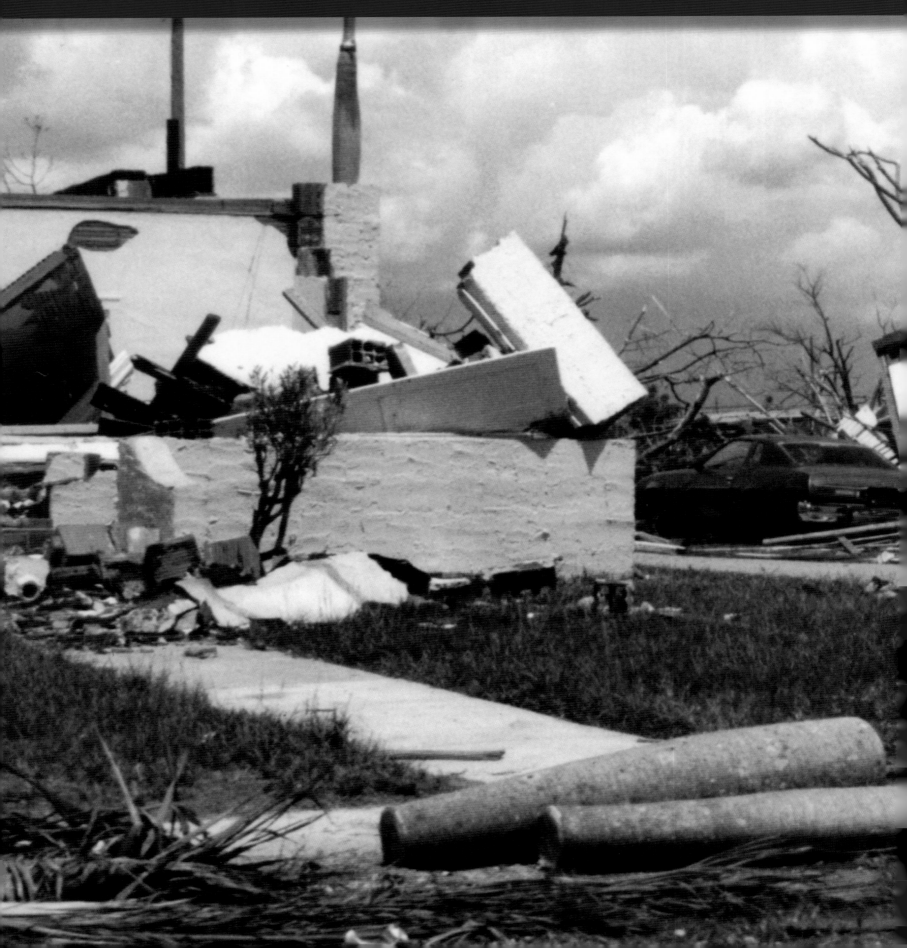

Blown Apart…Brought Together

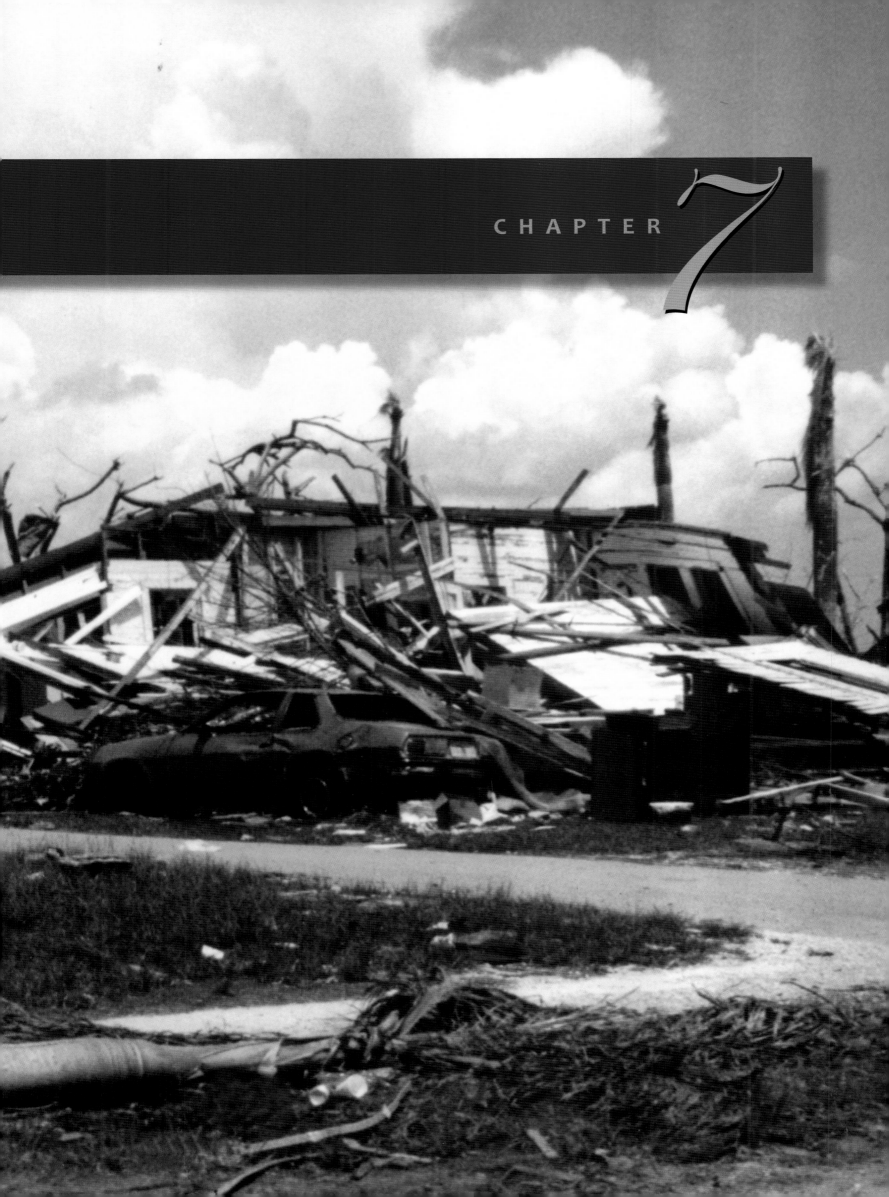

"Hurricane Andrew was a defining moment. In an instant, everything about the hospital and community changed. You really don't know how you are going to react until it happens and then you have to rise to the occasion."

Wayne Brackin
Administrator, Homestead Hospital
1992

The finances and future of the three hospitals in South Dade endured another challenge in the summer of 1992. For Miamians, the season began with the typical rites of passage — afternoon rains, mosquitoes and hurricanes. Weathercasters offered tips on hurricane preparations and complacent citizens ignored them. It had been 27 years since a hurricane had hit Dade County and more than half of the area's residents had never been through such a storm. The last threatening storm, David, in 1979, became the "big one" that never was.

So when a tropical wave stirred off the coast of Africa, no one gave it much thought. On Thursday, August 20, the storm had a name, Andrew, and Miamians waited for it to disappear north. The fateful turn never came. By Sunday, August 23, the winds reached 80, then 90 and then 110 miles per hour. The hurricane of Miami's nightmare was knocking at its door.

Forecasters predicted a path through downtown Miami, Aventura and Miami Beach. A last-minute wobble, however, put the track south. Some were thankful that Andrew would bypass most of the densely populated coastal areas and, instead, unleash its fury on sparsely populated South Dade.

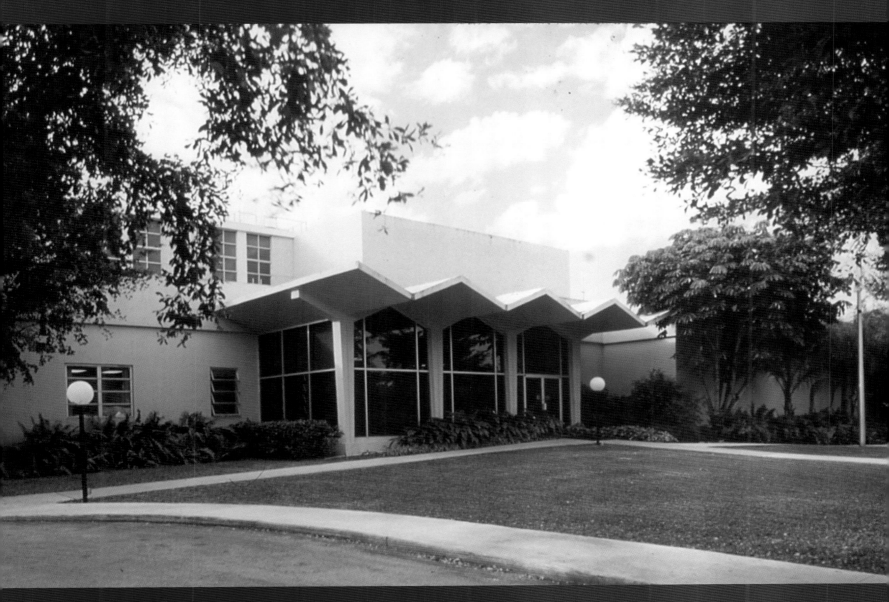

Hurricane Andrew's southern wobble put Homestead Hospital in the middle of the storm's path.

Stormy Times

The course left Homestead Hospital right in the middle of the worst of it. Wayne Brackin, the young administrator, was faced with the task of preparing for the storm, surviving it and recovering. He called a Sunday management meeting at 10 a.m. to put the hurricane plan in motion and convey to everyone the potential severity of what was ahead. Because the storm was so close, the hospital could not evacuate patients and needed to have a few days of supplies on hand. "I remember a sense of urgency on Sunday," said Bo Boulenger, then assistant administrator. "We recognized that so much had to be done in such a short period of time."

The hospital handled the emergency room cases and started discharging the inpatients it could until only about 70 remained. Employees checked the generator, cleared the grounds of debris, arranged to empty the dumpsters, prepared food and stocked up on ice. Medical teams also decided where to put patients, including oxygen-dependent ones and the approximately 35 pregnant women who came to the hospital that evening. Homestead also accepted 15 patients from nearby nursing homes.

By nightfall, the hospital shut its doors. Those inside tried to get some sleep. A little after 4 a.m., Hurricane Andrew struck Homestead with the full force of 150-miles-per-hour winds and gusts as high as 164 miles per hour. The winds, sounding like a relentless train barreling down the tracks, knocked out the hospital's electrical power. The emergency generator kicked in, causing flickering lights and blasting alarms. When the windows started breaking, employees hastened to move patients to safer areas. "As the wind picked up and the windows started to rattle, we decided to get all patients in the hallway," remembered Gail Gordon, R.N., then director of nursing. "The windows in 312, 315, 303 and 317 all broke during the height of the storm. While this was happening, we were moving half of the third floor to the east side of the building and providing constant reassurance." After all the third-floor patients were out of their rooms, employees moved those on the second floor.

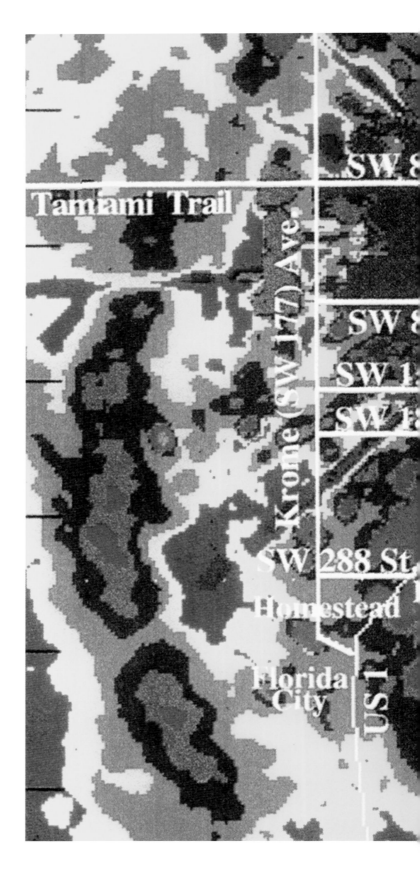

ℬy nightfall, the hospital shut its doors. Those inside tried to get some sleep. A little after 4 a.m., Hurricane Andrew struck Homestead with the full force of 150-miles-per-hour winds and gusts as high as 164 miles per hour.

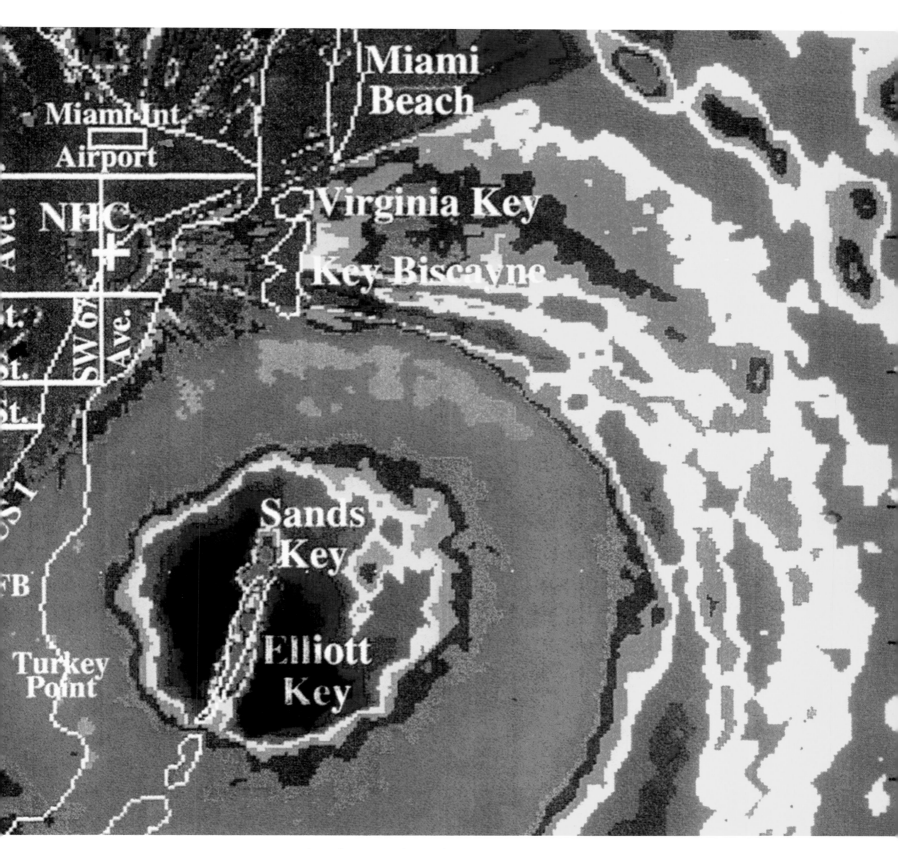

In the early-morning hours of August 24, 1992, the storm slammed South Florida with vicious winds.

"It looked like we had been through a nuclear holocaust."

Bo Boulenger

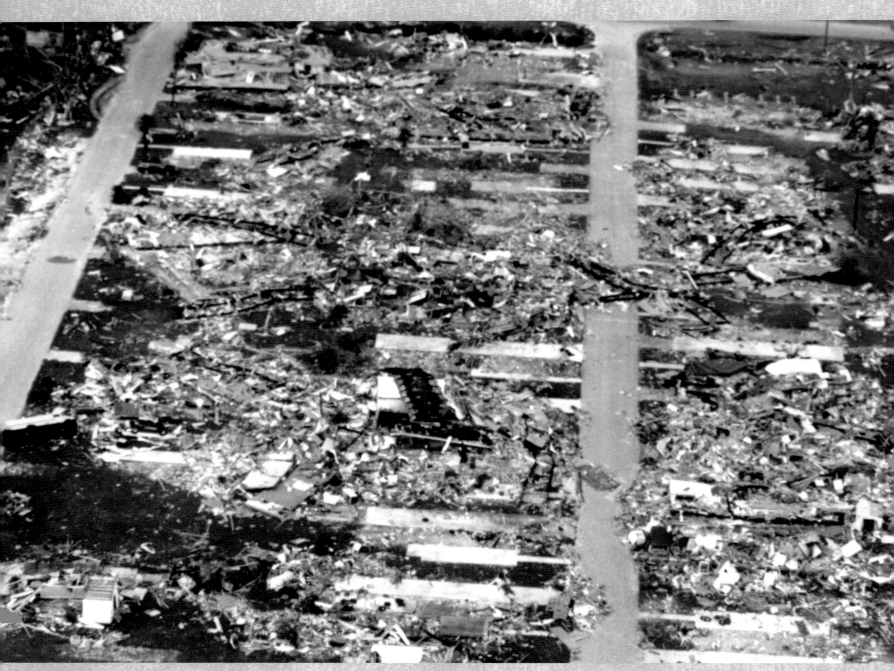

Hurricane Andrew left total destruction in its wake.

The doors of the empty rooms were marked with tape, a makeshift but effective system to guarantee no one was forgotten. "Getting the patients moved out of their rooms took a good 45 minutes during the storm," Boulenger remembered. "There was such a bizarre terror in the air; it was almost like being in a hospital during a war."

Doctors and nurses delivered 17 babies that evening, working by generator-powered lights. The nursery took in water, and resourceful staff members quickly transferred the babies to a room with no windows. Exterior doors clattered, threatening to blow in. Employees responded by grabbing what they could — pre-cut plywood, rope and piping — to try to secure them. Water gushed in through openings and the smell of salt wafted through the hospital. "The hardest thing was that it was night-time," Mr. Brackin said. "We really could not see what was happening. We heard the glass breaking, the wind pounding and part of the roof blowing off, but it wasn't until the morning that we truly understood the scope of the devastation."

In much of Homestead, Andrew left total destruction. When the winds quieted in the early-morning hours on Monday, dazed employees went outside to survey the damage. "It looked like we had been through a nuclear holocaust," Mr. Boulenger recalled. Many had the added burden of worrying about their own homes and what faced them when they returned.

For Baptist Hospital and South Miami Hospital, the storm proved harrowing but both were spared the full force of the winds. The hurricane preparations were similar — pregnant women arrived at the hospitals to ride out the storm, staff secured extra food and supplies, and employees cleared the grounds. Fears of widespread destruction proved unfounded. South Miami's skybridge swayed and shook but remained intact. The yet-to-be-completed home for Miami Vascular Institute at Baptist Hospital, two floors being built on top of the existing Surgery Center, sustained damage to mechanical infrastructure. Trees blew down, roof tiles flew off and roofs leaked. On the whole, however, both hospitals were battered and bruised but able to function. South Miami's employee newsletter proclaimed that the hospital was "Andrew Proof." Baptist's declared "Andrew zero, Baptist won."

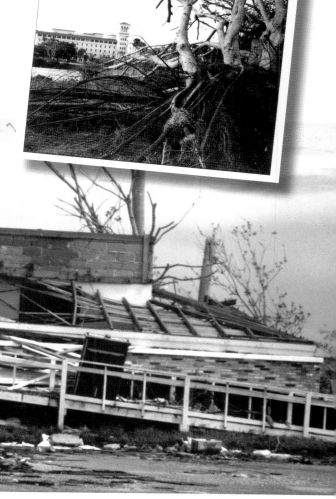

VOCAL CHORD

Published quarterly for employees and friends of Baptist Hospital of Miami

October 1992

Andrew zero, Baptist won

SATURDAY, AUGUST 22, 1992
Vice President Lee Huntley is on call when Channel 4 reports that Hurricane Andrew will make a direct hit upon Miami early Monday. He asks PBX to notify all department heads and managers to come to the hospital Sunday for an emergency hurricane preparedness meeting…

While the Kendall area survived much of Andrew's wrath, residents farther south were not so lucky.

Within a few days, electricity started being restored and streets began to clear. Over the next few months, employees began rebuilding their own homes, while simultaneously caring for countless patients. An estimated 1,500 employees at Baptist Hospital alone suffered major damage to their homes. Eighty employees, 31 of them nurses, resigned immediately, most choosing to relocate outside Dade County.

With strained resources throughout the southern part of the county, the patient census was high, particularly in the emergency rooms. The circumstances were exhausting and overwhelming. "The orderly process just disappeared. We had no history on most of the patients," said Diane Bolton, R.N., then director of critical care nursing at Baptist Hospital. "At one point we had eight nurses sleeping on the floor in a 15-by-15 space… Everyone went miles above and beyond."

With strained resources throughout the southern part of the county, the patient census was high, particularly in the emergency rooms. The circumstances were exhausting and overwhelming.

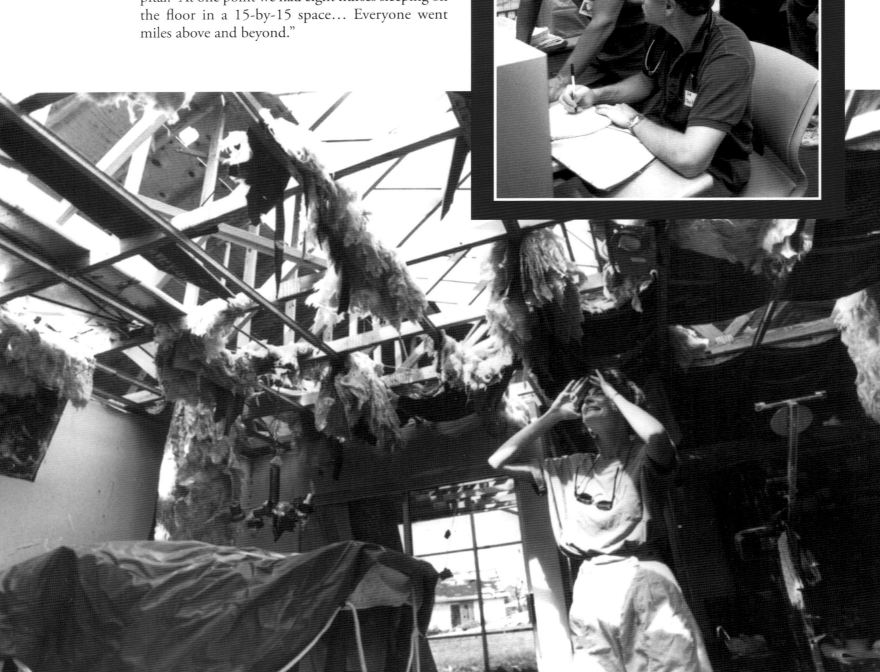

At Ground Zero

The scene at Homestead Hospital was even worse. In the wake of the storm, more than 300 dazed residents found their way to the Emergency Room, seeking treatment for storm-related injuries. The hospital was running on generator power but without city water. "I remember lugging gallons of water up four flights of stairs to run the rooftop generator," said Bill Duquette, then the laboratory director. "It was grueling but we had no choice." This posed an especially challenging problem when the aging generator soon failed. Without the necessities — power and water — the hospital would need to close.

During the post-storm hours, hospital administrators worked to evacuate Homestead's patients, quite a job considering that the surrounding community lay in ruins. Private ambulances transported patients to Broward County. Metro-Dade buses shuttled newborns to Miami Children's Hospital. "We were really in survival mode," Brackin said. "We abandoned procedures and just did the next thing in front. We had to get our patients out, close the hospital and make the necessary repairs to reopen."

By Monday evening, the hospital closed. The staff turned their efforts to recovery and repair. The goal was to do enough to get the hospital functioning. Administrators secured two backup generators. Workers replaced the ceilings in six patient rooms, patched the roof and replaced window glass. Employees carried in jugs of water and supplies. Physicians mopped the floor. Family members of employees pitched in, too, clearing debris and patrolling the area. "I quickly realized that the community's needs were so acute," Brackin said. "We put all our energy into just doing what we had to do to get the hospital up and running."

Mr. Brackin held daily managers' meetings to keep everyone up to date on recovery efforts. Often he perched atop an outdoor picnic table to address employees. The gathering also worked as a morale booster. With strong and caring leadership, Brackin made sure everyone moved forward. "He really instilled camaraderie and a sense of family," Gail Gordon said. "There was a sense that we were all in this together. We were all equal and that stemmed from the top."

On Monday, August 31, just one week after Andrew hit, Homestead Hospital reopened for business — but it was hardly business as usual. While the logistical accomplishment was amazing, the hospital grappled with the challenge of providing care in a changed community. Before the storm, Homestead had finally turned around its financial situation, earning more than $875,000 for the fiscal year. With the demographic changes in the community, however, profits quickly turned to losses.

In the months following the storm, Homestead Hospital treated thousands of patients without insurance — many of whom were transient construction workers. They streamed into the Emergency Room, using it as an ad hoc system of primary care. Before Andrew, the ER handled about 75 cases a day. The number grew to 300 right after the storm. Six months later, the volume averaged 120 patients daily. The numbers outside emergency care were even more dramatic. Before Andrew, about 11 percent of Homestead patients were uninsured. Immediately after the storm, the number reached 30 percent, before settling at around 22 percent a year after the hurricane. That cost the hospital nearly $3 million.

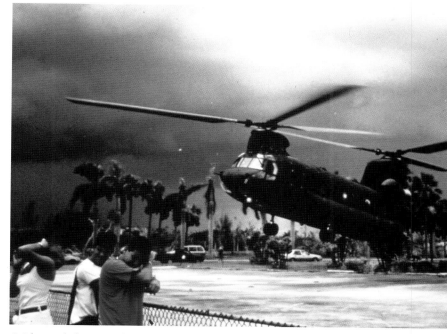

Military helicopters landed regularly at Baptist Hospital, bringing the injured to the Emergency Room.

The hospital looked to state and federal agencies for financial relief. The government promised to compensate Homestead but delayed action. After a prolonged battle with the Federal Emergency Management Agency (FEMA), Homestead did receive some help to offset the cost. But it was ultimately not enough. The increase in uninsured care was only part of the problem. The Homestead community lost one-fourth of its population, as many simply picked up and left. Private physicians joined the exodus, shuttering their offices and clinics which further burdened the hospital.

Ironically, Homestead Hospital would have been better served if it had closed for a year or more to rebuild and collected business interruption insurance. "Our finances were certainly impacted by our decision to stay open. We lost a lot of money," Brackin said, "but our hospital's founding mission was to provide healthcare to South Dade and it was our job to remain true to that philosophy." With Homestead Air Force Base destroyed and closed indefinitely, Homestead Hospital was the area's largest and most important business. It employed 600 people and had an annual payroll of $13 million. "We were probably the only building with our lights on within 20 miles of darkness," Boulenger remembered. "People used to tell me that when they saw the lights, it was a beacon of hope." By staying open, Homestead Hospital made an important statement that the community would rebuild and thrive once again.

The emotional toll on employees at Homestead and neighboring hospitals was significant. They had to balance increased patient loads with family pressures. Many were displaced from their homes. They relocated farther north or, in some cases, lived with co-workers. It was a time when everyone pitched in to help each other. Employee assistance funds at South Miami and Homestead reached more than $400,000 through individual and corporate donations. At Baptist Hospital, it grew to more than $500,000 within three months of the storm. "Everyone was absolutely fantastic, terrific, in terms of supporting the community and each other during this crisis," wrote Fred Messing, Baptist Hospital's chief operating officer, in an employee newsletter. "We are family. If anything ever proved that, Andrew did."

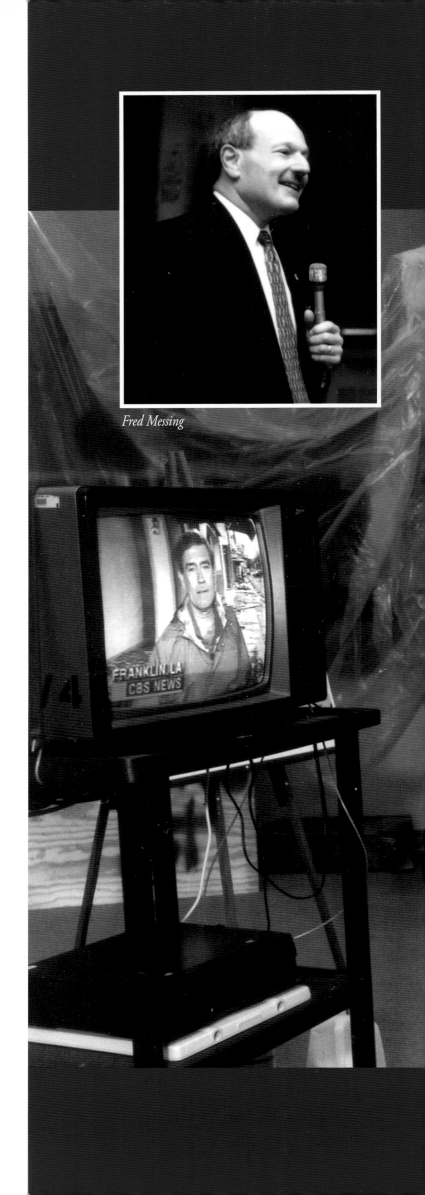

Fred Messing

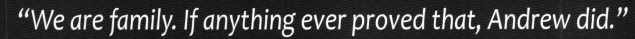

"We are family. If anything ever proved that, Andrew did."

Fred Messing
Chief Operating Officer, Baptist Hospital
1992

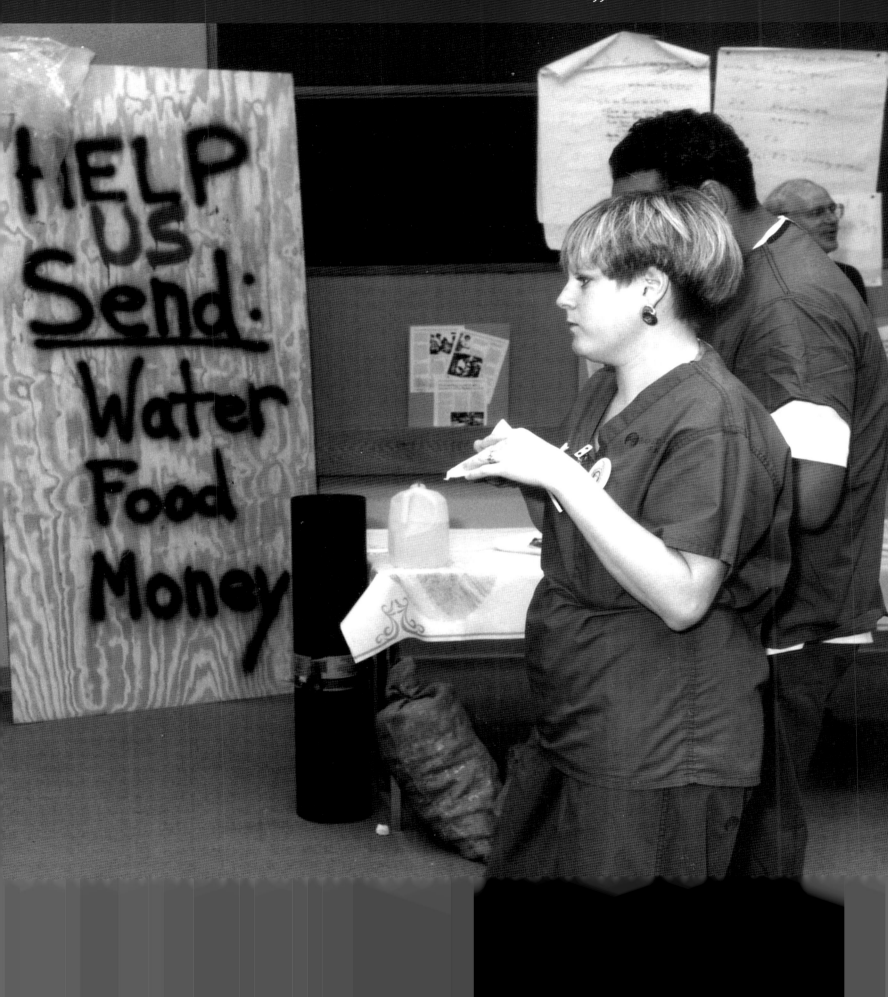

Out of the Clouds

Slowly but surely normalcy returned — especially for Baptist Hospital and the Kendall community. The hospital used the experience as a learning opportunity. It took direct steps to ensure smoother operations for future storms. Plans began to install shutters on all the openings and build emergency water wells. Administrators, weary of the high demand for construction materials after a storm, secured vendors outside of South Florida to provide rebuilding supplies.

Post-Andrew, the hospital also enjoyed targeted growth. Baptist began directly marketing its services to international patients, especially those from Latin America, who could come to South Florida for medical care. Miami Vascular Institute's new building opened, complete with state-of-the-art procedure rooms and cardiac rehabilitation facilities. Baptist Outpatient Center marked its fifth anniversary with a record of progress. When the Center opened in 1988, it averaged 4,200 procedures monthly. By 1993, the number reached 14,200.

Plans coalesced for a second medical arts building, the East Tower. A $19 million project, the building would include physician offices, an expanded home for Baptist Outpatient Center, a wellness center and physical therapy services. To manage the growing operations, leaders reorganized Baptist's structure to form Baptist Health Systems of South Florida. The change reflected the organization's broadening scope.

The new development and expanded services fit the trends in the medical industry — less inpatient care, more emphasis on outpatient services and hospital-physician partnerships. Like hospitals across the nation, Baptist Hospital's inpatient occupancy was declining. In 1992, the average rate of occupied beds was 80 percent. By 1994, the number was 72 percent. As a result, the hospital had to be financially savvy. "In this new age of managed competition, hospital survival will relate to how well hospitals can reduce their operating expenses," said Brian Keeley at the time. "Baptist is taking aggressive action now so it can avoid the problems that are being experienced by other Dade County hospitals." Administrators looked at ways to save money — from negotiating with vendors and conserving energy to reducing overtime.

Like Baptist Hospital, South Miami HealthSystem experienced growth amid challenges. As residents of surrounding communities put their lives back together, they looked toward the hospitals for more services. The Child Development Center at South Miami Hospital opened to provide diagnostic and early intervention services to the families of children with developmental delays. Homestead dedicated its new Emergency Room in honor of James Archer Smith, opened an on-site childcare center for employees and completed renovations that began before the storm. Leadership changed with Wayne Brackin assuming the role of chief operating officer for South Miami HealthSystem and Bo Boulenger, who had been vice president at Homestead, taking over as head of that hospital.

But the post-storm climate proved trying for the two hospitals. The Homestead community's recovery was slow, with two steps forward and one step back. Some signs were positive. Miami Dade College was set to expand its Homestead campus. The federal government decided to reopen a trimmed-down Homestead Air Force Base as a mixed-use civilian and military airport. Developer Ralph Sanchez and the city finalized details for a motorsports track that would serve as a permanent home for the Miami Grand Prix auto race. Despite these projects, abandoned houses and destroyed buildings were still an all-too-common sight.

South Miami HealthSystem's bottom line was suffering and in February 1995, it laid off 85 employees. The organization hoped the cuts would help the hospitals cope with the financial losses associated with the hurricane and managed care contracts. "There was not one precipitating factor," Wayne Brackin said during the layoffs. "It was an assessment of what it will take to be competitive in a managed care environment."

Staff morale was low as department after department was asked to do more with less. Many wondered how the hospitals would survive and just what their future held. It was a time of turmoil and uneasiness.

1993

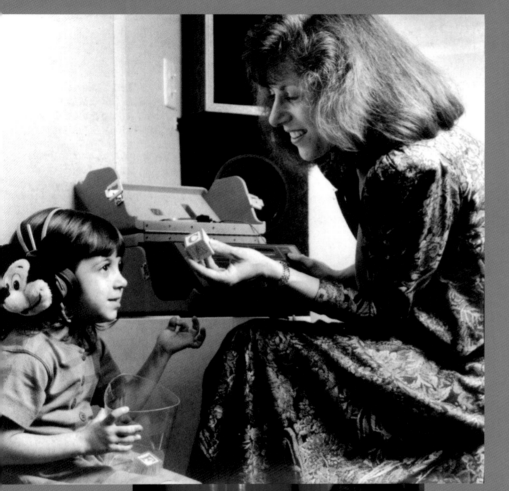

The Child Development Center

With one of the busiest maternity programs in South Florida, South Miami Hospital placed special emphasis on the care of infants and children. In 1993, the hospital emphasized this focus by opening the Child Development Center. Under one roof, families received a range of diagnostic services and treatments for their children — from physical and occupational therapy to developmental pediatrics and psychotherapy. The atmosphere was supportive and nurturing. Children stacked blocks, climbed stairs, pushed buttons and listened to music with the purpose of improving skills and developing muscles. It was the only community hospital-based program of its kind in the area.

Today, South Miami Hospital's Child Development Center, part of the hospital's Center for Women and Infants, continues the founding mission. "Parents come to us with concerns regarding their child's development. Through an interdisciplinary approach, we provide assessments and offer an individualized plan," said Carmen de Lerma, M.D., medical director. "Our purpose is to help children reach their full developmental potential. It is very satisfying to know the difference we have made in the 12,860 families we have helped over the years."

Becoming One

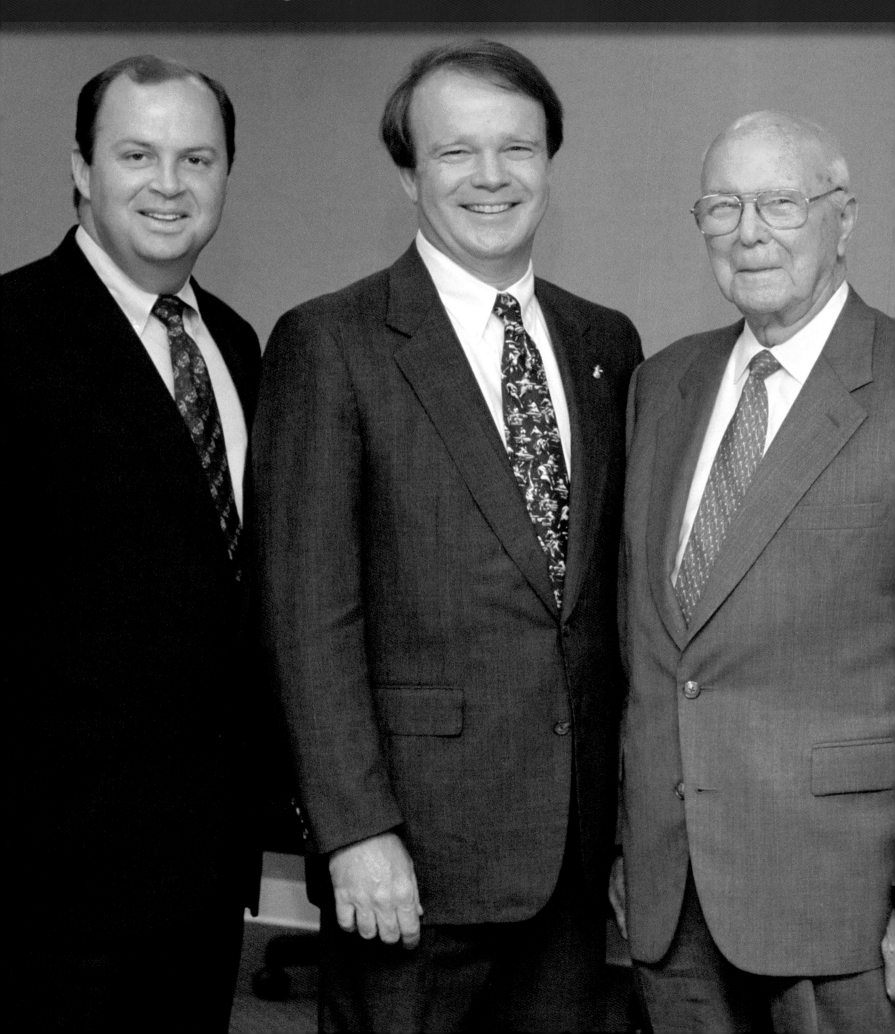

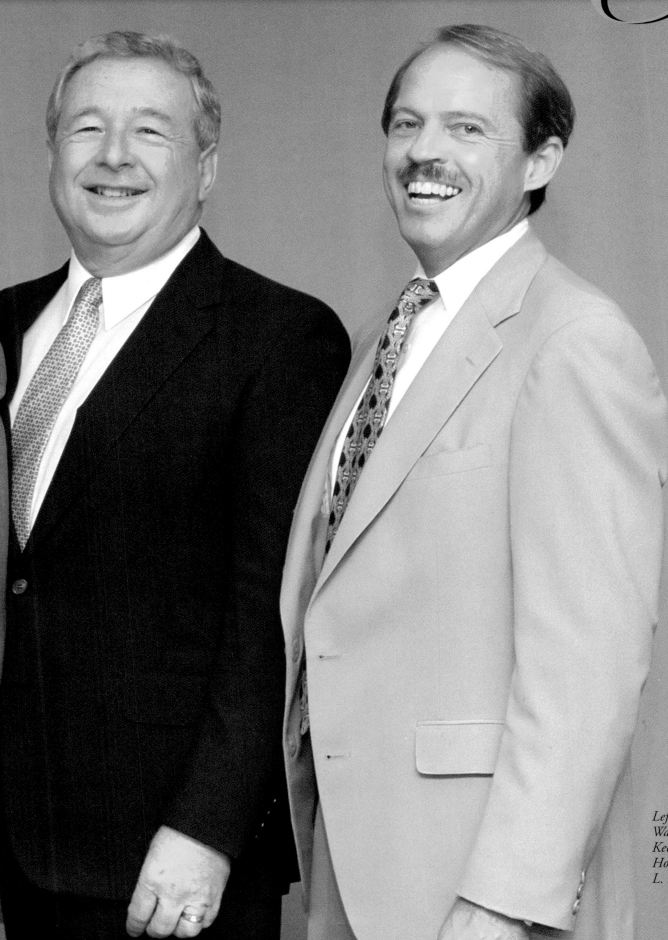

CHAPTER 8

Left to right:
Wayne Brackin, Brian E.
Keeley, Robert B. Cole, the
Honorable Judge Robert
L. Dubé and Ralph Lawson

"We can thrive and that's what we're going to do. But careful attention has to be paid to every detail. Everything we do must be strategic and extremely focused to ensure that it contributes to our mission."

Brian E. Keeley
President and CEO, Baptist Hospital
1995

By 1995, the construction dust was settling in the southern part of the county. Residents were recovering from Hurricane Andrew. They developed new routines, adjusting to new homes and new surroundings. For those at South Miami and Homestead Hospitals the return to normalcy came amid difficult circumstances. As expected, layoffs and financial problems created an atmosphere of gloom. The operating losses continued to mount, reaching more than $10 million for the fiscal year. The proud community hospitals were facing perhaps the worst times in their histories.

In an era of consolidation, alliances and mergers, a natural solution emerged — to sell South Miami HealthSystem. This was not easy to contemplate. Many at the hospitals had deep personal connections to their institutions. Both were grassroots places, founded by people in the community to serve the community. It was hard to imagine that they might be in the hands of a larger corporation, one that might even have its headquarters in another city. Emotions aside, the situation dictated action. Just what the action should be resulted in countless meetings, heated debates and controversial choices.

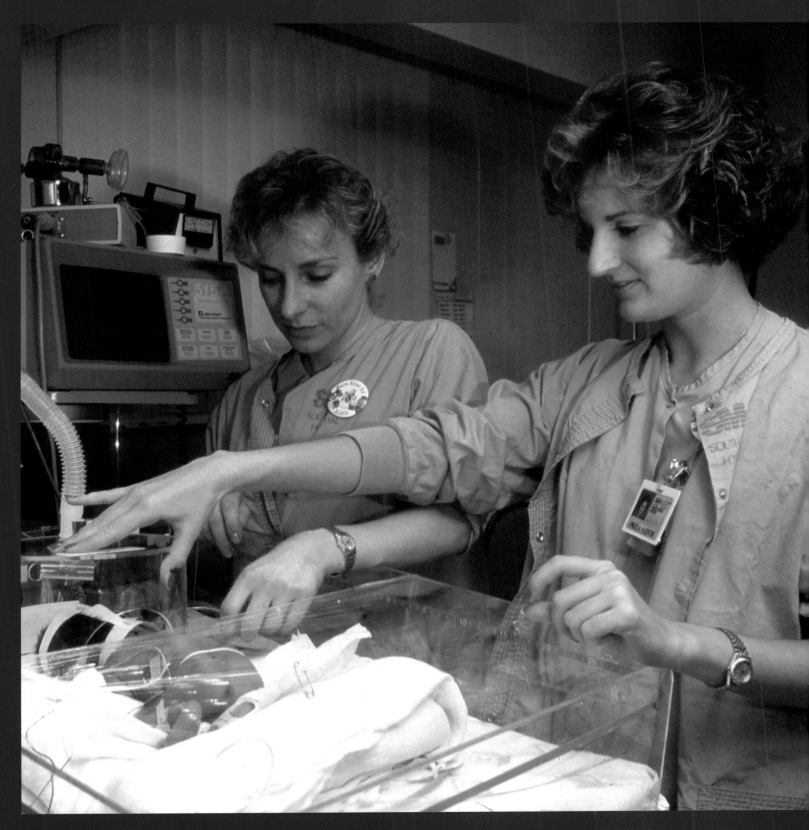

South Miami Hospital's maternity services included caring for premature infants.

A False Start

As early as November 1993, Baptist Health and South Miami HealthSystem started talking about forming a partnership. Two of the most visible not-for-profits in the area, they shared a similar mission. Leaders from both sides recognized the value of working together in some way — expanded service areas, more patients and purchasing power.

Baptist had already begun tentative steps at creative alliances to help improve its financials. The hospital, working with a network of physicians, formed a kind of managed care company. The purpose was to offer South Floridians a network of doctors and Baptist Hospital physicians a network of patients. In addition, Baptist was buying and managing primary care physician practices with the hope of building a profitable service and generating referrals to the hospital. "Integration was kind of a buzzword," Mr. Keeley said. "We were linking services and building partnerships, but it was all very new. We were working in unchartered waters."

South Miami's initial talks with Baptist fell through. South Miami then began serious court-ships with several for-profit corporations that had a strong presence in South Florida. In early 1994, Columbia Healthcare Corporation, a Texas-based industry leader, proposed a merger. (It became Columbia/HCA a few months into 1994.) The company hoped to add South Miami to its growing South Florida roster. Its goal, Columbia Chairman Richard Scott said in an earlier interview, "isn't to have one hospital in a market. It's to have significant market share."

But negotiations stalled and other for-profit companies, most notably National Medical Enterprises and OrNda, entered the picture. (Both companies later became part of Tenet Healthcare Corporation.) Those at South Miami and Homestead remembered for-profit representatives visiting the hospitals and making assessments. "It was obvious to everyone that we were at risk and needed to be taken over," remembered Gail Gordon, R.N., then Homestead's director of nursing. "These men in business suits, clearly from the for-profits, kept touring the hospitals. It made everyone uncomfortable." At South Miami Hospital, the uncertainty was particularly painful. "Here we were a critical presence in our community serving a critical need," said Board member James Stewart, M.D., "but unless we found help, we would soon be unable to pay our bills."

Despite its uncertain future, South Miami Hospital continued its tradition of quality patient care. This photo shows the Radiation Therapy Department, c.1993.

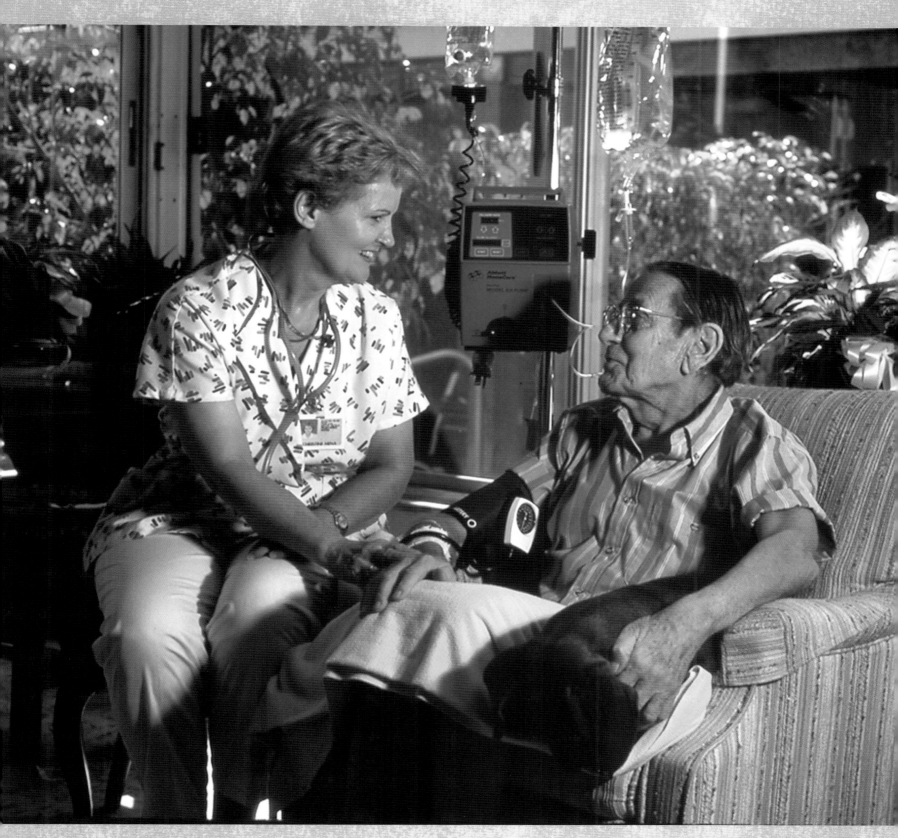

South Miami Hospital's home health service brought nurses, therapists and home health workers into the home. The program, founded in 1987, offered those recently released from the hospital security and convenience. Today, Baptist Health Home Care treats more than 2,300 patients annually.

The companies made attractive proposals to South Miami HealthSystem. "They had a big checkbook," said Board Chairman The Honorable Judge Robert L. Dubé, "and we certainly needed that." The for-profits wooed hospital leaders with dinners and impressive projections of profits. Representatives from South Miami traveled out of state to some of the for-profits' other hospitals to observe how things were run. "I remember that the companies promised us that we would be their flagship hospital," said Melvin Mackler, M.D., a member of South Miami Hospital's Board of Directors. "They talked about investing money in the hospital and buying all this equipment."

For CEO John Geanes and other South Miami Hospital administrators, the for-profits presented answers to an otherwise troubling financial future. Month after month, Mr. Geanes faced a frustrated Board of Directors with dismal revenue reports. With no end in sight, the outside companies offered immediate help.

While some were considering the for-profits, others wanted to take a step back and revisit the hospital's core mission. The discussions were heated and full of controversy. Hospital leaders and administrators were divided.

In an impassioned plea, Board member Allan Feingold, M.D., boiled down the future to a basic question: What was the purpose of the hospital? "I saw it as a moral issue," he remembered. "A for-profit company has to answer to shareholders and that should not have a place in medicine. Our primary purpose was to care for our patients and that goal was simply not compatible with profit margins."

The argument was a powerful one. "We realized we were not simply making a decision based on the hospital's economic needs," said Joseph Traina, M.D., a South Miami Board member. "We could not think only in terms of the business side. We had to look at the larger picture and consider the kind of hospital we wanted South Miami to be."

Beyond the philosophical issue, several Board members felt that the for-profit presentations were exercises of salesmanship. At the time, the companies were creating a large presence buying hospitals but had not yet established a track record. The lack of substance made some uncomfortable. "I think it was a case of if it looks too good to be true, it probably is," said James Loewenherz, M.D. "There was a lot of talk about significant amounts of money, but we were not sure what it really amounted to."

Some feared that a company with shareholders and leaders thousands of miles away would not be sensitive to the local community. "I had a real fear that the for-profits might decide to buy the hospital and then close it down. They had a history of doing that in other places," said lawyer Domingo Rodriguez, a Board member. "They really did not have to answer to our community and they admitted that in front of the Board."

"*A* for-profit company has to answer to shareholders and that should not have a place in medicine. Our primary purpose was to care for our patients and that goal was simply not compatible with profit margins."

Allan Feingold, M.D.
South Miami Hospital Board of Directors

Looking Toward Kendall

With a Board consensus against a move toward the for-profits, South Miami again turned to the not-for-profit Baptist Health. Talks resumed with more urgency. The South Miami Board directed Drs. Loewenherz and Mackler to negotiate with Baptist leader Brian Keeley. Mr. Keeley, who had spoken with the hospital leaders before, was impressed with the candor and honesty of the two physicians. "I realized that everyone was pretty serious in wanting to work together," he said. "So I was prepared to drop everything and do this."

The men met in Dr. Loewenherz's office waiting room and over breakfast at a local restaurant, Deli Lane Café, and began hammering out the details — even sketching points on a napkin. Both parties were well-prepared. Baptist Hospital already had done due diligence on South Miami Health-System and Keeley was well-versed on the financial details. While the idea was novel to Baptist Hospital, mergers and consolidations in the hospital industry were part of the national landscape. Mr. Keeley drew on his knowledge of national trends to guide him.

For South Miami, the negotiating points were clear. Baptist needed to show its commitment to South Miami and Homestead Hospitals financially and allow them to maintain their cultures and autonomy. This was especially tricky with South Miami. The hospital was a rival of Baptist. It was established in the same year and only three-and-a-half miles away. While many physicians enjoyed privileges at both hospitals, the staff and institutions often competed for patients and services. Some wondered just how the longtime competitors could become partners. How could true integration succeed?

To Keeley, the issue was challenging but manageable. He had watched Ernie Nott navigate the local hospital scene with ease, building friendships with South Miami's leader Ray Poore and Doctors' Hospital administrator Joe McAloon. The men saw themselves as part of a larger community, even meeting for lunch monthly, dubbing the gathering the Macy's-Gimbels club, after the rival department stores. Mr. Keeley learned from this spirit and brought that to the discussions with South Miami. "I always saw South Miami as a competitor but it was a friendly competition," he said. "We shared many similarities. Many of our doctors worked at both hospitals. We were not enemies."

The mutual respect between both hospitals' Board chairmen, Robert Cole and Robert Dubé, also helped Baptist and South Miami find common ground. The two men, lawyers by training, were honest and direct. They met a few times one-on-one in the South Miami Hospital auditorium to discuss the merger, and in the process developed trust. "I think we built a personal connection," Judge Dubé remembered. "I never thought that there was any salesmanship to what Mr. Cole was saying. He looked me in the eye and was always straightforward and that made a difference."

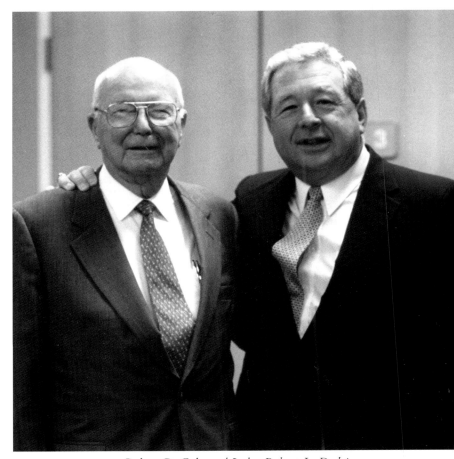

Robert B. Cole and Judge Robert L. Dubé

With a collaborative spirit, a merger agreement took shape. Baptist would immediately loan South Miami Hospital $10 million from its reserves — $6 million to pay off a 30-day loan that the hospital took from one of the for-profits, National Medical Enterprise, and $4 million for the hospital's working capital. Baptist also agreed to assume $70 million in debt and invest a minimum of $25 million in both hospitals over the next six years, including constructing a medical office building at South Miami Hospital. Beyond the financial details, Keeley and Baptist Hospital leaders insisted that they supported preserving the identity and culture at South Miami and Homestead.

At Homestead, there was less concern. The hospital was smaller and farther away from Kendall. It never competed directly with Baptist. Its purpose was to offer South Dade residents a healthcare option closer to home. In addition, Homestead employees were used to being managed by an outside party; other companies had run Homestead for more than 10 years. "I think the idea of assimilating to Baptist was easy for us," said Administrator Bo Boulenger. "We were already supported by a larger hospital — South Miami — so it was just an extension of that."

The physicians and employees at South Miami, however, approached the merger with more trepidation. They were fearful that Baptist would dictate policies and procedures without involvement and consultation. "We had our own way of doing things," Dr. Stewart said. "Any merger would have to protect our family culture and professional traditions." On the practical level, South Miami employees were concerned that jobs would be consolidated. They wondered if they would have to report to a supervisor at Baptist. "We were concerned about our positions in the new organization," remembered Kathy Sparger, R.N., then South Miami's vice president of patient services.

To quell those fears, the merger documents called for each hospital's medical leadership, Board of Directors and administrative team to remain in control of policies at their respective institutions. South Miami and Homestead Hospitals kept their own names, a significant and symbolic gesture to indicate independence and respect for storied histories. Even more important, each hospital kept most of its staff in place, including senior leaders and nursing officers. While John Geanes left, Wayne Brackin, a familiar face to both South Miami and Homestead employees, took over as South Miami Hospital's chief executive officer. Brackin was a popular leader with a strong presence at the hospitals. Bo Boulenger, who at age 34 already had 10 years of experience in hospital leadership, remained in his post at Homestead. "There was not a sense that Baptist Hospital was going to come in and clean house," Brackin said. "Brian Keeley did not say, 'I want and need my own people.' That is extraordinary in this kind of situation. I think by keeping the leadership intact, he reassured everyone at the two hospitals that this was going to be a collaborative process."

Indeed, it was both the decisions and personality of Brian Keeley that helped smooth the rough edges. Even-tempered and insightful, Keeley was the visionary behind the merger. "He saw the future better than anybody," said Kyle Saxon, a lawyer who worked on the merger. "There were very complicated issues — real estate, finance, billing, compliance, licensing and insurance — and he put together a team of highly qualified executives to handle them."

Keeley was also known to many at South Miami. He was businesslike and professional but without airs. His thoughtful and systematic approach to merger-related issues made the physicians and employees comfortable — a major contrast to the whirlwind surrounding the for-profits that had courted South Miami. "We had the sense that Brian Keeley was a good man, an honorable guy," Dr. Mackler said. "We knew him and respected and trusted him. It was important because some of the characters surrounding the corporations looking at South Miami did not always feel as above-board."

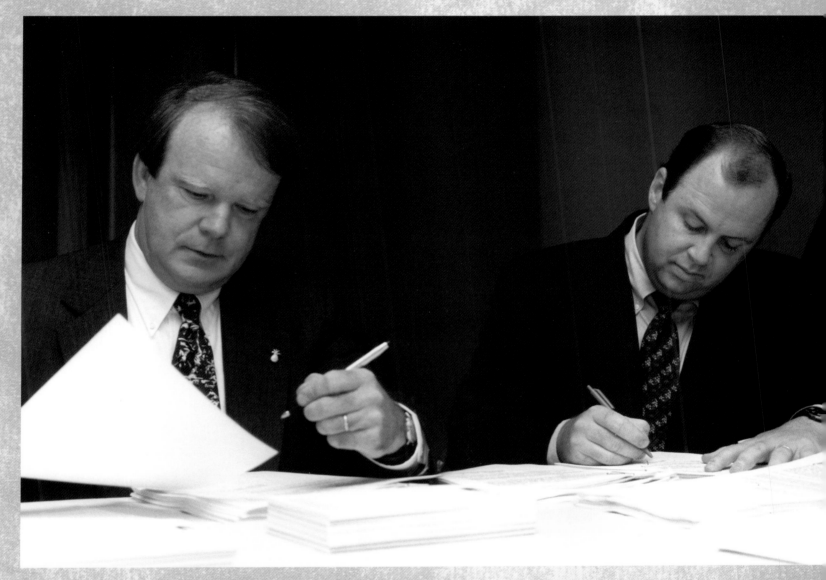

Brian Keeley and Wayne Brackin sign the merger agreement.

"*B*rian Keeley saw the future better than anybody. There were very complicated issues — real estate, finance, billing, compliance, licensing and insurance — and he put together a team of highly qualified executives to handle them."

Kyle Saxon
Lawyer who worked on the merger

The Final Step

On April 13, 1995, South Miami approved the merger with Baptist. The move came despite some last-minute intrigue. A few days before the final vote, Columbia/HCA sent a letter to South Miami's Board of Directors and Foundation offering to better Baptist's deal by about $30 million. In addition, it raised questions about Baptist's intention for South Miami, claiming that it might close the hospital — a point that Brian Keeley strongly contested. "For us to close South Miami is nonsense," Keeley told a newspaper. "There is a very strong desire on the part of the medical staffs to combine the two hospitals to take advantage of their strengths and to maintain local community control."

The letter's intent failed miserably. To those at South Miami, it felt underhanded and simply reinforced the decision to remain a not-for-profit. "Columbia/HCA wanted to make the argument that they could offer more money, but this was not a money deal," Dr. Loewenherz said at the time. "It was about collaboration." The letter hoped to disrupt a decision that followed countless hours of careful negotiation. "It damaged their position," Dr. Mackler explained. "It confirmed the resolve of the Board of Directors and the Foundation that we were doing the right thing by remaining true to our not-for-profit mission." So, with enthusiasm, the merger went from an idea to a vote to a reality.

Brian Keeley became president and chief executive officer of Baptist Health Systems of South Florida. Fred Messing, who had been Baptist Hospital's chief operating officer and executive vice president, took over as the hospital's CEO. To build this large, new organization, Keeley and other leaders had to consolidate some areas while separating others. They had to develop a corporate structure. Most importantly, they had to create a new culture in which employees would feel that they worked for Baptist Health, not simply their home hospital. "I remember that it was a real question just how to organize this thing," Keeley said. "I looked for a model where hospitals had integrated and talked to people." He also turned to Baptist Health's Board Chairman Robert Cole for support and guidance.

Mr. Cole had been on the Baptist Board since 1962 and was familiar with the intricacies of overseeing a hospital. He had vast legal experience and a sharp intellect — a quiet wisdom that steered the discussions. As the complicated details of the merger were worked through, Cole was one of the key players. "He was the driver of the merger at the Board level," Keeley remembered. "His expertise, gained from years on the Board and his professional success as general counsel to construction company Lennar, helped guide us through just how to bring the three hospitals together."

The strategy for integrating the three hospitals developed. In its simplest form, clinical matters and the day-to-day care of patients remained at the individual hospitals. Everything that was non-clinical, from marketing to payroll, became centralized. The distinction allowed the hospitals to continue to run as they had. "I realized that, given the situation at South Miami, I had to have

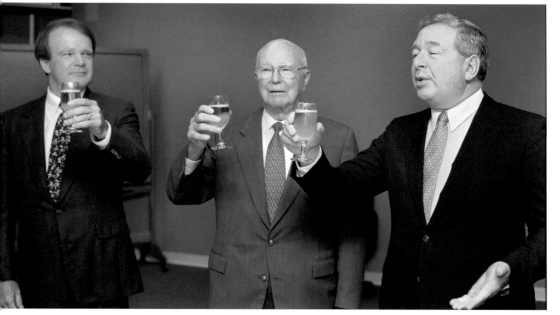

Brian E. Keeley, Robert B. Cole and Judge Robert L. Dubé toast the completed merger.

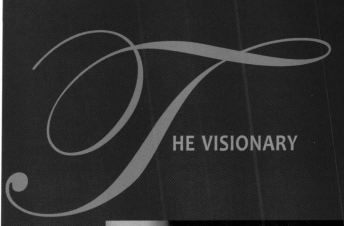

laser focus on streamlining what I could," Keeley said. "We were strengthening our market share, consolidating our corporate functions and increasing our purchasing power. This would save money in operations. We would be more efficient, but I also had to trust the employees at each hospital to do what they do best — care for patients."

To ease the transition, Chief Nursing Officers Kathy Sparger, R.N., (South Miami) Charlotte Dison, R.N., (Baptist) and Gail Gordon, R.N., (Homestead) began meeting together to bring the bedside caregivers onboard. After an initial uncertainty about who was reporting to whom and wondering if one person had any greater authority than another, the three women built a relationship based on mutual respect. The gatherings had both practical and symbolic purposes. "We worked hard on standardizing care where we could, while taking into account each hospital's culture and patient mix," Ms. Gordon said. "We were the first of any department to meet in such a way and I think we became a model of collaboration. The leadership at the corporate level recognized us and held us up as a way to do it together."

The physicians also played a key role in uniting behind a singular organization. The medical staffs at both South Miami and Baptist merged, while maintaining their own executive committees. (In 2004, the staff separated once again when it became evident that a joint group was too large to function effectively.) At South Miami, doctors realized that a partnership with Baptist offered both financial help and certain expertise. "Baptist as an organization brought a fiscal discipline to our hospital and that was something we lacked. They knew how to run things efficiently — billing, collections and certainly managed care contracts," Dr. Stewart said. "They also invested in our hospital. We had deferred maintenance and needed equipment and they provided that." The physicians, especially those at South Miami, concluded that the merger was a marriage of strengths.

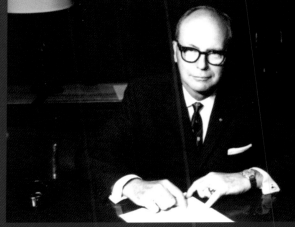

Robert B. Cole

In his 35 years on the Board of Trustees, Robert B. Cole was part visionary, problem solver and legal advisor.

He grew up in Orlando and graduated from the University of Florida with bachelor's and law degrees. He moved to Miami in 1935 to join what became the law firm of Mershon, Sawyer, Johnston, Dunwody & Cole. One of his clients was Arthur Vining Davis and the connection led him to Baptist Hospital.

Mr. Cole joined Baptist Hospital's Board in 1962 and became its chairman in 1985. He also chaired the Baptist Health Board of Trustees, beginning in 1993. He held both leadership positions, rarely missing a meeting or event, until his death at age 83 in 1997.

He used his analytical mind to guide the Baptist Hospital Board and, later, Baptist Health. Colleagues remember that he could read 400 pages of legal documents and find 20 typos. "Mr. Cole was a financial genius, a man with great vision, a man who could solve almost any problem," CEO Brian Keeley said. "He was the person I always turned to for counsel and advice. He was a real mentor."

Mr. Cole's abiding respect for employees guided his tenure. He led the effort to build an on-site employee daycare center at Baptist Hospital. "Some people questioned the fact that we wanted to put a substantial amount of money into an on-site daycare center when few businesses offered such employee perks. They said, 'We're in the hospital business, not the daycare business,'" Mr. Keeley said. "But Mr. Cole was truly an employee advocate. He knew that if you wanted an exceptional workplace, you needed exceptional employees. And he knew that to attract great people, you needed to meet their needs."

Mr. Cole also had a special appreciation for nurses. He established the Robert B. Cole Distinguished Nursing Lecture Series — an annual event that honors Baptist Health nurses and gives them the chance to learn and celebrate together. The lecture series continues today and is supported by his son, Richard Cole.

When the issues were complicated, especially when it came to the merger with South Miami Hospital, the circumspect Board chairman questioned and pushed. "Mr. Cole was tough as nails," Chief Financial Officer Ralph Lawson remembered. "He questioned everything. At one point he came up to me and actually apologized. He said he wasn't asking questions because he wanted to complicate the deal. He was doing it because he wanted to do the right thing. It was this commitment to intellectual honesty that made him a great man."

Introducing the new
Baptist Health Systems of S. Florida

Baptist Health Systems and South Miami HealthSystem are pleased to announce the merger of the two healthcare organizations, forming one of the largest and most respected not-for-profit hospital systems in Florida.

The new Baptist Health Systems of South Florida includes Baptist Hospital of Miami, South Miami Hospital and Homestead Hospital. It also encompasses a broad range of affiliated physicians' offices, outpatient facilities, medical equipment and supply companies, skilled nursing care, and home health care services.

All with the same not-for-profit mission of community service. The same local control by voluntary community leaders. And the commitment to medical excellence and personalized care you've come to know and trust.

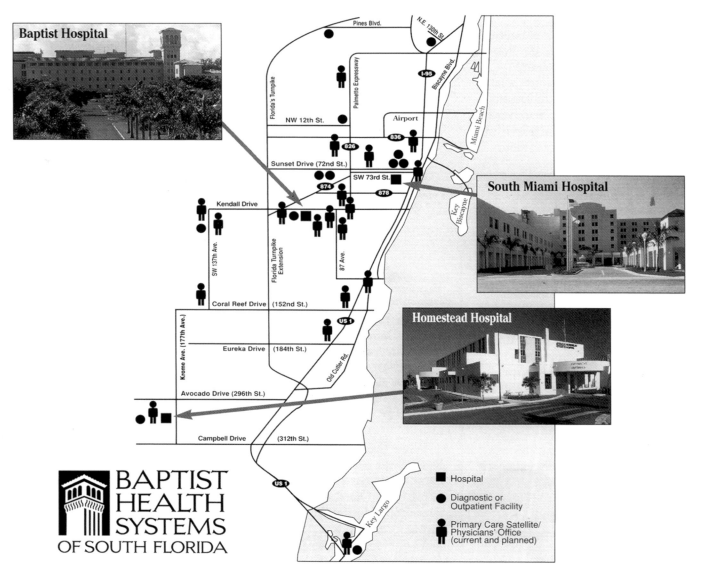

Baptist Hospital

South Miami Hospital

Homestead Hospital

■ Hospital

● Diagnostic or Outpatient Facility

Primary Care Satellite/ Physicians' Office (current and planned)

BAPTIST
HEALTH
SYSTEMS
OF SOUTH FLORIDA

BAPTIST HOSPITAL OF MIAMI – 8900 N. KENDALL DRIVE, MIAMI / SOUTH MIAMI HOSPITAL – 6200 SW 73RD STREET, MIAMI / HOMESTEAD HOSPITAL – 160 NW 13TH STREET, HOMESTEAD / MIAMI VASCULAR INSTITUTE, BAPTIST REGIONAL CANCER CENTER, BAPTIST NEUROSCIENCE CENTER, AND BAPTIST HOME CARE – 8900 N. KENDALL DRIVE, MIAMI / BAPTIST HEALTH CLUB, WOMEN'S HEALTH RESOURCE CENTER, AND BAPTIST OUTPATIENT CENTER – 8950 NORTH KENDALL DRIVE, MIAMI / BAPTIST WALK-IN MEDICAL CENTER – 9000 SW 137TH AVENUE, MIAMI / BAPTIST HEALTH CENTER – 8301 NW 12TH STREET, MIAMI / DIAGNOSTIC CENTER FOR WOMEN – 6140 SW 70TH STREET, MIAMI / BAYSHORE MEDICAL EQUIPMENT – 13020 NE 8TH AVENUE, NORTH MIAMI / SMH REPRODUCTIVE MEDICINE PROGRAM, SMH CENTER FOR WOMEN'S MEDICINE, AND SMH TRANSITIONAL CARE CENTER – 6200 SW 73RD STREET, MIAMI / SOUTH MIAMI AMBULATORY SURGERY CENTER – 6250 SUNSET DRIVE, MIAMI / SMH HERNIA INSTITUTE – 6280 SUNSET DRIVE, MIAMI / SOUTH MIAMI HOSPITAL HOME HEALTH – 9350 SUNSET DRIVE, MIAMI; 88005 OVERSEAS HIGHWAY, ISLAMORADA / FAMILY MEDICAL SUPPLY – 9999 SUNSET DRIVE, MIAMI / MIAMI OSTOMY CENTER – 8377 PINES BOULEVARD, PEMBROKE PINES / SMH OUTPATIENT CENTER – 160 NW 13TH STREET, HOMESTEAD

Building a Culture

As the merger became official on June 1, 1995, leaders began defining a discernible Baptist Health culture — what Mr. Keeley labeled the core values and salient features of the organization. They included integrity and ethical business standards, a strong commitment to a not-for-profit mission, which the hospitals all shared before the merger, and developing a family-friendly workplace with benefits such as on-site childcare and flexible shifts. Most importantly, Baptist Health became focused on the concept of service excellence. Executives instilled a passion for customer service at each hospital and that became a Baptist Health hallmark.

"Service excellence makes someone who goes to another hospital say, 'Wow, things really are better at Baptist,'" Keeley wrote in the employee newsletter at the time of the merger. "It is not only having the technical skills to do your job, but the people skills to make patients, families and co-workers feel special and valued." He promoted the idea that Baptist Health was in a service industry and its patients were essentially customers. In the coming years, Baptist Health developed tangible ways to measure how it was serving its "customers" and became well-known in the industry for its attention to compassionate service.

The merger meant other changes as well. The corporate leadership team standardized human resources policies so employees would receive the same benefits and have the same expectations regardless of where they worked. The information technology team began upgrading the computer systems so that the campuses were connected. It was all part of creating synergy, what Keeley defined as "a wondrous process of two or more entities working together to produce a combined effect greater than any one of them can achieve on their own." The word became a rallying cry of sorts for Baptist Health employees.

In retrospect, the merger succeeded because all of the parties came in line — business leaders, physicians and bedside caregivers — and a common culture emerged. It was not easy. It involved some pull and push, compromise and concessions. Some remained skeptical and unconvinced that the individual hospitals would retain their special cultures. But ultimately, each hospital and its employees found a place and a comfort level. The merger became a covenant based on necessity and potential. "I think everyone realized that as the larger organization thrived, everyone improved," Wayne Brackin said. "It was a rising tide that lifted all the hospital boats."

Within a few months, the rising tide looked to grow again. Baptist Health Systems of South Florida turned to a small community hospital in the Florida Keys for opportunity and expansion. The partnership would help create the largest not-for-profit healthcare organization in South Florida.

"*Service excellence makes someone who goes to another hospital say, 'Wow, things really are better at Baptist.' It is not only having the technical skills to do your job, but the people skills to make patients, families and co-workers feel special and valued.*"

Brian E. Keeley
President and CEO
Baptist Health Systems

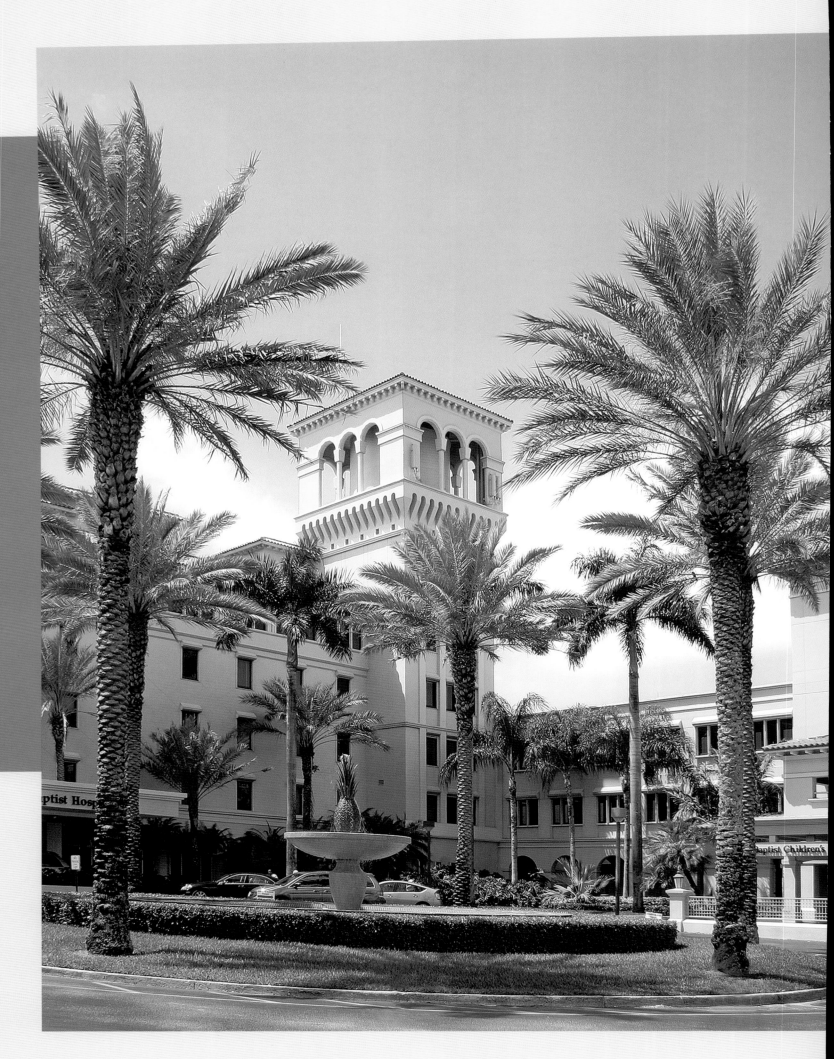

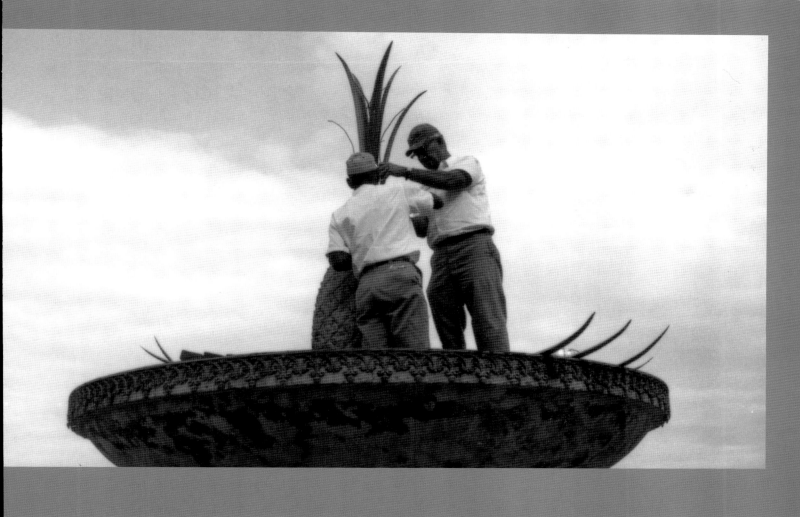

Pineapple Fountain Art

The pineapple fountain at the entrance to Baptist Hospital is a nationally recognized piece of artistic history. In 1995, the sculpture earned a place in the Art Inventories Catalogue compiled by the Smithsonian American Art Museum. The bronze pineapple, a Baptist landmark since the hospital opened in 1960, was sculpted by an unidentified artisan working for the hospital's architect.

When Arthur Vining Davis donated the land for Baptist Hospital, one of his conditions was that a pineapple fountain stand at its entrance. He never explained the reason for his request. At one time, he owned a pineapple plantation so perhaps he had an affinity for the fruit. Regardless of his motives, the pineapple, a European symbol of hospitality, is a fitting greeting for hospital visitors — and ultimately inspired Baptist Health's well-known logo.

A Hospital in the Keys

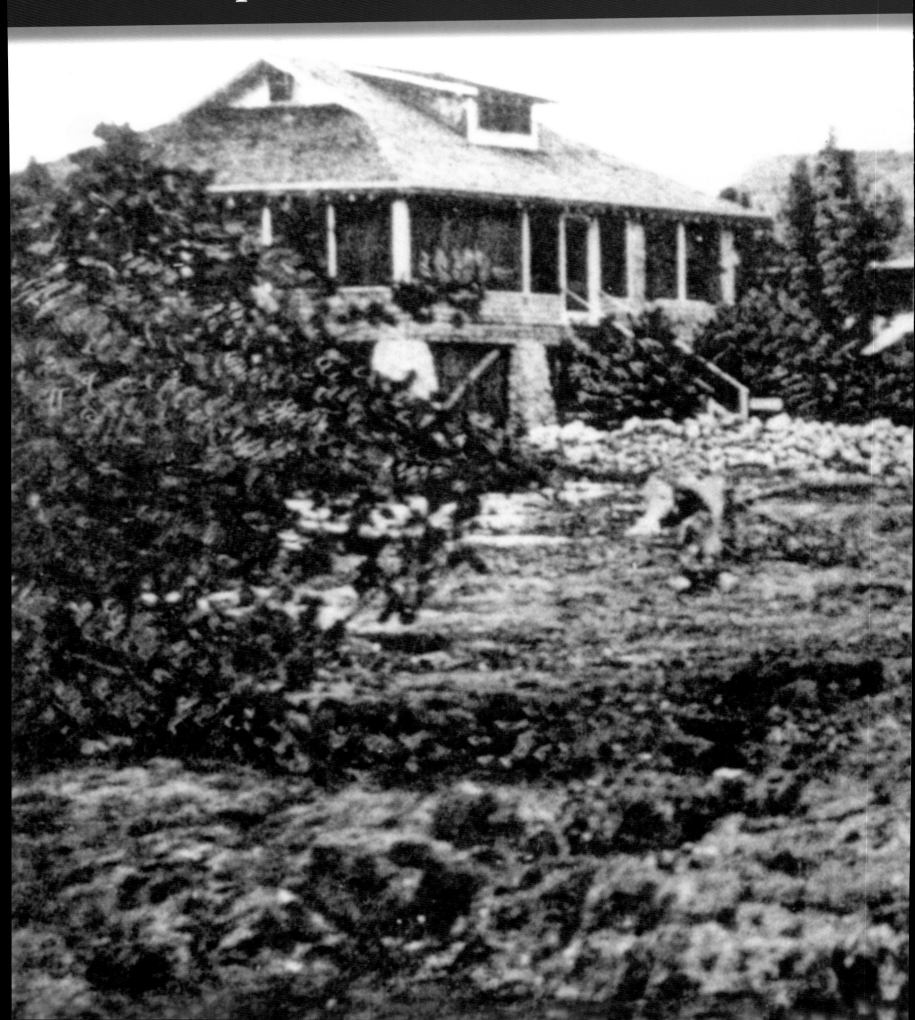

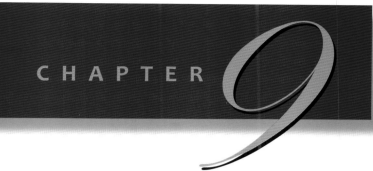

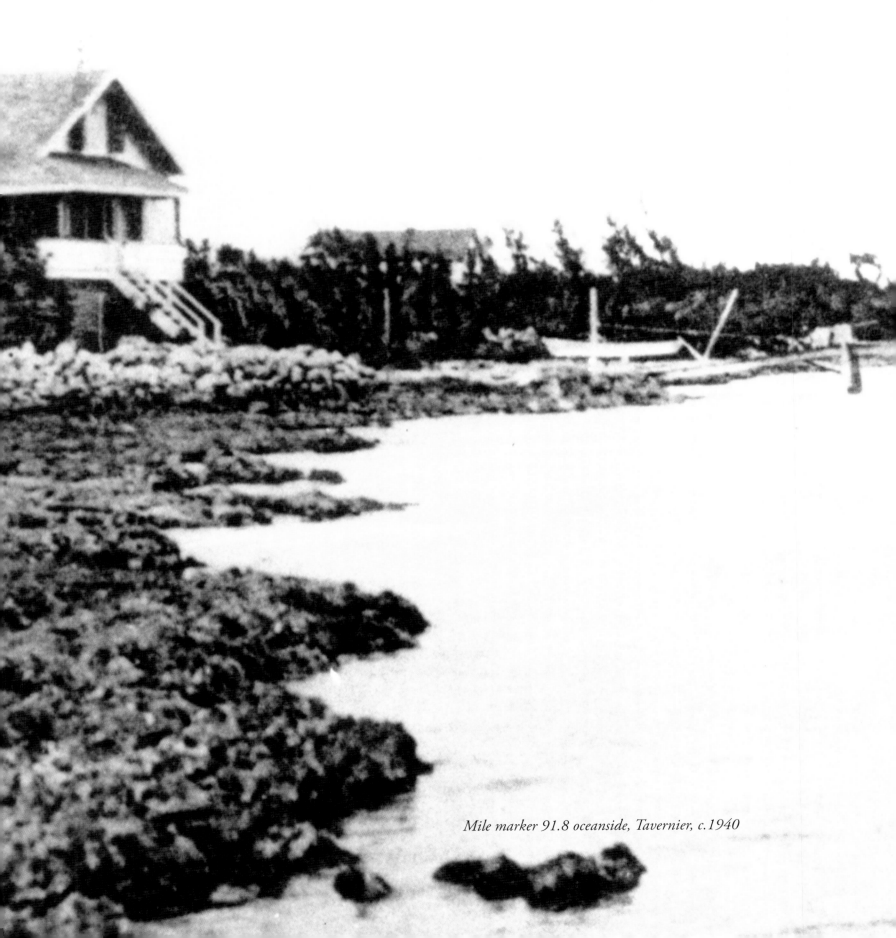

CHAPTER 9

Mile marker 91.8 oceanside, Tavernier, c.1940

"Something outstanding doesn't always have to be large in size or proportion. Most every community can boast of one or more small organizations which contribute substantially to the best interests of everyone concerned. In the Upper Keys area such an organization is Keys Community Hospital."

The Keynoter *newspaper*
describing the hospital
1968

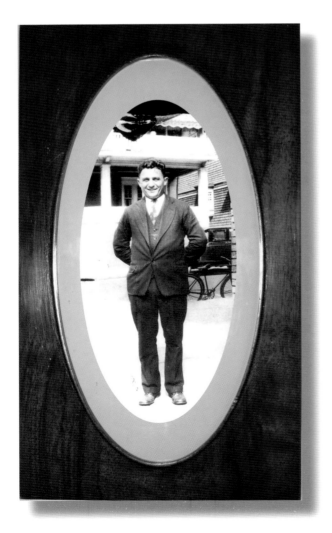

Nathaniel Levin was a pharmacist at Barskey's Drug Store in Philadelphia while working his way through medical school. He later settled in South Florida and helped establish Overseas Hospital.

In the late 1950s, Nathaniel Levin, M.D., came to the Upper Florida Keys, the area that stretched south from Key Largo to Long Key. The Russian immigrant lived in South Florida and bought a second home in the community. An avid fisherman and swimmer, he wanted to fully enjoy the water. He visited the Keys with his family whenever he could and embraced the lifestyle.

As a doctor, he became the go-to man for the area's medical ills. At the time, residents and visitors had few options for treatment. They could travel south to Key West or north to Homestead. But Dr. Levin was in their backyard. They would knock on his door and the doctor would see patients on his porch. Recognizing a community need, in 1962 Dr. Levin organized a nine-bed hospital, called Overseas Hospital, on property he owned next to his home.

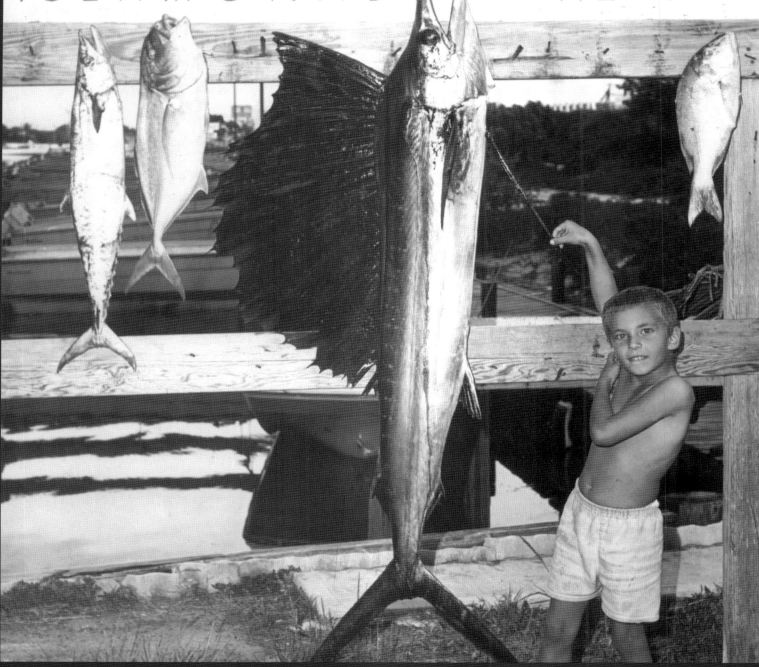

In the 1950s, people visited the Upper Keys to fish and enjoy the water.

An Immigrant Builds His Life

Dr. Levin was a true American success story. He grew up one of seven children in a close but poor family. After emigrating from Russia in the early 1900s, the family started a new life in Columbus, Ohio, and ultimately settled in Philadelphia. Nathaniel's father, Elimayer (changed to Max after arriving in America), was a tailor.

Life for the Levins was difficult. The children, strong and street-smart, worked in various jobs to help the family. Nathaniel (called Nate) was an amateur boxer and worked as a riveter building ships. By age 18, he had joined the Merchant Marines and sailed to North Africa.

Nate returned to Philadelphia from his overseas adventures ready to embrace his studies. He had been the only one of the Levin children to finish high school. After pharmacy school, he worked his way through medical school at Temple University and completed an internship in otolaryngology — an ear, nose and throat specialty.

With an adventuresome spirit and desire to serve, he enlisted in the U.S. Navy during World War II. His service included time in the Florida Keys patrolling for German submarines — his introduction to the subtropics. After the war, he built a practice in Miami and spent his leisure time on Plantation Key.

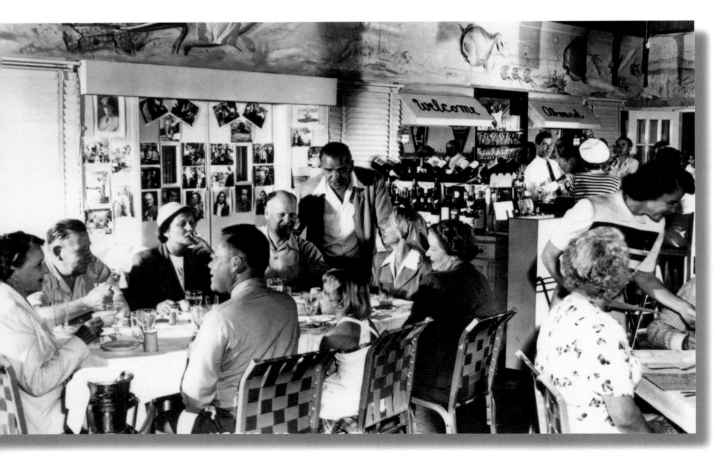

The Caribbean Club in Key Largo, built by entrepreneur Carl Fisher, was a popular draw for Keys visitors. In this 1950s photograph, guests enjoy the club's restaurant.

$\mathcal{W}$ith an adventuresome spirit and desire to serve, he enlisted in the U.S. Navy during World War II. His service included time in the Florida Keys patrolling for German submarines — his introduction to the subtropics.

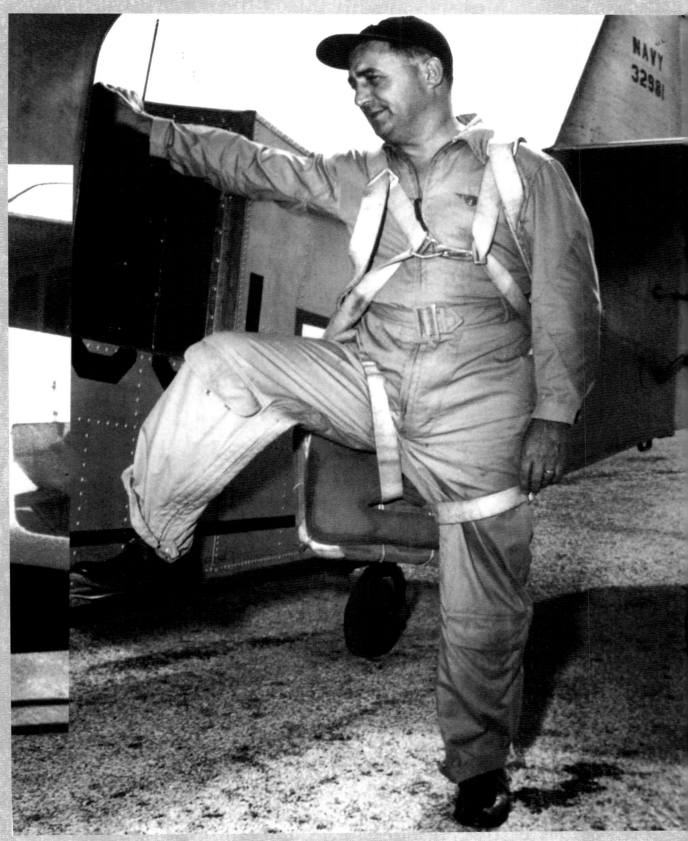

Commander Nathaniel Levin, U.S. Navy Amphibians in World War II

Far From the City

Plantation Key began as a small community just south of Tavernier. Like most of the Upper Keys, its population was a collection of fishermen and residents who worked in tourist-related industries. The nearest city was 90 miles south in Key West.

For much of its early history, Plantation Key was primarily inhabited by Indians. The 1870 census reported two families as its residents. Joseph and Mary Sawyer farmed the fertile land. Richard Sawyer (no relation), a seaman, lived on the key with his wife and five children. Coconut palms and pineapples were plentiful, and soon others joined the Sawyer families in creating a makeshift community.

The surrounding settlements, including Tavernier, Matecumbe Key, Indian Key and Key Largo, were similarly inhabited by a handful of homesteaders. For them, life was about agriculture, water, coexisting with Indians and surviving hurricanes. In 1905, railroad magnate Henry Flagler made a bold and daring edict. He publicly announced his intention to extend his railroad from Miami all the way to Key West. Like the South Florida mainland, the area changed with the coming of the railroad.

To build a railroad over water was an engineering challenge. Flagler committed more than 2,500 men and $20 million to the project, approximately 40 percent of his total Florida investment. Though some derided the idea as "Flagler's Folly," daily train service from Miami to Marathon began in 1908. Stations dotted the route in Key Largo, Rock Harbor, Tavernier, Islamorada and Marathon, and the railroad sparked development. Post offices, small general stores and community docks had sprung up by the depots. Over time, settlers built hotels, boarding houses and fishing clubs.

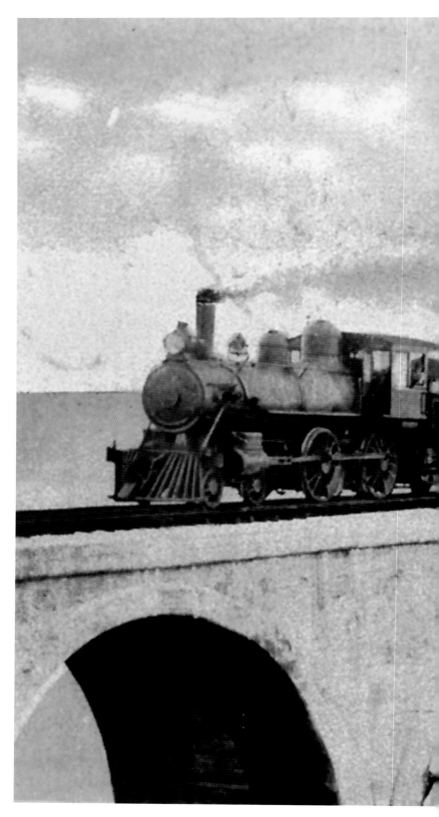

This postcard shows Henry Flagler's Special, the first train crossing over Long Key Viaduct, c.1909.

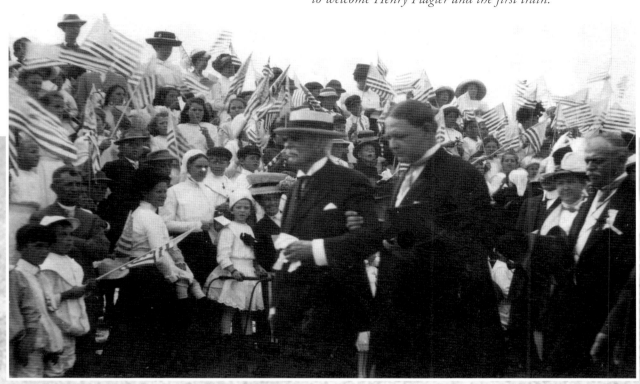

On January 22, 1912, 10,000 people gathered in Key West to welcome Henry Flagler and the first train.

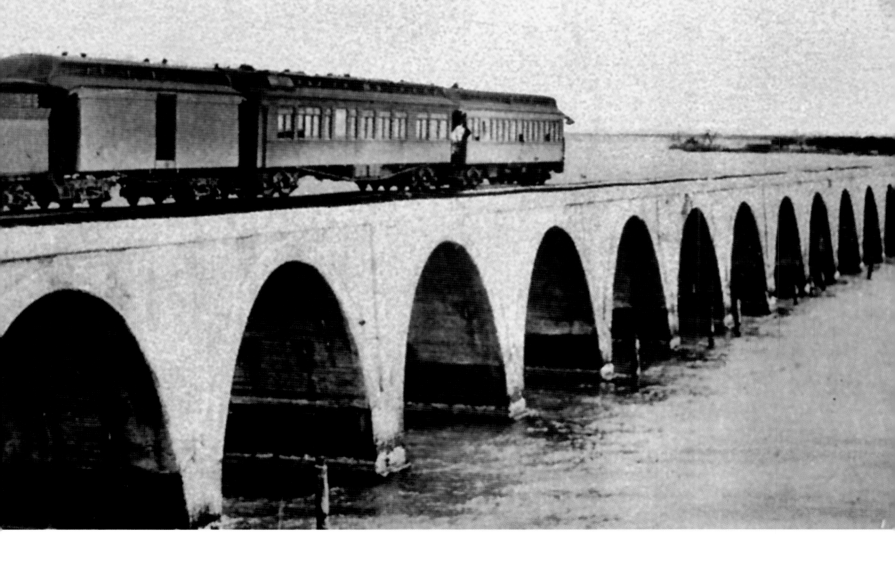

A Road Comes South

The Upper Keys received another boost with construction of the Overseas Highway. The 1920s brought a frenzy of real estate activity to South Florida, and Keys leaders wanted a piece of the economic growth. Their communities were still a small collection of permanent residents. The 1920 census put the population of Tavernier at 91, Plantation Key at 53, Marathon at 100 and Islamorada at 180. The areas relied heavily on winter tourists, who arrived by the railroad.

With the introduction of the automobile, visitors would be able to come by car — if there were a road. Monroe County and Dade County worked together to construct what became known as the Overseas Highway. The highway opened in sections, a haphazard combination of roads, bridges and a ferry system that transported people and cars. As local boosters had imagined, it stimulated

growth. Subdivisions popped up with fanciful names such as Atlantic View, Angler's Park, Sunset Cove and Palma Sola. Developers gobbled up land with the hopes of capitalizing on the boom-time conditions. Charles Sexton, for example, purchased land surrounding the Key Largo train depot to build a "Venice of the Keys." By 1925, he had a hotel, store with a post office and restaurant.

Still, the disorganized nature of the Overseas Highway was a hindrance to development. The ferry service was slow, unreliable and expensive. By 1930, officials formed plans to build bridges between the islands, eliminating the ferries. The timing was right. The land boom had gone bust and the nation was entering the Great Depression. The public works project would bring much-needed jobs. A group of unemployed World War I veterans came to the Keys to start construction.

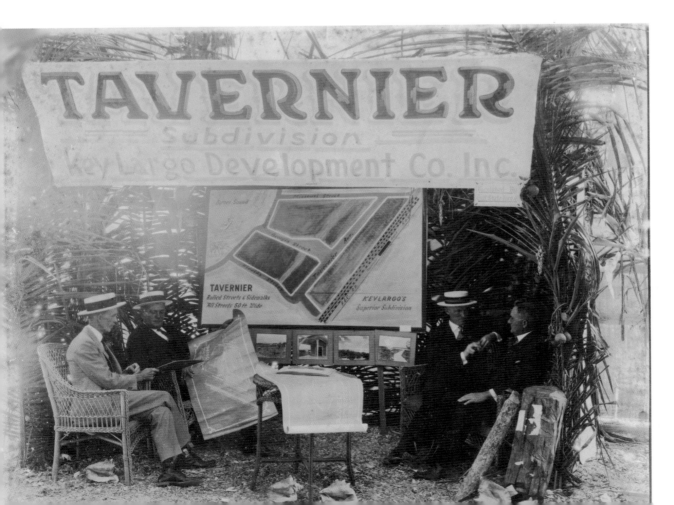

The Florida land boom brought development to the Florida Keys, including Tavernier, the site of today's Mariners Hospital.

With the introduction of the automobile, visitors would be able to come by car — if there were a road. Monroe County and Dade County worked together to construct what became known as the Overseas Highway.

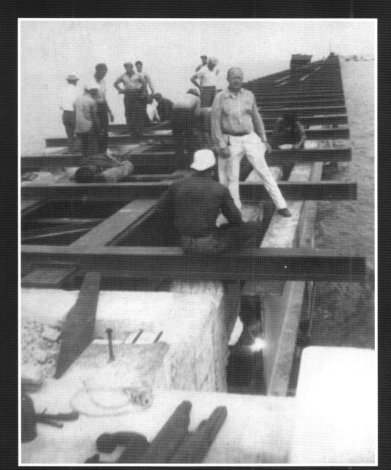

Right: Converting a railroad bridge to a vehicle bridge

Bottom: The Overseas Highway at Sugarloaf Key, c.1929

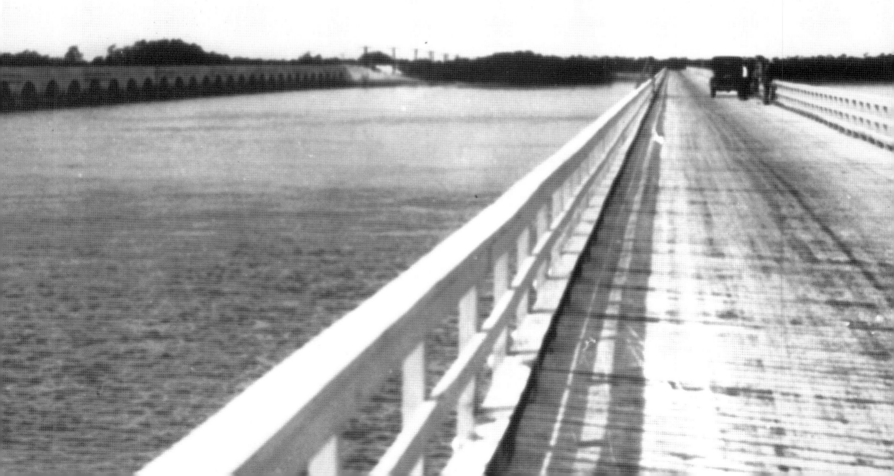

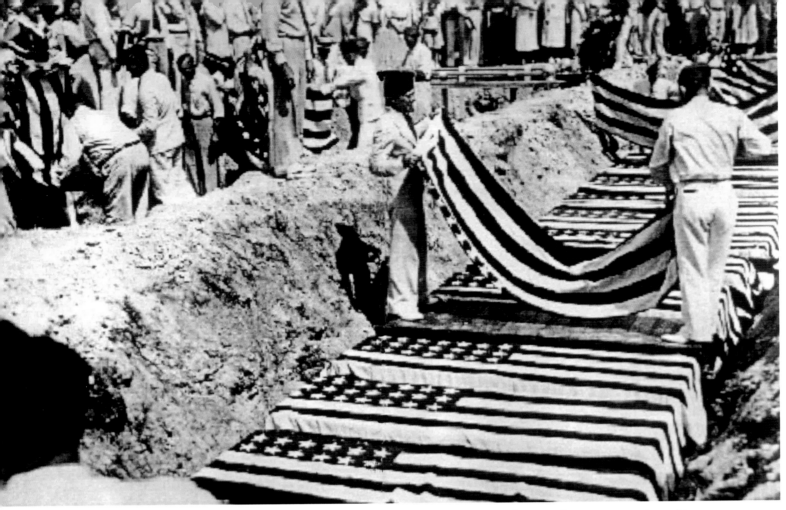

The veterans who died during the 1935 hurricane were buried in a mass grave at Woodlawn Park Cemetery in Miami.

By 1935, about 700 veterans were working on the highway until tragedy struck. On Labor Day, 1935, Miamians received word of an approaching hurricane. Officials sent a train to the Upper Keys to evacuate the highway laborers, but a broken cable delayed the train's departure and it arrived at Islamorada in the middle of the fury. Raging water swept across the island, tossing the steel railway cars as if they were toys. Rescue workers later found most of the train sprawled across broken tracks on its side.

The category five storm, with 200 mph winds and a storm surge of 15 to 18 feet, devastated the Upper and Middle Keys, killing 428 people, more than half of them veterans. The storm destroyed 42 miles of Henry Flagler's mythical "railroad that went to sea," and it would not be rebuilt. While much of the Upper and Middle Keys portion of the Overseas Highway lay in ruins, government officials planned to repair and complete the road. By March 1938, vehicles were traveling the length of the Florida Keys.

With easy access by car and boat, the Upper Keys became a tourist draw. Charter fishing developed into one of the area's most important industries. Several fishing clubs and hotels opened. The installation of a water pipeline in 1942 brought fresh water into the Keys. That same year public electricity came to the area. Before that, privately owned generators and small plants supplied occasional power to some participating residents. The first public high school also was planned. In 1951 Coral Shores School on Plantation Key opened. Students no longer had to transfer to Key West, Homestead or Miami to receive a high school diploma. As the new decade began, the Upper Keys was blossoming into a full-fledged community. Its approximately 1,000 residents had a highway, water, power and a new high school.

This postcard shows the keystone monument that commemorates the victims of the 1935 hurricane. It still stands today in Islamorada.

With easy access by car and boat, the Upper Keys became a tourist draw. Charter fishing developed into one of the area's most important industries. Several fishing clubs and hotels opened.

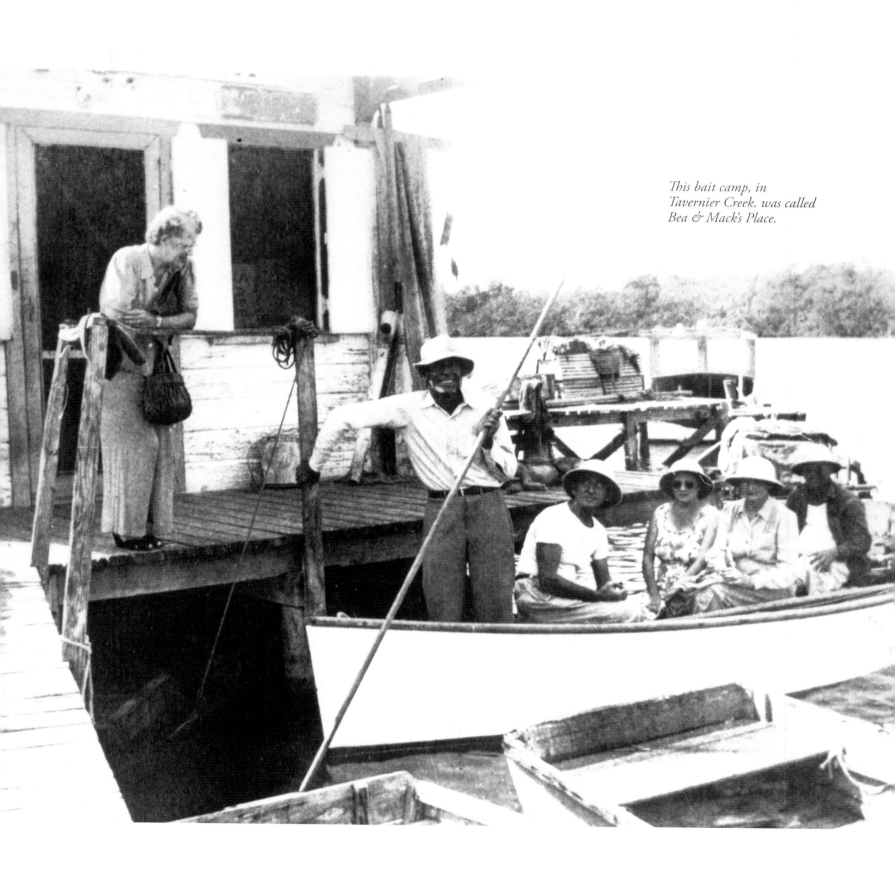

This bait camp, in Tavernier Creek, was called Bea & Mack's Place.

A Hospital Comes South

Despite the emerging infrastructure, medical care remained spotty. As in Homestead, residents were served by nurses. Frances Tracy and Mrs. George Brown, both nurses, cared for the community in the 1930s and 1940s. With no nearby pharmacies, they used a mixture of intuition and home remedies to treat patients. Miami doctors who had weekend homes in the Keys would bring medications and offer their services.

After World War II, residents worked to establish a permanent medical facility. In 1951, citizens, including Nurse Tracy, organized a Florida Keys Clinic Board to create reliable, full-time medical care on the islands. With their efforts, Harvey Cohn, M.D., a surgeon at Miami's Victoria Hospital, opened an office in Tavernier in 1953. Dr. Cohn, a native of Maine, had visited the Upper Keys to fish. The Board helped convince him to relocate his office to Tavernier, where he became the only doctor between Homestead and Key West.

Initially a jack-of-all-trades, Dr. Cohn was loved and respected. He served as doctor, nurse, receptionist and janitor, and even cared for some animals. His wife, Dorothy, was a registered nurse who helped as well. The Florida Keys Clinic was housed in two cramped rooms that had been used as a school. In 1959, he moved his practice to Plantation Key. Over time, a pharmacy and dental office also opened.

Medical services were less than adequate, however, until Dr. Levin got involved. A well-known surgeon in Miami, Dr. Levin was in charge of ear, nose and throat, and head and chest surgery at Dade County Hospital in Kendall. He also worked at Jackson Memorial, Mount Sinai and the newly opened Baptist Hospital, and was an associate professor at the University of Miami. He spent his leisure time in the waters off the Florida Keys. "He loved the area," said son Joel Levin, M.D., a Baptist Hospital plastic surgeon. "He took care of people who came by the house. He knew that the community needed more."

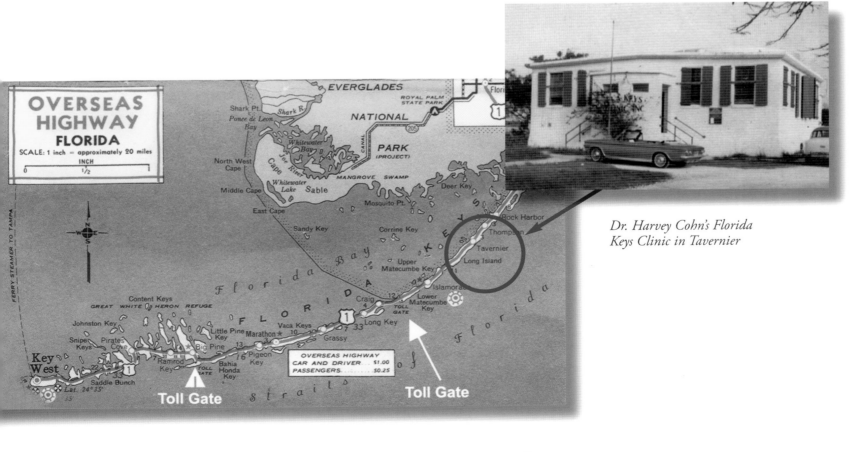

Dr. Harvey Cohn's Florida Keys Clinic in Tavernier

> *"Driving from the mainland onto the famed Overseas Highway is far from a journey into the wilderness, leaving civilization behind. The visitor or resident need be no more than 20 minutes traveling time from a hospital."*
>
> The Keynoter *newspaper*
> 1962

In 1962, Dr. Levin began transforming land he owned in the High Point subdivision on Plantation Key into a small hospital. His wife, Sylvia, worked on furnishing and decorating it. Stanford Setnor, M.D., a Syracuse University medical school graduate with extensive surgical experience, helped manage the hospital and received one-fifth interest in it.

In early May 1962, the Overseas Hospital accepted its first patient. The nearly 5,000-square-foot building had nine beds, two modern operating rooms and an X-ray department. Five nurses cared for patients alongside Dr. Levin and Dr. Setnor. Internist Jack Reiss, M.D., and Miami-based oral surgeon William Schiff, DMD, were called in to treat patients as needed.

The hospital was built to accommodate more beds. By October, 1,000 square feet housing four beds, storage, and dining and kitchen facilities were added. The 1962 opening of the 36-bed Fishermen's Hospital in Marathon in the Middle Keys meant that residents were now served by two hospitals. "No longer does the winter visitor need to be concerned about the lack of medical facilities in the Keys," the local newspaper, *The Keynoter*, proclaimed. "…Driving from the mainland onto the famed Overseas Highway is far from a journey into the wilderness, leaving civilization behind. The visitor or resident need be no more than 20 minutes traveling time from a hospital."

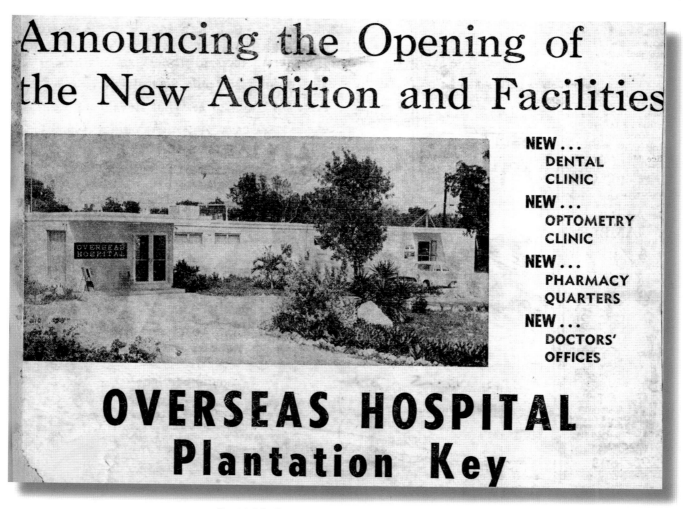

By 1964, Overseas Hospital was an important part of healthcare in the Upper Keys. This March 1964 advertisement for the hospital appeared in The Keynoter.

A Controversy Comes South

By 1966, the hospital's name was changed to Keys Community Hospital to reflect its mission. Dr. Levin no longer wanted to be involved in day-to-day management and sold his interest to Dr. Setnor. The 14-bed hospital was now solely Setnor's and he became its public face. Longtime employees remember that he was a constant presence, overseeing every detail, from treating patients to ordering supplies. He even monitored activities on the night shift, telephoning the nurses for updates.

Dr. Setnor also was the center of controversy. The local newspaper reported that, on several occasions, the hospital turned away patients who could not pay. Setnor emphatically denied the charge. There were misconceptions, the owner argued, about the hospital's for-profit status, which prevented it from receiving state funds to help care for the indigent. "Doctors in private hospitals are more than willing to donate their services but money must come from somewhere to pay for the penicillin, blood, laundry and the costs of the operating room," he said at the time. "An operation today, for example, required the services of five people — which represents five salaries."

To counter the growing public relations issue and plan for the hospital's future, community leaders formed the Keys Community Foundation. Led by neurologist Frederick Bond, M.D., the Foundation sought to have the community purchase the hospital and make it not-for-profit. Then, fundraising and government support could help finance a much-needed expansion that would broaden services.

By 1966, Stanford Setnor, M.D., was the sole owner of Keys Community Hospital.

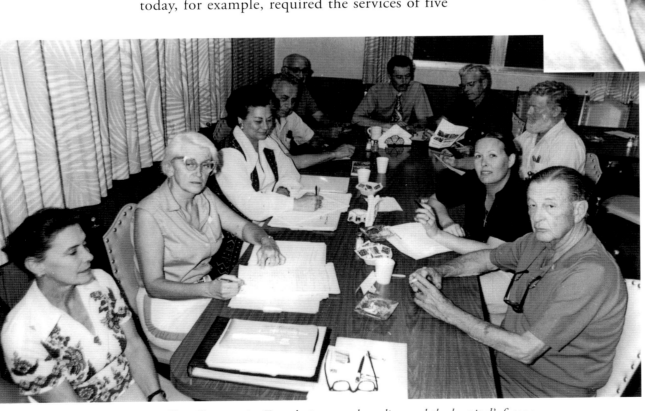

At this 1973 meeting, Keys Community Foundation members discussed the hospital's future.

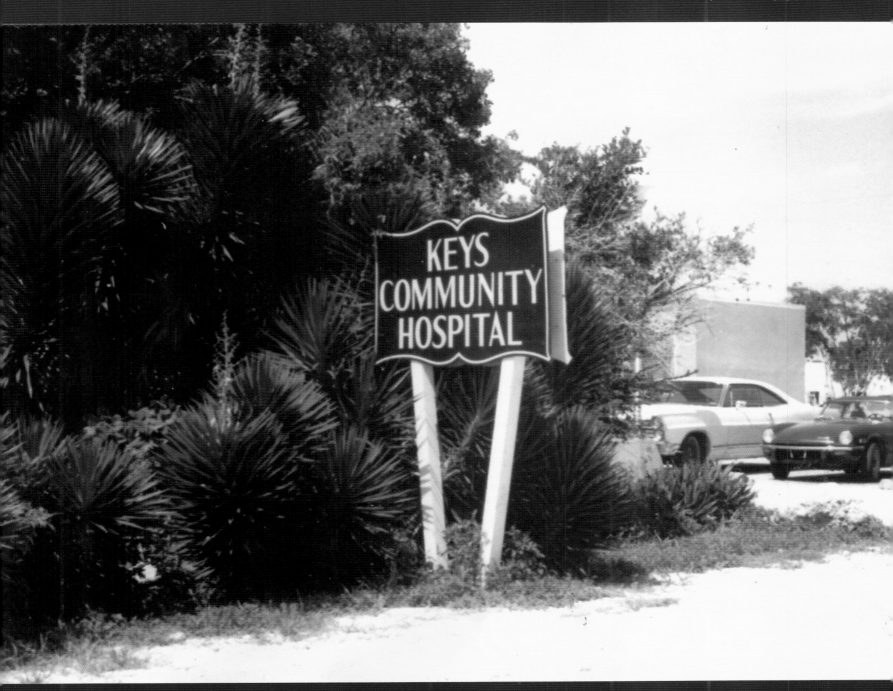

"*Nothing* but good can come from the current efforts to bring about community ownership of the Keys. Upper Keys folks have a distinct advantage in that an existing facility can be bought and expanded to meet the ever-increasing needs of a growing community."

Editorial
The Keynoter *newspaper*

In 1966, the hospital's name was changed to Keys Community Hospital.

The Foundation's effort drew support. "Nothing but good can come from the current efforts to bring about community ownership of the Keys [hospital]," *The Keynoter* newspaper concluded in 1967. "Upper Keys folks have a distinct advantage in that an existing facility can be bought and expanded to meet the ever-increasing needs of a growing community." It looked to Fishermen's Hospital as a model. The community-backed hospital provided a range of services. "Can there be any doubt that the present medical needs in the Upper Keys are any less great than what Marathon experienced a few years back?" the editorial asked.

Dr. Setnor, a polarizing figure, was unable to keep the hospital going on his own. With financial and community pressure mounting, he had little choice but to consider selling. In late 1967, the Foundation hired outside consultants to explore what the community wanted to do with the hospital. After sampling 294 households, about 5.5 percent of the Upper Keys population, the consultants reported that 80 percent supported taking community ownership of the hospital and maintaining it with yearly membership fees. The alternate proposal of assuming community ownership through a taxing district was less popular.

When the consultants presented their findings in April 1968, Foundation leaders decided to move forward with community ownership. They started planning how to delicately handle Dr. Setnor and diminish his role as the hospital's visible leader. Strategizing about fundraising was another priority. Appraisals put the purchase price at about $200,000. "It might take seven years to reach the goal," Dr. Bond said, "but I see no reason why the community won't rally behind the hospital."

In May 1968, the Foundation's efforts took a step forward. The group quietly pushed Setnor to the background and spearheaded the hiring of a full-time administrator. Robert Lee, fresh from a post at the National Institutes of Health, came aboard. Lee had a master's degree in hospital administration from the Medical College of Virginia and experience in hospital management. Before his time at the National Institutes of Health, Lee was chief administrator of North District Hospital in Pompano Beach. During his tenure there, the hospital expanded from 62 to 204 beds.

Keys Community Hospital had an experienced professional administrator to handle the next phase. "This is the best thing to happen to the hospital since I became associated with the Foundation," Dr. Bond said. But the Foundation leader had no illusions of the financial task ahead. "It will require the efforts of every member of the Board, an auxiliary, as well as community support and understanding if we are to be totally successful in this campaign."

Despite Dr. Bond's and the Foundation's intentions, the fundraising effort stalled and the hospital's future was in limbo. In January 1969, Lee left, citing a better opportunity elsewhere. Privately, however, Lee raised questions about Dr. Setnor's continued presence and the hospital's finances. Some community leaders again pushed for a special taxing district to finance community ownership. But the proposal was controversial and complex. Ultimately, the Keys Community Hospital Foundation came out against the plan, and residents voted down the proposed district in a November 1969 election. It was a case, as the newspaper reported, of "no one ... voting for anything that might even mean more taxes."

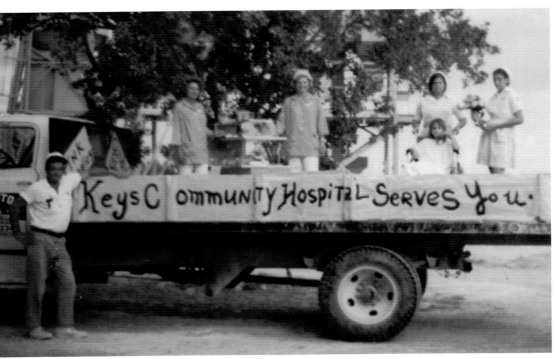

The Ladies Auxiliary posed on this float for a community parade.

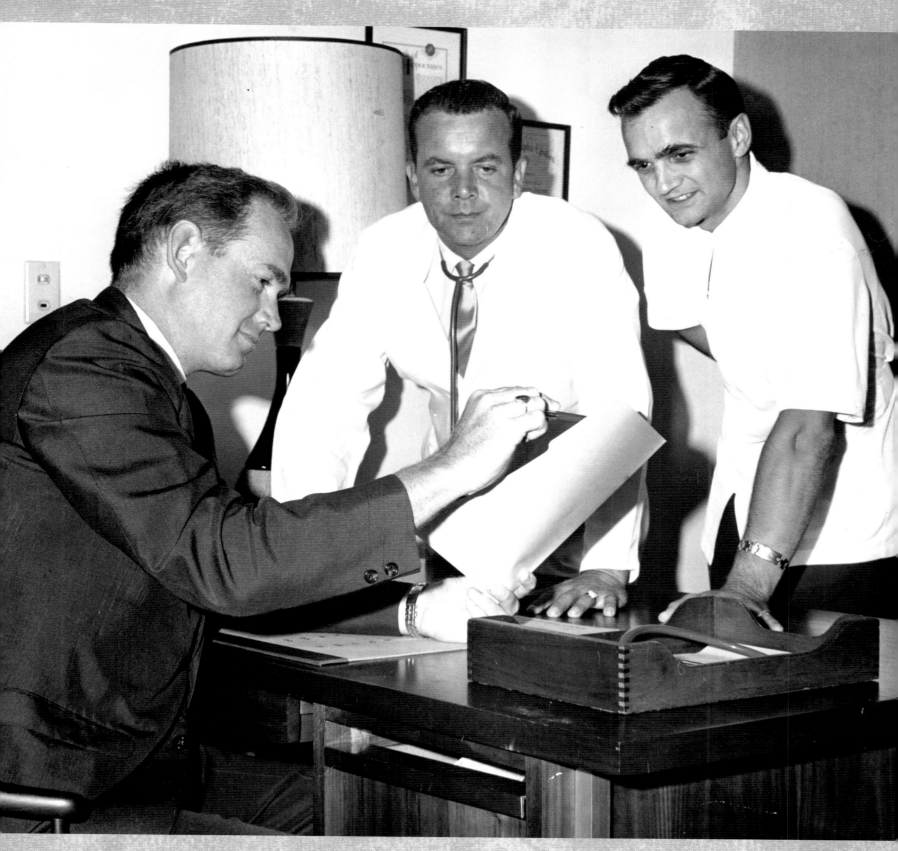

*Administrator Robert Lee meets with doctors Glenn Ross, M.D., and
Alex Amadio, M.D. Lee came to Keys Community in 1968.*

A New Owner

After the proposal's defeat, Setnor sold Keys Community Hospital to American Medical Affiliates, Inc. (AMA), which operated eight nursing homes in Pennsylvania, New Jersey, Maryland and Florida. It represented the company's first foray into hospital ownership. AMA announced an expansion plan that included a new wing. "Our entire program will be directed at creating a more complete medical facility in the Upper Keys, one which we hope will better accommodate the needs of this fast-growing community," said Joseph Aylsworth, executive vice president.

Plans called for a nearly $1 million addition that would bring the total number of beds to 42, a four-bed coronary care unit, two new operating rooms, an expanded emergency room, physical therapy rooms, doctors offices, dining room, conference room and a dental clinic. Room rates were to rise as well. Semi-private rooms would increase from $45 to $48 and private rooms from $52 to $58. AMA brought in its own administrator, Ralph Settle. The hospital's sale and new direction left Dr. Setnor's role unclear. Rumors had him resigning, leaving the Keys and moving to Costa Rica. While Setnor denied the rumblings, he did note the difficulty of his role as the hospital's leader. "One thing I learned is that you can't be a good guy and also run a hospital," he said. "The two just don't go together."

The optimism created by new ownership and expansion was short-lived. Within a few months, hospital leaders announced the closing of the emergency room at night and on weekends. The issue, naturally, was money. The hospital had to absorb the cost of staffing the emergency room — something that it could not handle, especially since many of the patients could not pay for services. "Anyone who thinks emergency room service makes any money is wrong," said Ralph Settle. "With increasing salaries, where do you stop boosting charges? Where do you stop losing money on indigents?"

The ER cutback again brought negative publicity to Keys Community Hospital. The closing added 20 to 25 minutes for an ambulance ride, a potentially deadly delay. AMA officials tried to spin the situation by reassuring that once the expansion was completed, resources would allow for a reopening. In February 1971, construction began on the hospital addition.

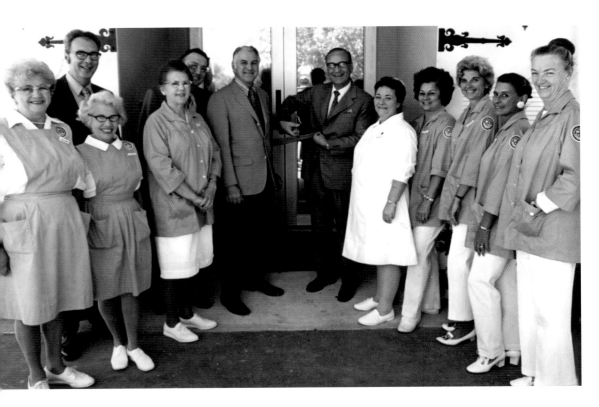

The new wing of Keys Community Hospital was dedicated on February 20, 1972.

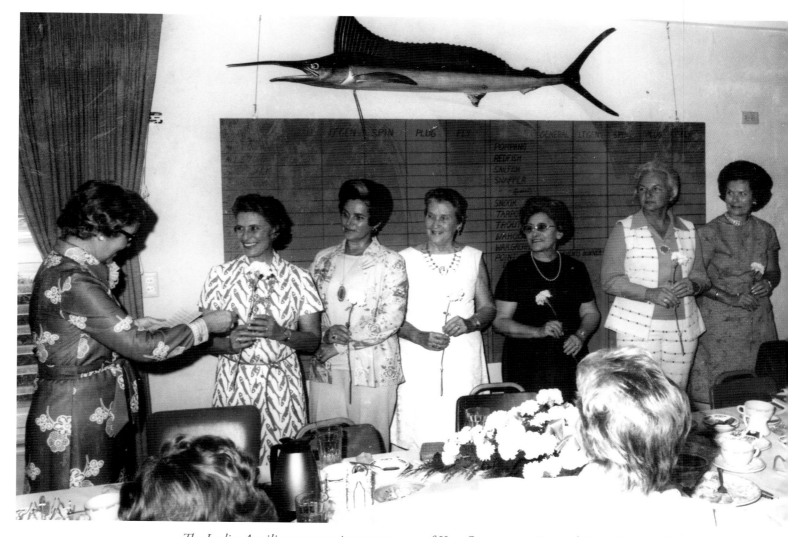

The Ladies Auxiliary was an important part of Keys Community Hospital. Members could be seen decorating the lobby, helping in the kitchen or comforting a patient. In this 1975 photograph, officers are being installed by South District Director Mrs. John Ewing. From left to right: Mrs. John Ewing, Mrs. H. Dalton Wood, Mrs. Chester Bright, Mrs. W.D. Haynie, Mrs. Peter Cipolla, Mrs. George Sands and Mrs. Lee Loumas.

When the project was completed a year later, those associated with the hospital hoped it marked a new beginning. "In just under 10 years' time, a little hospital in the Upper Keys has lived through periods of unheralded praise and stormy controversy," *The Keynoter* reported. "Now, almost at full maturity and in the process of overcoming growing pains, Keys Community Hospital presents a significant milestone compatible with the growth and development of the Upper Keys."

It took a few months and public pressure but AMA finally reopened the emergency room by the end of the summer of 1972. But the problems continued. The hospital administrator position was in constant flux as AMA struggled to earn a profit. By 1974, the hospital had its fourth leader in three years. Newspapers reported that local doctors were questioning AMA's billing practices and finances. Some in the community clamored to revisit the idea of making the hospital not-for-profit.

After a little more than a decade of operation, the future of Keys Community Hospital remained very much in doubt. "We all should do some heavy personal thinking on exactly what our hospital means to us," said an editorial in *The Reporter*. "For us to be without any hospital is unthinkable... If we have complaints, they should be brought out and aired and resolved and corrected. A rumor campaign can only hurt us all." The community agreed on the need for a hospital. The problem was just how to run it successfully.

1970

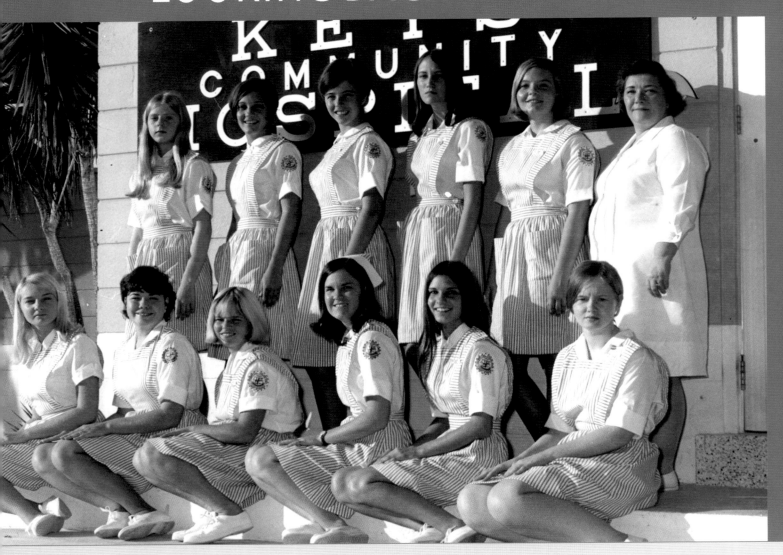

Candy Striper Volunteers

The Candy Stripers were teenage girls who volunteered at Keys Community Hospital. The group, formed in 1968, was sponsored by the Ladies Auxiliary. Membership was open to Coral Shores High School students ages 15-18. The Candy Stripers followed strict behavior guidelines and worked after school and weekends at the hospital. They supplied an extra pair of helping hands, assisting nurses and patients. Other local hospitals, including Homestead, Baptist, South Miami and Doctors', had similar volunteer groups.

The CODE of a "CANDY STRIPER"

I WILL BE--

1 DEPENDABLE... I'll do what I agree to do. If I can't make an assignment, I'll let my supervisor know ahead of time.

2 ANXIOUS TO LEARN... I'll try to know all I can about the hospital, its rules, and its services. If I don't understand, I'll ask questions.

3 QUIET... I'll walk and talk quietly so as not to disturb patients.

4 COURTEOUS... I'll <u>listen</u> to others, <u>think</u> of others, <u>help</u> others.

5 NEAT and CLEAN... I'll be well-groomed...clean in person and in dress.

6 PLEASANT... I'll have a friendly <u>smile</u> for everyone...and a sense of humor.

I WILL NOT--

1 DISCUSS PATIENTS in or out of the hospital, or discuss illness <u>with</u> patient. <u>Everything</u> I see or hear on duty I will keep CONFIDENTIAL.

2 TRY TO GET FREE MEDICAL ADVICE from doctors for myself or others.

3 CHAT or VISIT WITH OTHERS except in the line of duty.

4 MAKE PERSONAL PHONE CALLS, EAT, DRINK, CHEW GUM OR SMOKE while on duty.

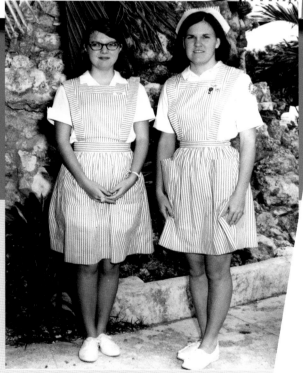

Left to right: Roxanne Baad, Beany Corley, March 11, 1970

WHY is a "CANDY STRIPER" IMPORTANT ?

Because she supplies that "extra pair of helping hands" that can make a patient's stay in the hospital more comfortable and pleasant-- an "added touch" to the trained services of the hospital staff.

The "Candy Striper" adds a "lift" no one else can supply-- because she's young, eager, enthusiastic... and <u>cares</u> enough to take <u>her</u> time to come and do her best to <u>help</u>.

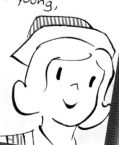

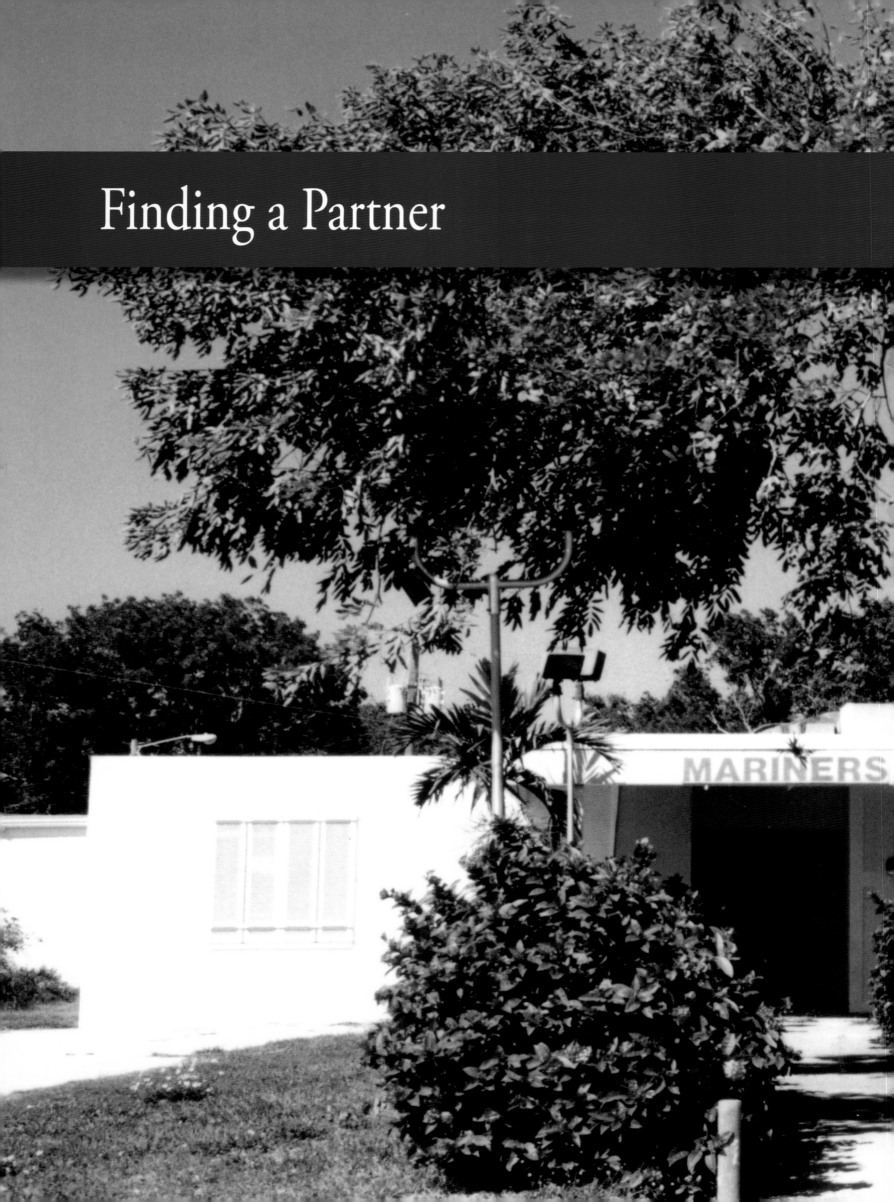

Finding a Partner

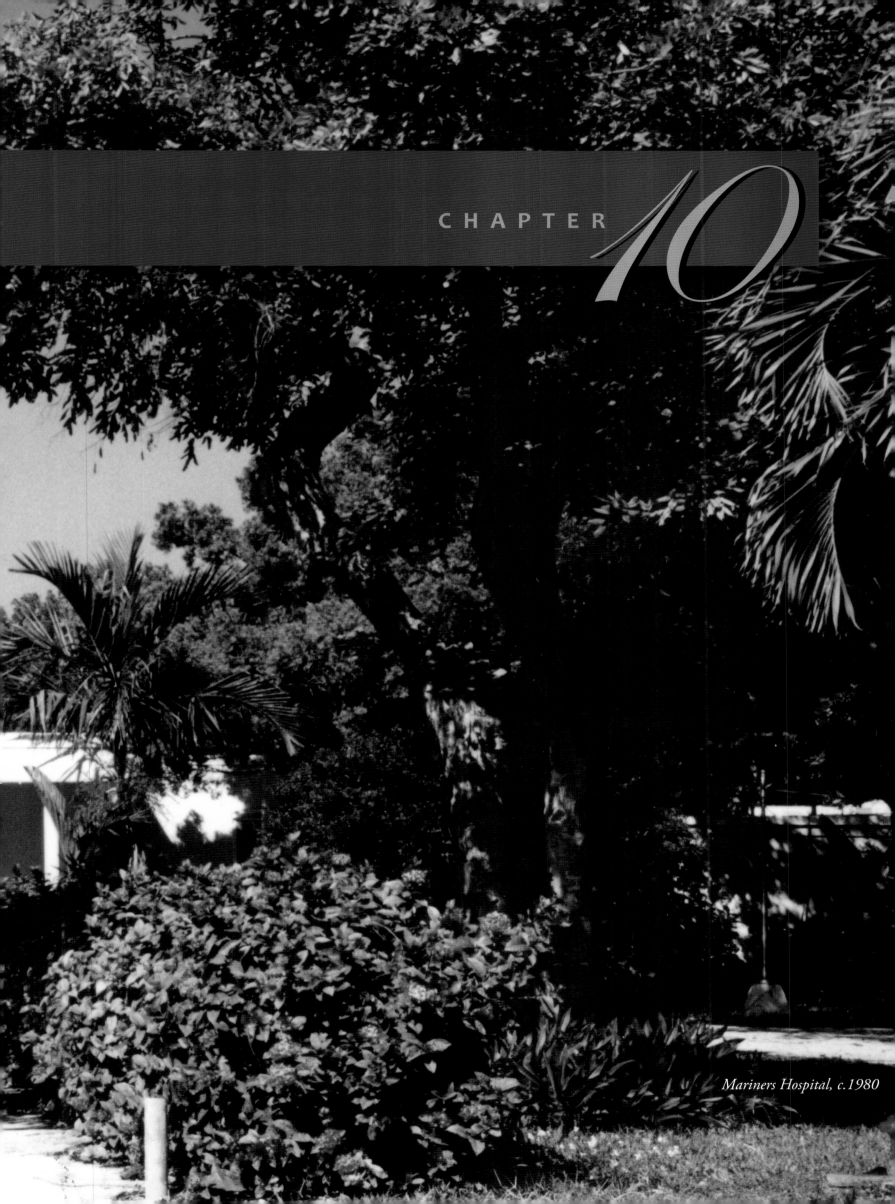

CHAPTER *10*

Mariners Hospital, c.1980

"Founded in a spirit of self-reliance and perseverance uniquely characteristic of the residents of Florida's Upper Keys, Mariners Hospital became a dream fulfilled on June 10, 1980. It is now a thriving, vital locus of quality health care for all who live, work and play in paradise."

Mariners Hospital brochure
1992

For those dedicated to Keys Community Hospital, there were no easy answers. Expenses continued to rise and bills remained unpaid. The formula seemed unworkable — the community wanted and needed the hospital but could not pay for it.

In early 1979, the situation took a dramatic turn for the worse. Keys Community Hospital faced a nearly $200,000 deficit. If the financial picture did not improve, American Medical Affiliates would shut down the hospital or convert it to a more profitable nursing home. Officials presented the grim scenario and asked the Monroe County Commission for financial help, setting a June closing date if the commission refused to act. "The key will be turned and the facility would close," Administrator Don Miller told a local newspaper.

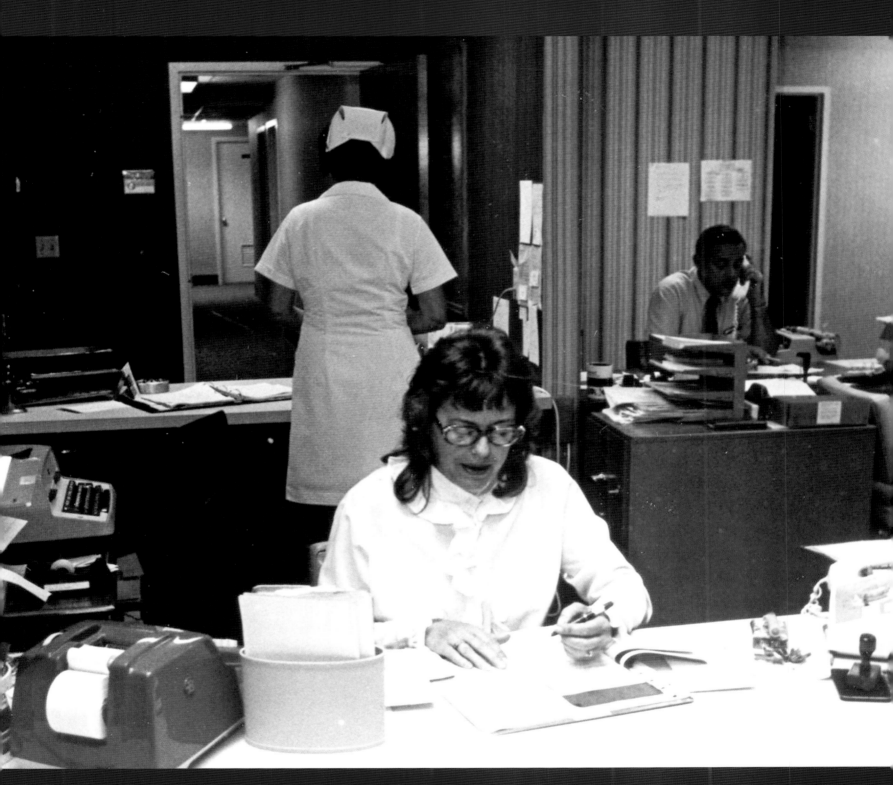

Employees at Keys Community Hospital, c.1979

Problems and More Problems

The problem was simply a lack of patients. Many Keys residents were leery of the controversial hospital. Since 1974, admissions had steadily decreased, dwindling to an average of 14 patients a day in the last six months of 1978. While the emergency room was busier, many of its patients were visitors who often lacked means or a commitment to pay the bill. Hospital critics cited a lack of medical specialties as a cause for the underuse. The hospital did not have some important services, including orthopedics and ophthalmology. Residents typically traveled to Miami for specialty care and often maintained relationships with physicians there. It was an endless cycle. People did not come to Keys Community because it was missing specialties, but hospital officials could not justify having those specialties without more patients.

When Administrator Miller brought the hospital's predicament to the County Commission, he described four possible solutions. The commission could subsidize the hospital by loaning it $150,000; AMA could sell the hospital to the county; AMA could sell the hospital to a private company; or AMA could convert the hospital to a nursing home. The commission wanted more information. County officials asked the not-for-profit Health Systems Agency (HSA) to study just how genuine was the hospital's community support. "If they're only coming to the hospital at the rate of 14 a day," County Commissioner Curt Blair said, "maybe the community doesn't want the hospital."

HSA appointed a task force of community leaders and medical professionals to look at options and put together a questionnaire for residents. The questionnaire asked residents about their experiences and thoughts concerning the hospital.

In the meantime, employees at Keys Community Hospital quietly cared for their patients and tried to ignore the uncertainty surrounding the institution's future. Employees brought their own pens and pencils to work because the budget did not allow for office supplies. Finances were so tenuous that when employees would deposit their paychecks in the local bank, they were never sure the hospital had enough money to cover them. "One week I went to the bank five days in a row before I was actually able to cash my check," remembered Roberta "Scooter" Fismer, R.N. "It seemed the money was going out as fast as or faster than it was coming in."

Despite this, the staff never really feared for the hospital's viability. "I don't think we all thought the hospital would close," said Cheryl Cottrell, R.N., chief nursing officer, who began work at the hospital in 1971 as a nursing assistant. "We believed that something would happen. We always seemed to survive the downturns."

By the end of February 1979, the task force released the survey's findings. Of the 584 permanent residents responding, 72 percent supported purchasing the hospital. HSA identified some underlying problems. Residents were apathetic toward the hospital, which operated without local input due to its out-of-town ownership. As expected, it also pointed to a lack of specialties at the hospital, and poor public relations and marketing efforts. Adding to the problem was the boom or bust nature of the Florida Keys, which produced an unpredictable seasonal population and, therefore, an unsteady stream of patients.

If the survey found an uninterested public, the publicity surrounding the hospital's potential closure certainly changed that. Letters to the editor of the local newspapers appeared each day. Most supported the hospital and implored residents to organize to save it. In April 1979, a "Save Our Hospital" committee formed, hosting meetings and open houses. "I don't know why we didn't see the concern before: maybe the community felt that American Medical Affiliates would continue to subsidize the hospital, or maybe June 1979 seemed a long way off," wrote Joan Kantrowitz, R.N., director of nursing, in a letter in *The Reporter*. "At any rate, I'm glad the concern is being shown now. Maybe I won't have to go job hunting…Maybe I can continue to help provide healthcare to my friends and neighbors, which is what I want to do."

"I don't think we all thought the hospital would close. We believed that something would happen. We always seemed to survive the downturns."

Cheryl Cottrell, R.N.
Chief Nursing Officer
Keys Community Hospital

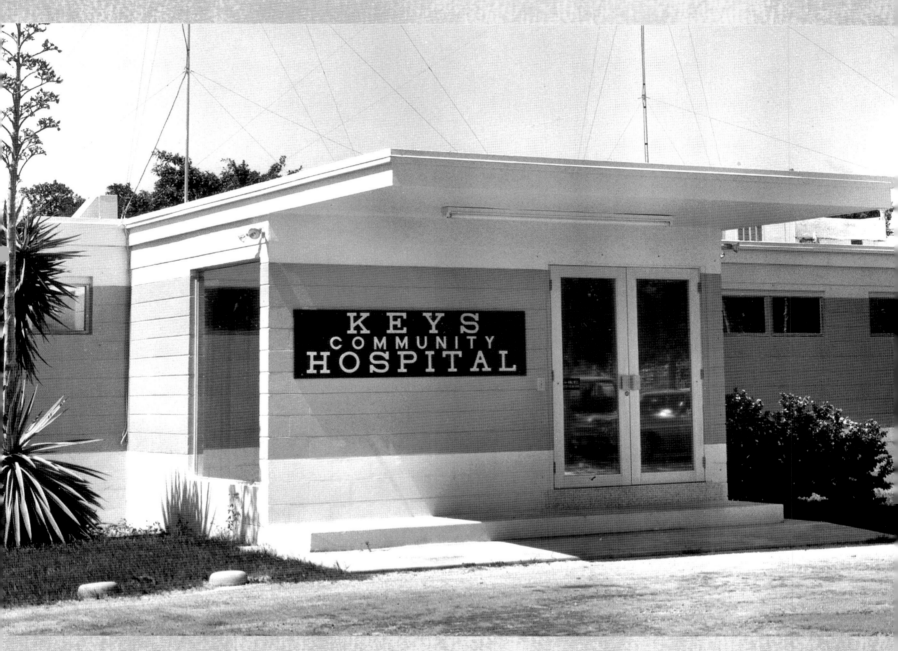

In 1979, the hospital's future was in doubt. Administrators contemplated closing its doors because of financial pressure.

A New Approach

By May 1979, Save Our Hospital was actively looking to purchase the hospital or find a way to keep it open. As the June "act or close" deadline approached, the Committee thought it had found an answer. Another for-profit company, Southern Health Services (SHS) in Atlanta, emerged as a potential buyer. Because negotiations were in progress, AMA postponed the close date. With a reputation for sound management, SHS operated seven hospitals and four nursing homes in three states. Equally important, the company believed in local involvement. At each of its hospitals, a Board of Directors made up of community residents oversaw policy and reported to the corporate office. Unfortunately, at the eleventh hour, Southern Health Services walked away, concluding it would suffer the same problems that had plagued AMA.

Despite the setback, the Save Our Hospital Committee continued its efforts. After countless meetings, it decided to create the not-for-profit Keys Hospital Foundation and purchase the hospital with money from tax-free revenue bonds. The Committee would then contract with Southern Health Services to manage day-to-day operations and appoint a local Board to offer local input. "What we are saying to the public is it is your hospital," said Save Our Hospital Committee member Ken Sorensen. "You can change it."

The plan gained support from the County Commission. With the details falling into place, one obstacle remained — getting the community's acceptance. "While the nitty-gritty details of purchasing the hospital take place... your role is not to sit complacently on the sidelines watching," an editorial in *The Reporter* declared. "Talk it up with your neighbors. Discuss it with your doctor. Tell him that when this project is on line you don't want to get shipped to a Miami hospital... If you truly believe we need a hospital in the Upper Keys, stand up and be counted."

However, another roadblock to the plan emerged. A February 1980 HSA report pointed to the patient numbers and questioned how, even with broadened services, the hospital could generate enough revenue to turn things around. After a series of public meetings that featured shouting matches, the Keys Hospital Foundation proposed a financial safeguard. The City of Layton, located at mile marker 68.5 on Long Key, agreed to authorize the bonds. This took the ultimate financial responsibility away from the Foundation. While community leaders continued working on the sale, they wanted to give the hospital a new identity. So they sponsored a name-the-hospital contest. The winner would receive $500. After sorting through hundreds of entries, Committee leaders chose Mariners Hospital — the suggestion of Key Largo resident Lyle J. Petty.

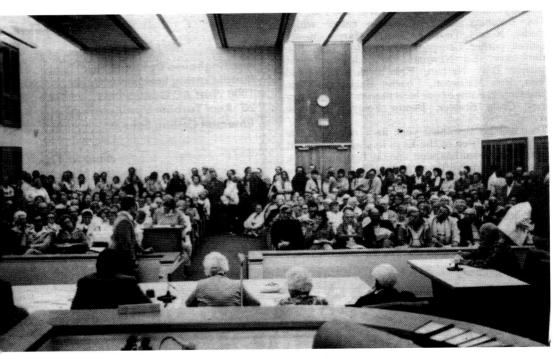

At a February 2, 1980, meeting at the Government Center on Plantation Key, residents came out in full force to discuss Keys Community Hospital.

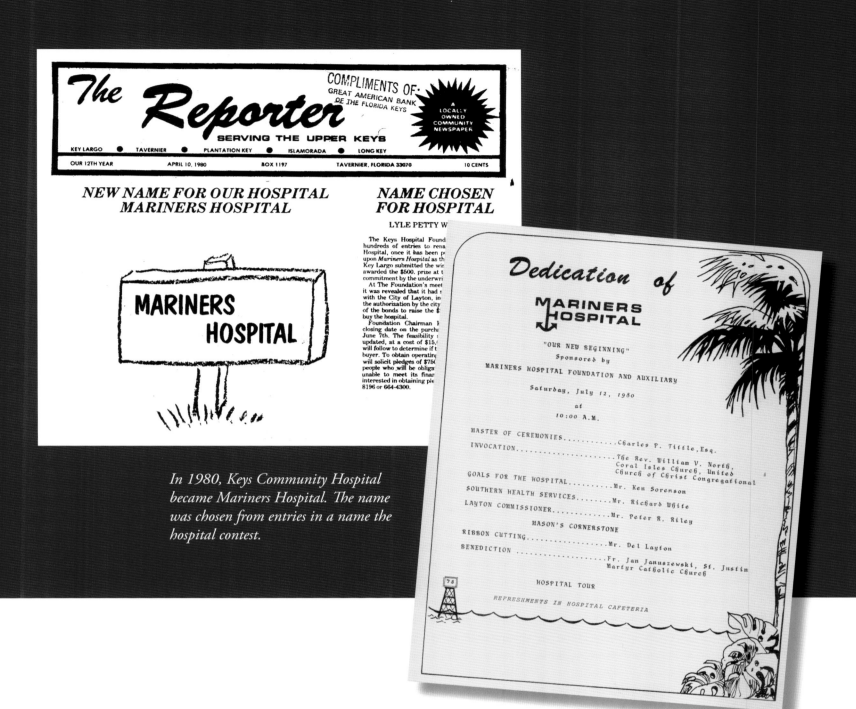

The Reporter
SERVING THE UPPER KEYS

KEY LARGO ● TAVERNIER ● PLANTATION KEY ● ISLAMORADA ● LONG KEY

| OUR 12TH YEAR | APRIL 10, 1980 | BOX 1197 | TAVERNIER, FLORIDA 33070 | 10 CENTS |

NEW NAME FOR OUR HOSPITAL MARINERS HOSPITAL

NAME CHOSEN FOR HOSPITAL

LYLE PETTY W...

MARINERS HOSPITAL

The Keys Hospital Found... hundreds of entries to rena... Hospital, once it has been p... upon *Mariners Hospital* as th... Key Largo submitted the win... awarded the $500. prize at t... commitment by the underwri...

At The Foundation's meet... it was revealed that it had ... with the City of Layton, in ... the authorization by the city ... of the bonds to raise the $... buy the hospital.

Foundation Chairman ... closing date on the purcha... June 7th. The feasibility ... updated, at a cost of $15,... will follow to determine if t... buyer. To obtain operating ... will solicit pledges of $75... people who will be obligat... unable to meet its finan... interested in obtaining ple... 8196 or 664-4300.

In 1980, Keys Community Hospital became Mariners Hospital. The name was chosen from entries in a name the hospital contest.

Dedication of MARINERS HOSPITAL

"OUR NEW BEGINNING"
Sponsored by
MARINERS HOSPITAL FOUNDATION AND AUXILIARY

Saturday, July 12, 1980
at
10:00 A.M.

MASTER OF CEREMONIES.............Charles P. Tittle, Esq.

INVOCATION.....................The Rev. William V. North, Coral Isles Church, United Church of Christ Congregational

GOALS FOR THE HOSPITAL..........Mr. Ken Sorenson

SOUTHERN HEALTH SERVICES........Mr. Richard White

LAYTON COMMISSIONER.............Mr. Peter R. Riley

MASON'S CORNERSTONE

RIBBON CUTTING.................Mr. Del Layton

BENEDICTION ....Fr. Jan Januszewski, St. Justin Martyr Catholic Church

HOSPITAL TOUR

REFRESHMENTS IN HOSPITAL CAFETERIA

On June 10, 1980, the newly christened Mariners Hospital became a community-owned, not-for-profit hospital. The ending of the saga was really the beginning. "The easiest thing in the world to do now is roll over and go to sleep," read an editorial in *The Reporter*. "The first battle may be over but the success of purchasing the facility can only be considered the opening salvo in a long fight. Unless the hospital operates in the black, we will have won the battle and lost the war." As the ink dried on the papers, the Foundation's leaders, including Ken Sorensen, Gordon Osborn, David Day and Charles Tittle, turned their attention to the work ahead — getting the community involved, recruiting doctors and improving the facility.

The theme for the July 12, 1980, dedication ceremony was, appropriately, "Our New Beginning." Plans took shape to expand the emergency room, upgrade the intensive care unit and bring in such new services as physical therapy. By the end of the first year, the patient census was up and the hospital was just about on budget. And the Board, elected by the Foundation, looked for even greater successes. "We want to do better than break even," said Mariners Board member Gordon Osborn.

MARINERS HOSPITAL CAN'T SAVE LIVES WITHOUT YOUR HELP!

SUPPORT THE MARINERS HOSPITAL COMMUNITY PLEDGE DRIVE TODAY

With locally pledged support in 1980, our community purchased Mariners Hospital now serving area health needs around the clock with 14 active staff physicians, including 5 surgeons, a 24 hour fully staffed emergency room, and comprehensive outpatient services.

Today, Mariners is reaching out into the community again. We need your generous pledge to keep our hospital growing. Based on your support pledged now, TIB, your community owned and operated bank, will lend Mariners the funds necessary to maintain our health care standards.

We've never called a pledge yet. The accounting firm of Price Waterhouse is confident that Mariners Hospital has a bright future ahead. Your pledge is a safe investment in the health of your family and your community . . . and it should never cost you a dime.

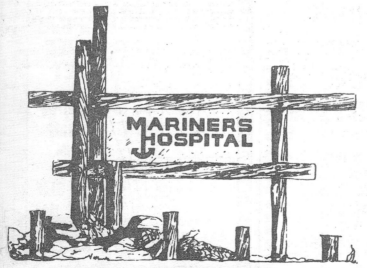

YES!

I WANT TO PLEDGE MY SUPPORT TO OUR COMMUNITY HOSPITAL. PLEASE HAVE A HOSPITAL FOUNDATION MEMBER CALL ON ME!

NAME_____

ADDRESS_____

MILE MARKER LOCATION_____

TELEPHONE_____

I WISH TO PLEDGE $_____

SEND TO: MARINERS HOSPITAL
50 High Point Road
Tavernier, Florida 33070

IF YOU BELIEVE IN MARINERS — HANG THIS POSTER IN YOUR WINDOW

After failed attempts at outside management, leaders wanted to run the hospital independently. They looked to the community for financial support.

Back to the Beginning

The transition would not prove to be smooth. By the summer of 1982, the hospital was at another crossroads after the Board of Directors terminated the management contract with SHS and brought it its own administrator and financial personnel. The Board concluded that the management company had disorganized business operations and inexperienced managers and had failed to pay some taxes. While Mariners was able to meet payroll, few long-term goals were achieved. "SHS wasn't prepared to take over the management of the hospital and as far as that's concerned, they never did get properly prepared for it," Mr. Osborn said in a report to the Board.

Mariners turned to the community for pledges of financial support. But this was only a stopgap solution. Something had to change fundamentally to give the hospital working capital and financial breathing room. Mariners advocates proposed a special taxing district to cover the debts and enable the hospital to buy new equipment and improve its facilities. Publicity surrounding the referendum vote reassured residents that the hospital would not receive a blank check. The taxing district had a narrow focus and was limited to three years.

On May 8, 1984, Upper Keys voters approved the special tax for Mariners Hospital by a two-to-one margin. The support was a testament to how far the small hospital had come. Through a revolving door of management, bad publicity and financial missteps, the community stood behind Mariners. The hospital had done its part, broadening services and now operating in the black. "It's a vote of confidence by the community for the dedicated healthcare professionals at the hospital," Board member Charles Tittle said.

The vote gave the Board some psychological and financial freedom. Continuing efforts to improve the facility, Mariners upgraded its diagnostic services, purchasing a CT scanner, and better maintained the physical plant. Most importantly, the hospital was operating at an impressive surplus. In 1986, Mariners earned $164,000, thanks to expanded services and greater community support. The trend continued through the next decade. As a not-for-profit, the surplus went back into the hospital for improvements. "Instead of keeping busy putting out fires," Board Chairman Chris Schrader said, "we can look forward to more positive things."

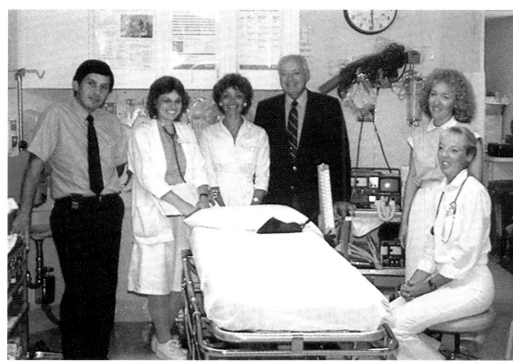

Mariners Hospital emergency staff, November 1987: (left to right) Nelson A. Terzian, M.D.; Phyllis Kelper, R.N.; Mary Stringer; Jerry Cox, M.D.; Debbie Blaida, R.N.; and Linda Gaspeny, R.N.

A New Building

The positive momentum brought the hospital to an unimaginable place — a new location and new building. With the hospital's survivability no longer in question, the Board of Directors began looking at a new home for Mariners. "We need more space," a letter about the effort read. "The hospital has expanded where and when it could, but has reached a point where it no longer makes good financial sense to do so. There isn't much room left for expansion, and the cost of a complete renovation would be comparable to the cost of building a new hospital." In October 1991, Mariners received a certificate of need from the state that allowed the hospital to construct a new facility.

The leadership team planned a fundraising campaign, entitled "Caring for the Community," with a $1.25 million goal. The idea was not necessarily to add more beds but make the hospital better fit the community's needs. More services were being performed on an outpatient basis, so the hospital needed space to meet the demand. In addition, visits to the Emergency Room neared 9,000 in 1990 — an increase of more than 36 percent in four years. The new building needed a modern ER.

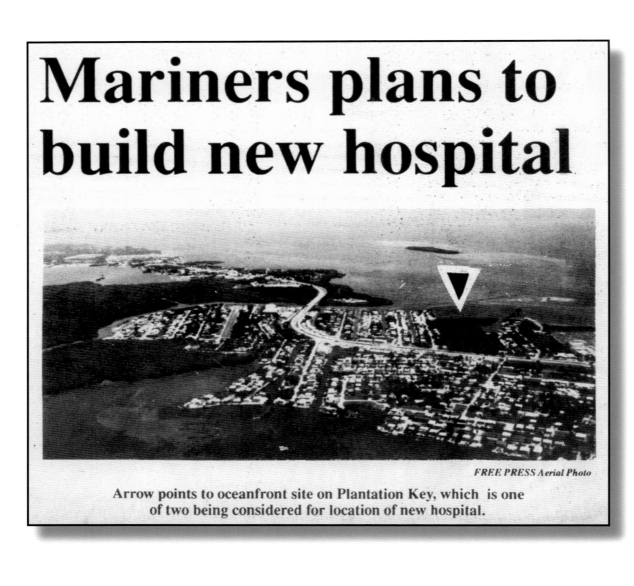

Mariners plans to build new hospital

FREE PRESS Aerial Photo

Arrow points to oceanfront site on Plantation Key, which is one of two being considered for location of new hospital.

By 1990, the Board of Directors was looking for a new home for Mariners Hospital. The hospital needed more space and a modern facility.

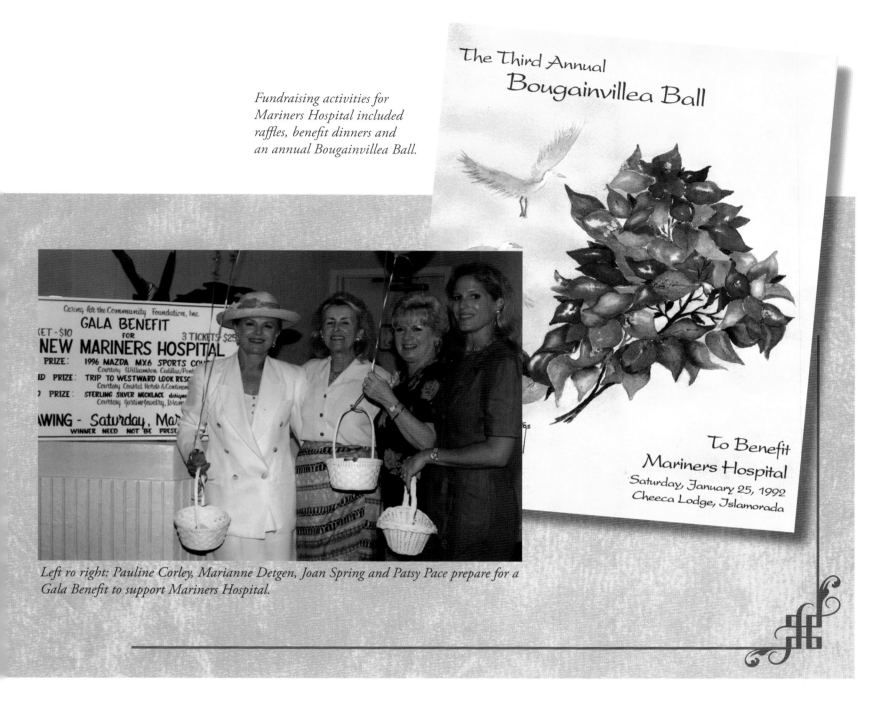

Fundraising activities for Mariners Hospital included raffles, benefit dinners and an annual Bougainvillea Ball.

The Third Annual
Bougainvillea Ball

To Benefit
Mariners Hospital
Saturday, January 25, 1992
Cheeca Lodge, Islamorada

Left ro right: Pauline Corley, Marianne Detgen, Joan Spring and Patsy Pace prepare for a Gala Benefit to support Mariners Hospital.

On April 24, 1992, Mariners Hospital paid $600,000 for a plot of land in Tavernier at mile marker 91.5. The site would be the future home of Mariners Hospital. Employees cheered when they got the news from Administrator Howard Anderson. They had contributed more than $50,000 to the fundraising campaign. "It felt exhilarating," remembered Cheryl Cottrell, chief nursing officer. "After so long, it was kind of an 'aha' moment. We realized we were really moving forward."

While hospital leaders had raised $700,000 by June, they still needed more money. They proposed another special tax that would have to be approved by Upper Keys voters. In a September 1992 referendum, residents approved the tax with the pro-ceeds going toward building the new hospital. But the issue did not end with the vote. In 1993, a group of residents, many from Ocean Reef in North Key Largo, protested the election. They argued that because the vote took place one week after Hurricane Andrew, residents were not well-informed about the issue or even in the area to cast a vote.

Some saw the objections as an organized way to avoid taxes. Regardless of the intent, after a few months of discussions and debate, the County Commission voted to rescind the tax. In an unusual move, the taxes were eventually refunded to residents. Hospital executives were discouraged but more committed than ever to building the new hospital.

Of Mergers and Money

Robert Luse was hired as the chief administrator of Mariners in January 1993, replacing Howard Anderson, who had left amicably several months earlier for another opportunity. Luse came with years of experience in hospital administration and was drawn to Mariners because of the excitement surrounding the new facility. "I remember thinking that this is very special — to have a community vote to tax itself so it could build a new hospital," he said. "When it fell through, I still knew that we had to complete the project. It was simply time to refocus our energy and effort."

With special taxes no longer an option, Mariners needed to fund the new building. The timing was important. The certificate of need would soon expire and, without it, construction could not move forward. The leadership team began exploring partnerships, affiliations and mergers with outside groups that could financially back the project. South Miami HealthSystems entered the picture by forming an alliance with Mariners in which it would help fund the new hospital. The ill-fated partnership fell apart; South Miami was mired in its own financial problems and was in no position to help another hospital.

Yet the Mariners Board recognized it could not build the new hospital without a partner. They turned to the Lower Florida Keys Health System, which owned and operated Florida Keys Memorial Hospital and dePoo Hospital in Key West. The Lower Keys System's public face was Roberto Sanchez, a strong figure who was full of big ideas. Sanchez assured Mariners that he could build the new hospital and efficiently manage it.

Some of the Board members had concerns about Mr. Sanchez's salesman style. "I remember he was always so forceful and positive," said Charlen Regan, who joined the Board in 1988. "It was as though he had all the answers, which made me uneasy. I wondered if he was open-minded enough to pull the hospital together." Despite the reservations, the Board kept negotiating. "We signed the agreement after some soul-searching," said attorney Jay Hershoff, who joined the Mariners Board in 1993. "We knew that we had to find a bigger player to help us build the hospital.

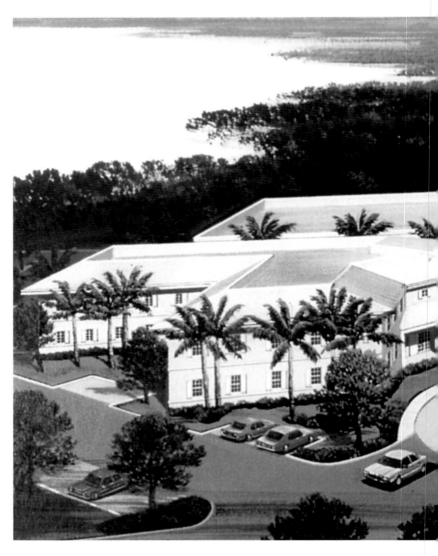

We looked at different ways to do it and this seemed like an appropriate step."

On April 4, 1994, the Mariners Board joined the Lower Florida Keys Health System for a ceremonial groundbreaking at the site of the new hospital. Typically, this would have ushered in cement trucks, hard hats and cranes as construction began. But things did not go as planned. Doubts about the deal lingered. The Board faced problems with the certificate of need, which had expired, forcing the hospital to apply for an extension. Questions also arose about a profit split with Lower Keys. "There was definitely some tension about the money and Sanchez moving some of our surplus out of our hospital and our area to the Lower Keys,"

"I remember thinking that this is very special — to have a community vote to tax itself so it could build a new hospital. When it fell through, I still knew that we had to complete the project. It was simply time to refocus our energy and effort."

Robert Luse
Administrator, Mariners Hospital

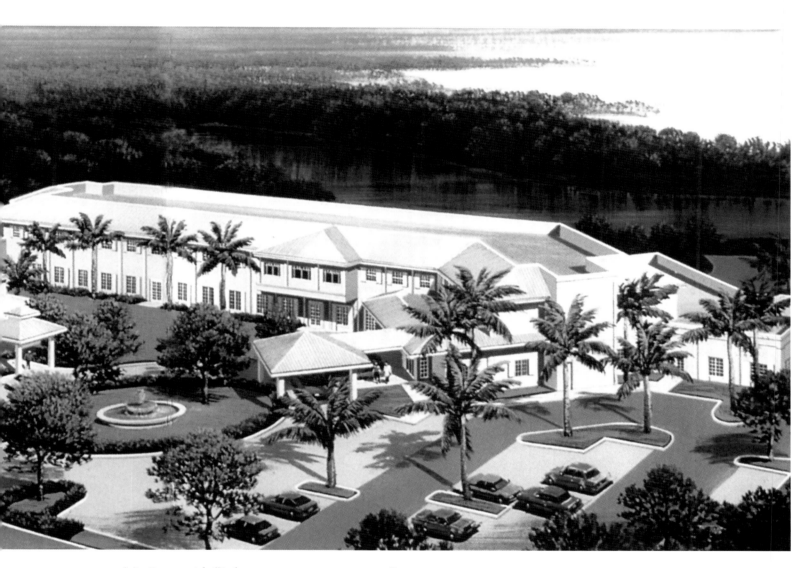

Mr. Luse said. "It became very contentious."

As the year ended, nothing was happening at the "new" Mariners. The relationship with Mr. Sanchez continued to deteriorate. It became obvious that Lower Florida Keys Health System was not able to meet its part of the deal. On December 6, 1994, the lease agreement with Lower Florida Keys Health System expired. Mariners turned its attention to another suitor who had lingered in the background — Baptist Health Systems. At the time, Baptist Health was in its first stages of growth, building some satellite facilities, including an outpatient and walk-in clinic at the Beacon Center and a family center in West Kendall. Baptist Health also was exploring a partnership with South Miami HealthSystems.

This illustration shows the proposed new Mariners Hospital. When Mariners and Baptist Health began their merger discussions, the idea of a new hospital became a reality.

Mariners' strengths fit Baptist Health's strategy. "We were a profitable hospital at the time. We ran efficiently and successfully," Luse said. "So we had a lot to bring to the table. We offered an attractive situation for Baptist's growth." The reverse was true as well. Baptist Health was a welcomed presence in the Upper Keys. After so many fits and starts with other companies and hospitals, Baptist Health, under the leadership of Brian Keeley, came to the negotiations with a reputation for honesty and integrity.

The Mariners leadership team was impressed. "Baptist Health is interested in serving our patients for tertiary care only," Luse said, after Keeley appeared before the Board in late December. "They do not want to come down and take over." Mariners employees, proud of their hospital and its friendly family atmosphere, did not want an outside organization, with its own culture, to come in and change the spirit at Mariners.

If the fiercely independent Keys community feared the presence of the more dominant Baptist Health, the need outweighed any misgivings. Mariners realized what Baptist Health brought to the equation, including financial stability, management expertise and, most importantly, the ability to carry out a construction project. "It was a marriage of necessity," Mr. Hershoff said. "We recognized that we really needed them, but from the beginning, we also knew that they would do what

they said they were going to do. We could tell that they were first-class and there was no skimping on quality. This was particularly important as we looked to build a new hospital."

As Mariners finalized plans with Baptist Health, Keeley's team was putting its finishing touches on the merger with South Miami. It was not until the Baptist Health and South Miami agreement was finalized in June that attention could turn fully to Mariners.

In December 1995, Mariners Hospital merged with Baptist Health. It was an exciting time for Mariners. "We can share and exchange resources that are almost unlimited," Luse said. "A patient will have an enviable list of options at their fingertips." Brian Keeley welcomed Mariners with reassuring and purposeful words. "This is a marriage, not a merger," he said. "The next, highest priority is to get your new hospital in the ground."

Mariners Hospital's Seth Horowitz, M.D., and Dennis Holstein are pictured with the hyperbaric chamber at the old hospital.

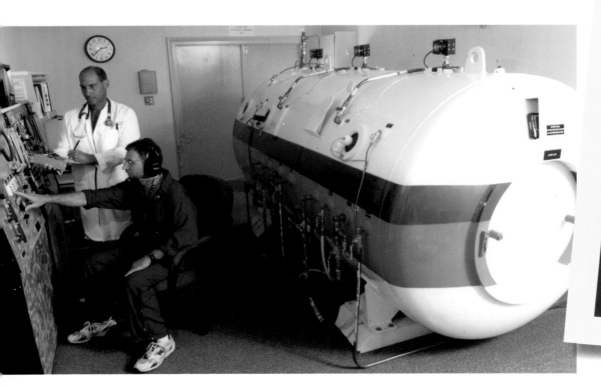

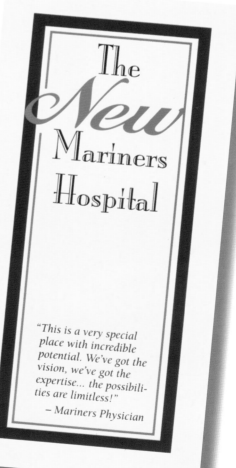

The *New* Mariners Hospital

"This is a very special place with incredible potential. We've got the vision, we've got the expertise... the possibilities are limitless!"

– Mariners Physician

"This is a marriage, not a merger. The next, highest priority is to get your new hospital in the ground."

Brian E. Keeley
President and CEO, Baptist Health

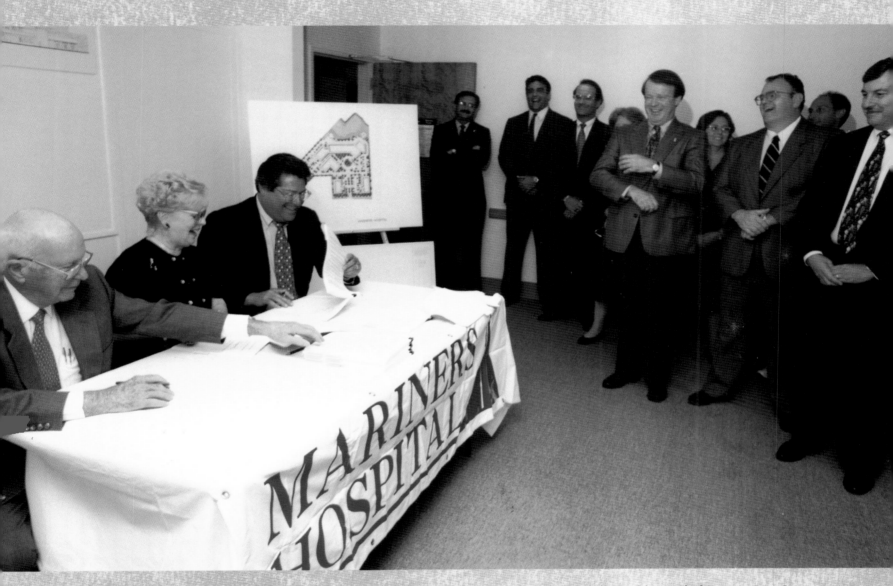

Robert B. Cole, chairman of Baptist Health Board of Trustees, Joan Spring, chairman of Caring for the Community Foundation, and Jay Hershoff, chairman of Mariners Hospital Board of Directors, sign the merger document.

Ups and Downs

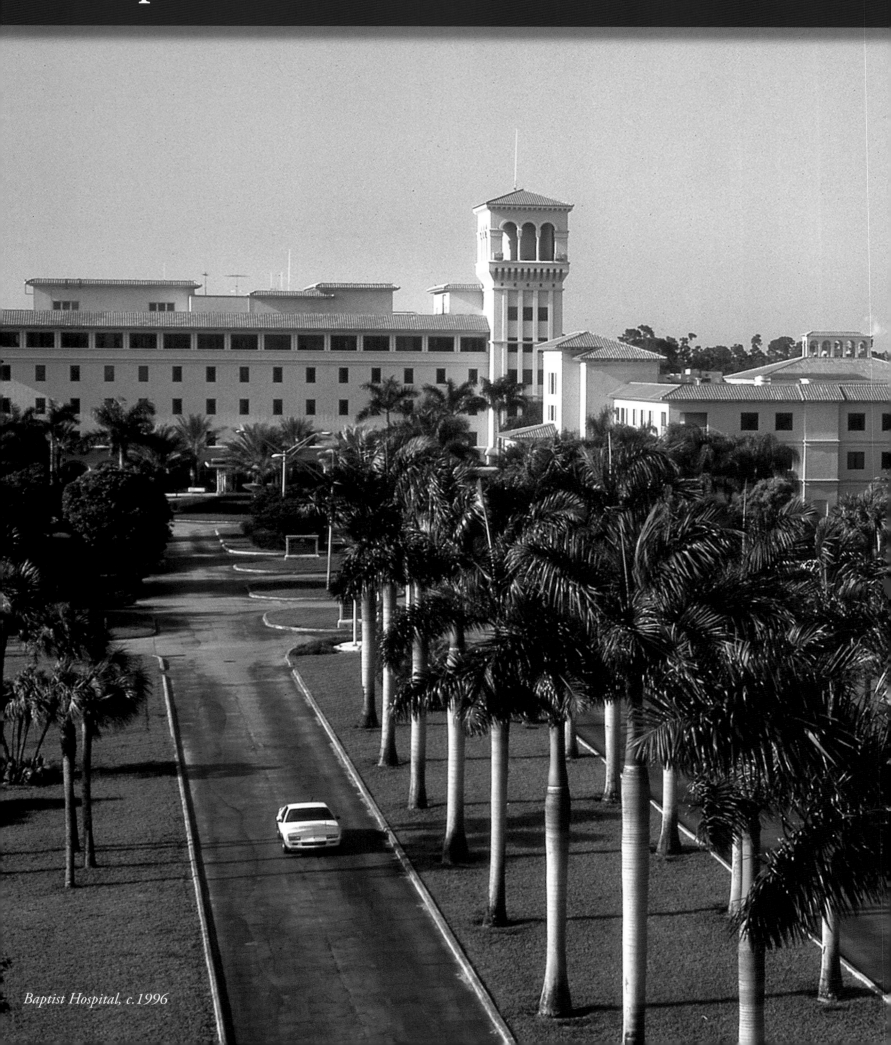

Baptist Hospital, c. 1996

CHAPTER 11

"We are faced with constant challenges, which is why our philosophy of clinical, service and financial excellence is so important. We are looking at ways of improving and it is absolutely a continuous process. But it's what has kept Baptist Health Systems on the leading edge."

Fred Messing
Chief Operating Officer, Baptist Health
1999

With the bumps and upheaval of the merger behind it, the newly expanded Baptist Health began its second year. The organization included more than 7,000 employees, 1,600 affiliated physicians, a half-billion dollars in revenue and a healthy bottom line. The consolidation of services and renegotiation of supply contracts to take advantage of large-scale discounts saved the hospitals an estimated $2.2 million. Both South Miami and Homestead were on the financial upswing, with profits predicted for South Miami by 1997. "We have everything in place to flourish," Chief Financial Officer Ralph Lawson said.

As a not-for-profit organization, Baptist Health could afford to be forward-thinking. The administrators did not have to answer to shareholders who demanded returns on investments. Instead, any "profits" supported Baptist Health and were invested in expansions, capital improvements and the overall mission. "Our view is not what will happen next year," Brian Keeley said in 1996. "Ours is a five- to 10-year horizon. We have a phenomenal advantage over the public corporations. Everything we do is with a long-term focus."

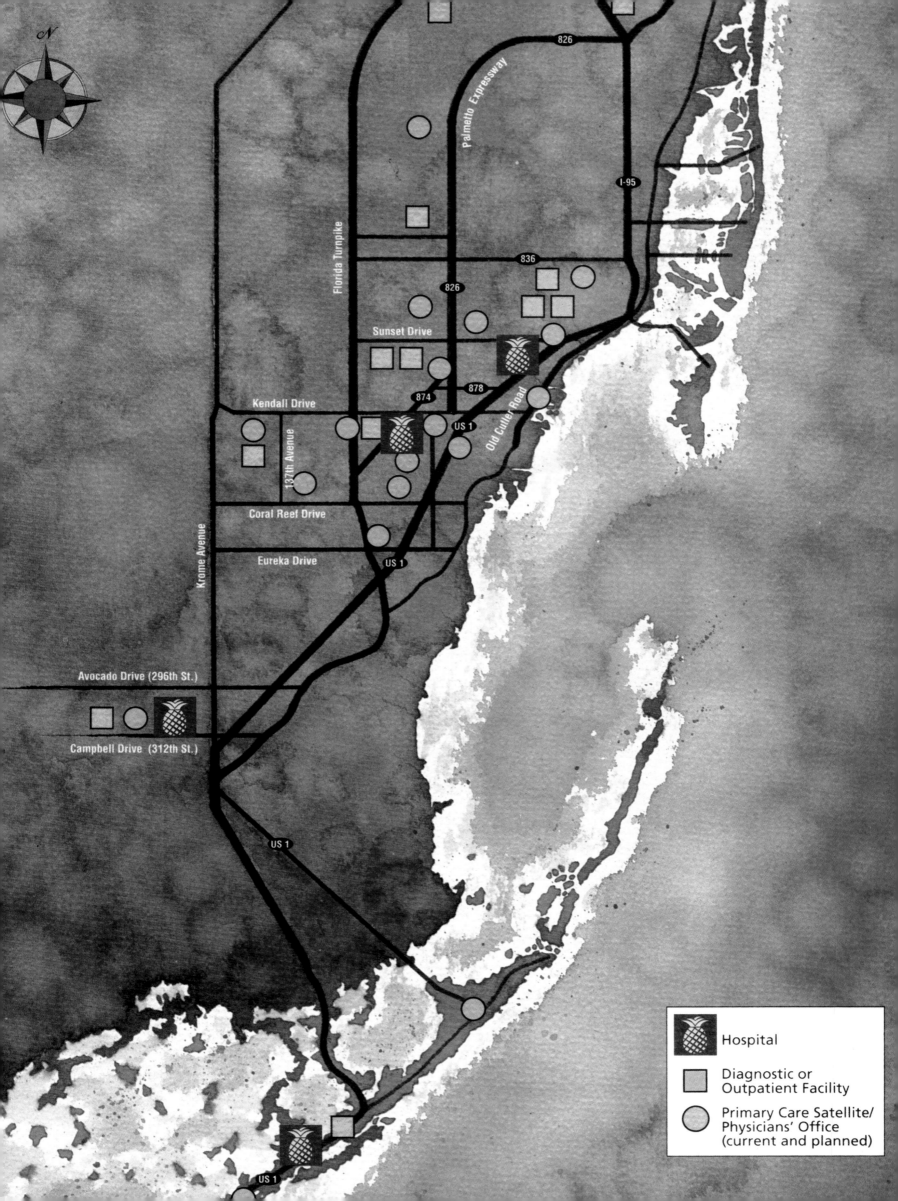

N

Palmetto Expressway

826

I-95

Florida Turnpike

836

826

Sunset Drive

874   878

Kendall Drive

US 1

137th Avenue

Old Cutler Road

Coral Reef Drive

Krome Avenue

Eureka Drive   US 1

Avocado Drive (296th St.)

Campbell Drive (312th St.)

US 1

US 1

Hospital

Diagnostic or
Outpatient Facility

Primary Care Satellite/
Physicians' Office
(current and planned)

Growth on All Fronts

Baptist Health turned to fulfilling its promise to the Upper Keys to build a new hospital. In early 1996, Mariners applied for a certificate of need to start construction. Administrators thought this was simply a formality. The state had already approved a certificate when Mariners first began planning the new facility in 1991. During all the false starts and almost mergers, the original certificate expired. State officials denied the reapplication, again raising questions about financing and the community's interest in the hospital.

The state's decision was puzzling. The financing was stronger now with Baptist Health's involvement than it was five years earlier. "Baptist is one of the most financially stable healthcare institutions in the state, and we clearly have the financial resources to fund this project," Mr. Keeley responded. "Simply put, we guarantee the funds to build the new hospital." Part of the holdup was a move by neighboring Fishermen's Hospital in Marathon. Fishermen's parent company, Health Management Associates Inc., objected to the certificate in a petition with the state, arguing that renovating the existing Mariners was a more efficient alternative.

The claims and counterclaims amounted to competitive posturing. Fishermen's shared some of Mariners' service area and was fearful that a new facility would threaten its financial health. Brian Keeley and his team saw the issue as a temporary obstacle. "We are going to build it," Keeley said. "I'm an eternal optimist." After a few months of discussions between Fishermen's and Baptist Health, the Marathon hospital dropped its objection. Fishermen's and Mariners agreed to a cooperative relationship, especially when it came to treating patients who could not pay for services. By the fall of 1997, construction was under way on the new Mariners Hospital.

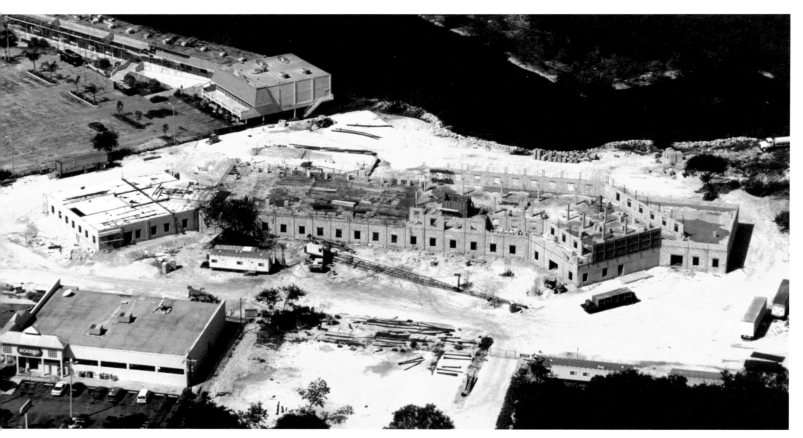

After several delays, construction on the new Mariners Hospital began in 1997.

Mariners Hospital...
LOOKING BACK

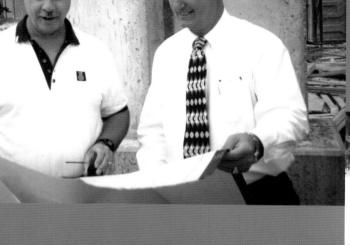

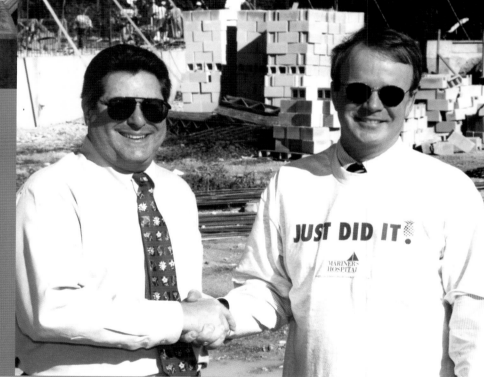

Above: Mariners Hospital CEO Robert Luse (left) and Florida Keys Electric Cooperative CEO Charles Russell

Right: Mariners Hospital Board Chairman Jay Hershoff and Baptist Health CEO Brian Keeley

The New Mariners Hospital

In a move that broke with Baptist Health tradition, leaders decided against a groundbreaking ceremony to mark the start of construction on the new hospital. "Mariners already had a groundbreaking for a building that never got going," said Brian Keeley, referring to a plan with another healthcare organization that never materialized. "I didn't want to do anything until we were under construction and sure that we would actually have a hospital." Baptist Health opted instead for a foundation-pouring ceremony that took place on November 6, 1997.

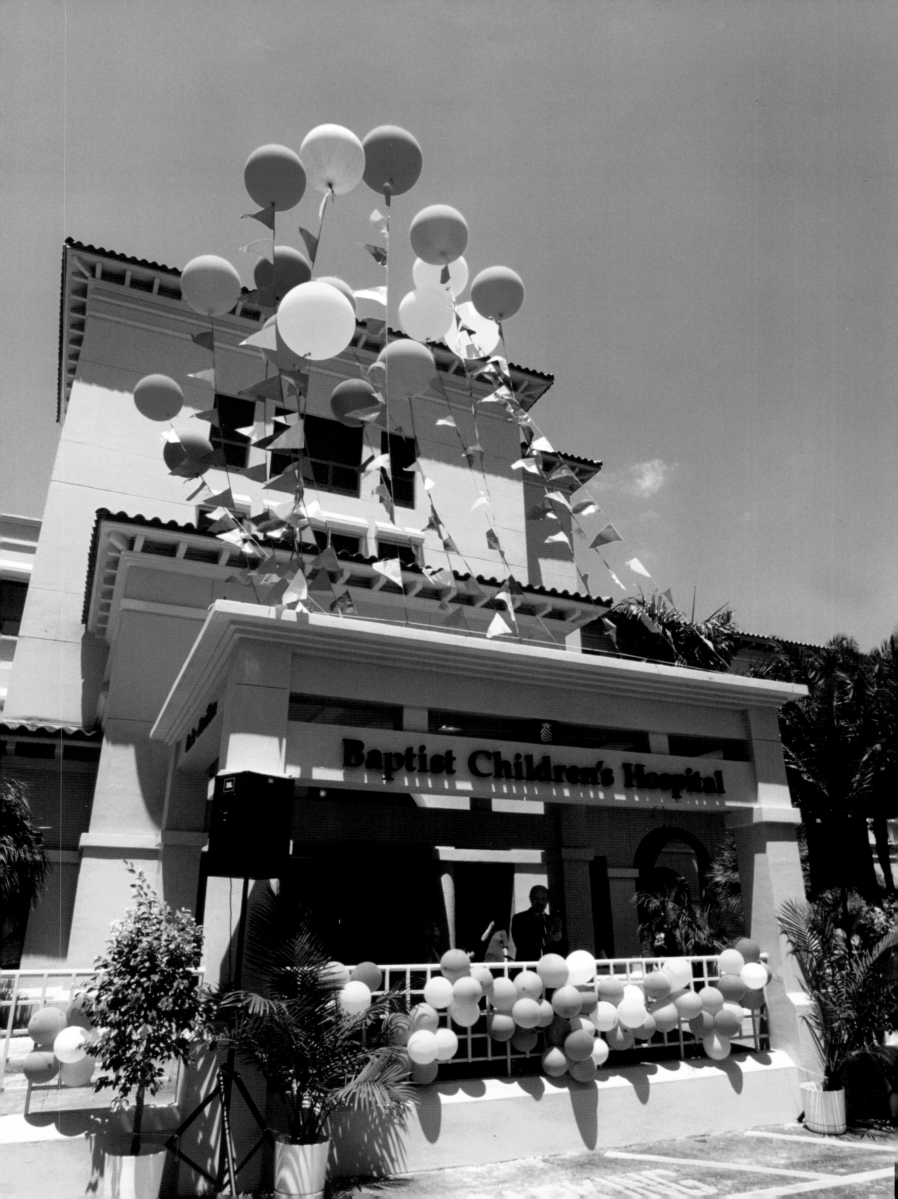

The hospital answered a growing need for pediatric services. In 1996, there were 19,000 visits to the Children's Emergency Center at Baptist and 6,000 pediatric outpatient visits.

That same year, the organization expanded by opening the 38-bed Baptist Children's Hospital on the Kendall campus as a hospital within a hospital. Services included a 24-hour Emergency Center, a range of pediatric specialists from hematology to surgery, a new Level III neonatal intensive care unit that could treat the most critically ill and premature newborns, and child life specialists who help children and families deal with the psychological side of illness. The hospital answered a growing need for pediatric services. In 1996, there were 19,000 visits to the Children's Emergency Center at Baptist and 6,000 pediatric outpatient visits. "Our children's services are of a uniformly excellent clinical level," said then Baptist Hospital CEO Fred Messing. "But we saw an opportunity to make them even better."

While Baptist Hospital had always treated children, Baptist Children's Hospital marked a philosophical change. At the new hospital, everything — both the medical and nonmedical — was created with the eyes of a child in mind. From a therapeutic playground equipped with toys to a staff with special training in pediatrics, the hospital was entirely dedicated to children. It was an important step in the growth and evolution of Baptist Health. "It has taken many years, the addition of exceptionally trained physicians and staff, the building of new facilities, the acquisition of state-of-the-art pediatric equipment and the creation of many new specialty services before we became comfortable calling ourselves a children's hospital," Mr. Keeley said when the hospital opened.

Beyond the expansion in the Keys and Kendall, Baptist Health grew in other areas. In the summer of 1997, Baptist Health relocated some of its corporate operations to an office building at 6855 Red Road in Coral Gables. Baptist Health planned to occupy three floors for finance, human resources, managed care, planning, and marketing and public relations. The move would free up some much-needed space at the hospitals.

To further integrate the medical staffs and build business, Baptist Health created DadeWell, a partnership that included more than 750 doctors at Baptist Hospital, South Miami Hospital and Homestead Hospital. The concept was to offer insurance companies a comprehensive roster of physicians and services that would steer policyholders to Baptist Health facilities. "We will improve the way healthcare is delivered by coordinating all components of healthcare across the spectrum," said DadeWell President and CEO Sergio Gonzalez-Arias, M.D., about the partnership. Baptist Health also formed Baptist Medical Group, which bought primary care physician practices. Baptist Health employees would handle everything from day-to-day billing to managing the offices. The idea was to give Baptist Health a high-quality primary care network and show a commitment to local physicians.

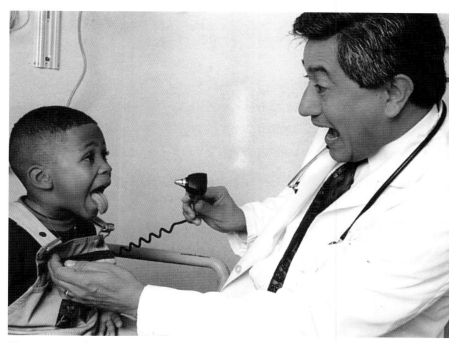

Francisco Medina, M.D., medical director of Baptist Children's Emergency Center, examines a young patient.

Facing page: Baptist Children's Hospital opened in 1997 to centralize pediatric services.

More than Brick and Mortar

With all of these pieces in place, Baptist Health focused on operations, ensuring high-quality care for patients, meeting the needs of a large and diverse workforce and providing physicians with the latest technology. The strategic vision also focused on maintaining and developing leaders with a vision. Thinking about what was next had propelled a single hospital into a full-service healthcare organization. Baptist Health looked at the landscape and found opportunity. In late 1996, construction began on the first Baptist Medical Plaza at 8750 S.W. 144th Street. The two-story, 32,000-square-foot facility would have physicians' offices, including a large pediatric practice, diagnostic services, a health resource library and an after-hours urgent care center.

The idea of a satellite facility was not new to Baptist Health. The organization had an outpatient occupational health center at the Beacon Center, and a Family and Education Center in Kendall. But plans for the suburban community near U.S. 1 and S.W. 144th Street were more ambitious. "Our goal is to make a range of services more convenient and accessible," Mr. Keeley said. "We will provide outpatient services that people often have had to come to a hospital campus to receive. It is the first of many that we will be building in the years ahead."

The concept evolved from what Corporate Vice President for Strategic Planning and Business Development Ana Lopez-Blazquez described as "where do we go from here thinking." The strategic team identified a clear trend in South Florida — thriving outpatient services. In 1996, there were more than 410,000 outpatient visits to Baptist Health facilities. This represented meteoric growth. In 1990, 18 percent of Baptist Hospital's revenues came from outpatient services. By 1996, with all Baptist Health facilities considered, the number exceeded 30 percent. "We recognized what was happening — that so much was going on beyond the hospitals," Ms. Lopez-Blazquez said. "We were ahead of the curve in identifying where the growth was."

Lopez-Blazquez, Keeley, Ralph Lawson and others also recognized the need to address another salient reality — overburdened emergency rooms. Visits to the ERs at the four hospitals exceeded 130,000 patients a year, with more than two-thirds of the patients going to Baptist Hospital. Long waits and crowded hallways became a disturbing and well-publicized feature of ER trips. "We looked at our numbers and our market and we started asking questions — how can we decompress the hospital campuses?" Lopez-Blazquez said. "We concentrated on a way to serve our patients more effectively by bringing some of our services out of the hospital and into the neighborhoods."

"*We* recognized what was happening — that so much was going on beyond the hospitals. We were ahead of the curve in identifying where the growth was."

Ana Lopez-Blazquez
Corporate Vice President for Strategic Planning, Baptist Health

Facing page: Baptist Hospital's 10-story, 135,000-square-foot Medical Arts Building East Tower provided outpatient services. It was part of Baptist Health's growing emphasis on outpatient care.

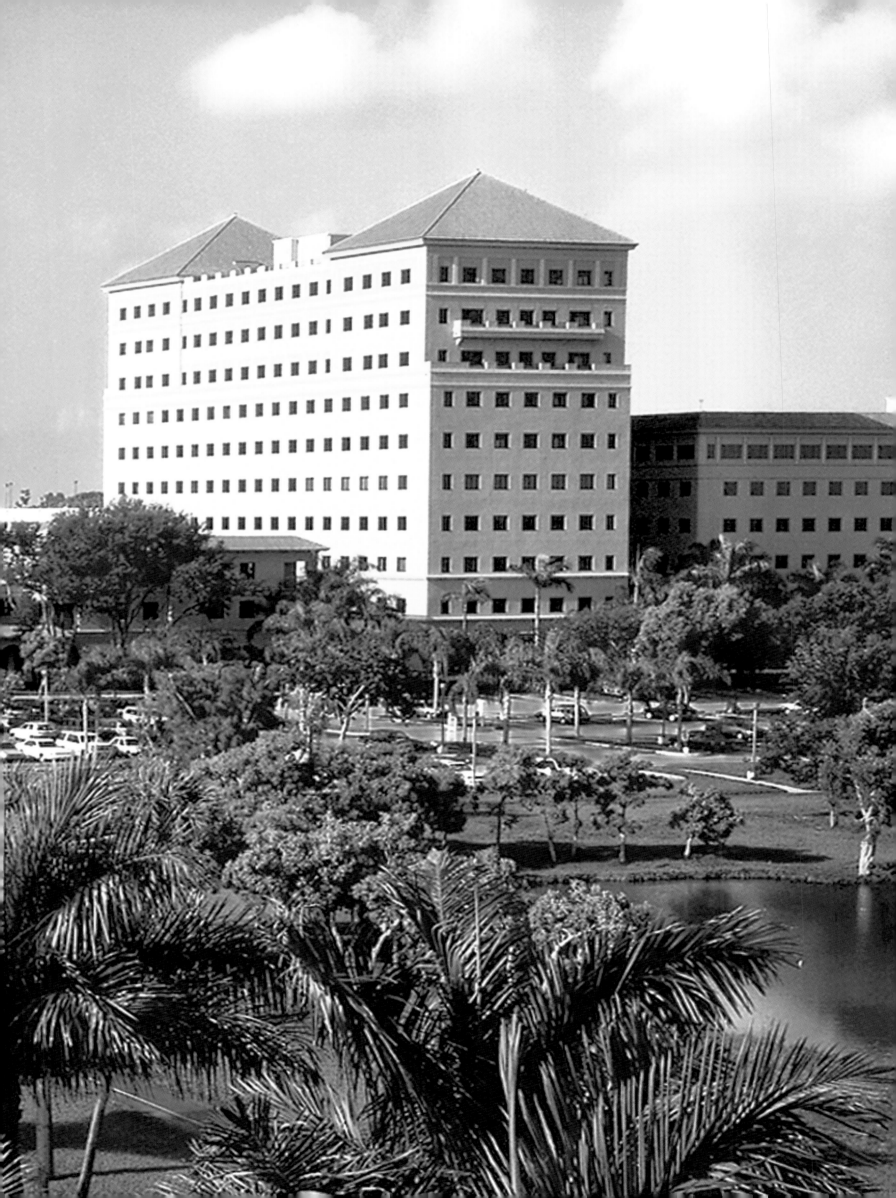

Baptist Medical Plaza at Kings Bay (later renamed Palmetto Bay) was an immediate success. In its first year, the staff performed 15,514 diagnostic procedures — 60 percent more than anticipated. The after-hours urgent care center logged 4,440 visits — 35 percent more than planned. Buoyed by that success, the strategic team planned new sites. In 1998, Baptist Health opened a satellite location for mammography at Burdines department store in Dadeland Mall. The unusual partnership, a first in Florida, put a new twist on making an important medical test convenient. The concept worked. Baptist Mammography Center finished the first year 31 percent above the projected number of patients. In June of 1999, Baptist Health added a medical plaza in Coral Gables at 320 Giralda Avenue. While the range of services at the new locations varied, the general concept remained the same: to make medical care convenient and easily accessible, close to where people live or work. "The outpatient centers succeeded beyond our most optimistic expectations," Lopez-Blazquez said. "We had a successful formula and, given how difficult medicine had become with managed care, they made a huge financial contribution to Baptist Health's overall bottom line."

In addition to taking advantage of an opportunity, the leadership team nurtured the concept to maximize success. The outpatient centers were built with a sound business plan at their foundation. Baptist Health planners chose the locations after careful study, reflecting the real estate adage of location, location, location. "We targeted areas where there was enough population with insurance, so we knew that the community could use and support the plaza," Lopez-Blazquez said. "We continued to grow our business where it made sense." Also crucial was the design and consistent branding of the Baptist Medical Plazas. "Our philosophy was that we had to bring people in. They had to want to come to our facilities, so the aesthetics were important," Mr. Keeley said. "We put in high ceilings and beautiful interior features. Our idea was to not just build it but build it great."

The outpatient medical plazas represented a bold direction for Baptist Health and its fiscally cautious Board of Trustees. The organization's trustees (each hospital also had its own Board of Directors) tended to consider all angles, especially the financials, before making a decision. Many Board members were longtime community leaders schooled, like the original Baptist Hospital leaders, in the values of discipline and diligence. Their support of the outpatient centers reflected a confidence in Brian Keeley and his team. "I think that the Board recognized that this was a smart move, not a reckless one," Ms. Lopez-Blazquez said. "We were well-prepared. We were well-run fiscally and this expansion fit in with our strategy."

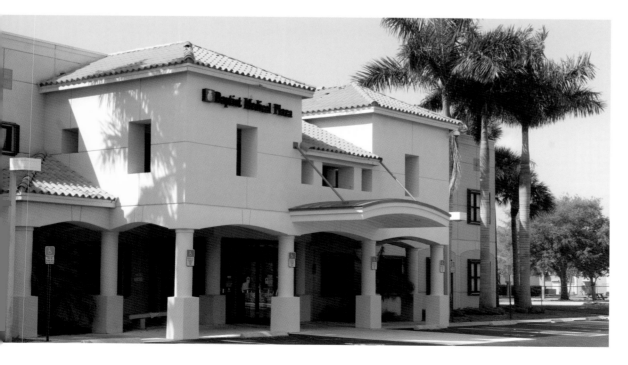

The Baptist Medical Plaza at Palmetto Bay, 8750 S.W. 144th Street, brought medical care into the neighborhood.

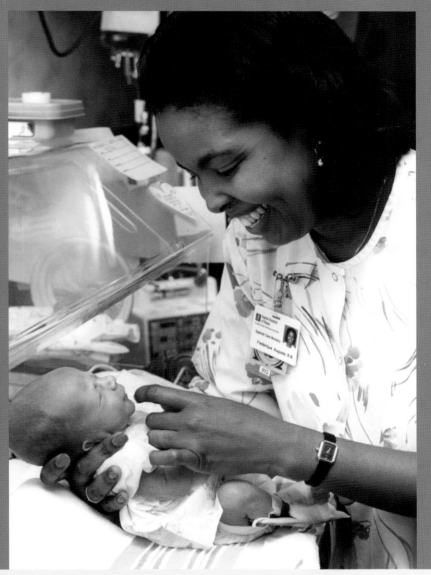

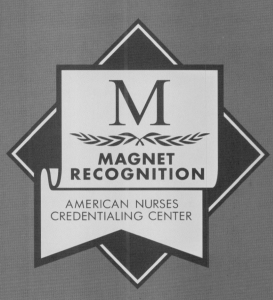

1998

Baptist Hospital...
LOOKING BACK

A Magnet Hospital of Excellence in Nursing Services

In 1998, Baptist Hospital became the first hospital in Florida and the 11th hospital nationwide to be awarded Magnet status for excellence in nursing by the American Nurses Credentialing Center — the leading nursing credentialing organization in the United States. Magnet status, a four-year designation, recognizes quality patient care, nursing excellence and innovations in professional nursing practice. To earn Magnet status, Baptist Hospital completed a comprehensive application process that included a two-day site visit. The nursing staff worked long and hard on the Magnet application. "It's been a 2 ½-year engagement. This is the wedding party," said Charlotte Dison, R.N., vice president and chief nursing officer, at the celebration for the honor.

Today, Baptist Health continues its place as a leader in nursing excellence. Baptist Hospital earned Magnet status again in 2002 and 2006. South Miami Hospital received Magnet recognition in 2004 and 2008. Doctors, Mariners and Homestead Hospitals plan to apply for Magnet recognition in 2012. "Magnet status is national recognition of the superior level of care provided by our nursing staff," said Deborah S. Mulvihill, R.N., corporate vice president and chief nursing officer.

A Tough Decision

While Baptist Health was achieving admirable results with its outpatient model and continued to look for more sites, it also considered adding another hospital. In August of 1996, Baptist Health signed a letter of intent to merge with Mercy Hospital, a 532-bed facility in Coconut Grove. On the surface, the partnership made sense. It would add a powerful link in the Baptist Health network and broaden its market share. Opened in 1950, Mercy was a Catholic hospital with a long history in South Florida and a large following with the area's Hispanic community. In 1995, Mercy treated more than 23,000 people in its Emergency Room and admitted more than 15,700 patients. "This is a natural fit," Mr. Keeley said at the announcement of the letter of intent. "It's like dating somebody for three months and suddenly you wake up the next morning and say, 'I'm in love.' The lights just clicked."

As the agreement began to take shape, however, a major roadblock emerged. Mercy, which was owned by the Sisters of Saint Joseph religious order, had limits on what procedures could be performed at the hospital, especially in terms of women's reproductive health services, such as surgical sterilizations and abortions. The restrictions left Baptist Health in a bind. Physicians feared that a merger would hamper their ability to offer women the full range of services. Community groups and women's activists protested the alliance as well, even threatening to boycott all Baptist Health facilities. It became a public controversy and Baptist Health leaders struggled to find a common ground between the religious covenant at Mercy and the desires of its physicians and surrounding community.

Niberto Moreno, M.D., performs minimally invasive surgery on a patient's heart at Baptist Hospital, c.1996.

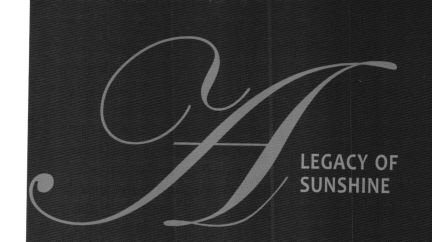

Teams from each hospital worked on the merger details. Baptist negotiated compromises, including one that limited the procedures in question to a center separate from all Baptist Health hospitals. In an attempt to find a middle ground, however, no one was satisfied and the opposition persisted. After nearly two years of debate and negotiation, the merger fell apart. In July of 1998, leaders from both organizations called off the partnership.

For Brian Keeley and his team, the end was disappointing. They had worked long hours and engaged in delicate and time-consuming discussions that had diverted manpower from other operations. "We took our eyes off all those other things," Keeley said in a 1999 interview. "After it was over, we said we needed to refocus back on the basics."

For the first time in many years, those basics proved challenging. The organization that had found success was facing a bleak financial outlook. In 1999, losses from operations exceeded $8 million. "This is unprecedented," Keeley told *The Miami Herald*. "We are the busiest we've ever been. We were blazing along, until this year. Now we are turning back patients and losing money off operations, which is almost impossible to do." While part of the problem was the managed care environment that left hospitals with unfavorable payments and the continuing cutbacks in Medicare reimbursements, Baptist Health also was saddled with some money-losing operations. Outside ventures, such as the Baptist Medical Group and physician partnerships, were not making money.

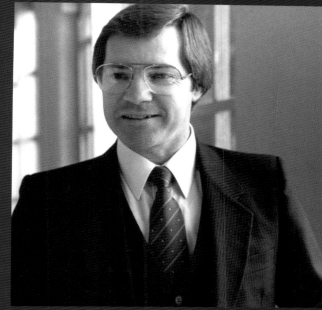

Rev. Robert W. Jakoby

The Sunshine Fund

In 1987, Bobby Bebber, the two-year-old son of Baptist Hospital engineer Phil Bebber, needed a life-saving liver transplant. The young boy and his family traveled to Children's Hospital in Pittsburgh for care. The Bebbers' plight inspired employees at Baptist Hospital who wanted to help their co-worker with expenses. Employees raised money with bake sales and a bowl-a-thon.

The Bebbers' plight also prompted a more official response — the creation of the Baptist Hospital Sunshine Fund. This pool of money started providing gifts and no-interest loans to employees facing a hardship. Employees donated money and Baptist Hospital matched each donation, creating a lasting fund for employee assistance. "I think employees will want to help other employees, knowing that at some point they too may have a critical need," said Pastoral Care Director Robert Jakoby, when the Sunshine Fund began.

The Sunshine Fund's greatest challenge and finest hour came in 1992, when Hurricane Andrew destroyed half the homes of Baptist Hospital's 3,000 employees. "The disaster of Andrew brought a blessing to the Fund," Chaplain Jakoby said.

Baptist Hospital Foundation donated $50,000, Georgia Baptist Hospital in Atlanta donated $100,000. Vendors and physicians added thousands. With the hospital match, the Sunshine Fund grew to more than $500,000 to help employees rebuild after the storm.

Today, the Sunshine Fund provides assistance to employees across Baptist Health. For every dollar donated by employees to the Sunshine Fund, Baptist Health kicks in $2. In budget year 2009, for example, 1,716 employees received a total of $2.3 million in no-interest loans and gifts.

So, Baptist Health cut back, streamlined and revised its strategy. Administrators closed the practice management department and dissolved the Baptist Medical Group. All the contracted physicians returned to private practice. Baptist Health also consolidated two home health agencies into one and restructured the physician partnerships, such as DadeWell, into more traditional HMOs to limit their financial impact. As expected, the changes brought anxiety. Many employees were left without jobs as positions were eliminated. Yet with Baptist Health's mindful attention to employees, the organization worked hard to relocate those affected by the closings. "One of the most wonderful things about working for Baptist Health Systems is that at any given time, there are literally hundreds of job openings from the Keys to Coral Gables," reassured Chief Operating Officer Fred Messing in

an employee newsletter. Ultimately, those who wanted to stay with Baptist Health found jobs in other departments.

In retrospect, Baptist Health had moved away from its core mission and proven track record. In an aim to keep up with the changing climate of medical care, the organization embraced areas outside of its expertise. "We were really taking the same steps that other large healthcare organizations were taking — physician partnerships and forming managed care groups — but I realized quickly that we did not truly understand those businesses," Mr. Keeley reflected. "We were great at delivering high-quality healthcare and keeping our employees and patients happy, but this was in a different realm." Having recognized the mistakes, Keeley acted. "I am not one to dwell on what ifs and what went wrong," he said. "We licked our wounds and moved on."

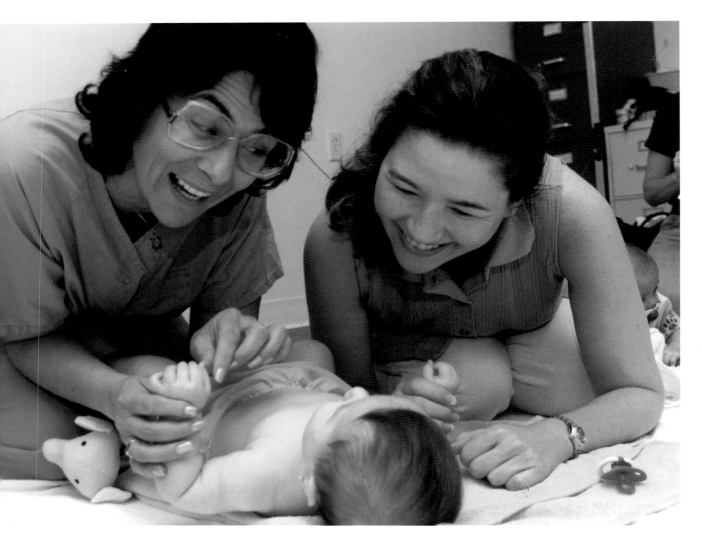

South Miami Hospital offered maternity care and classes such as infant massage. In this c.1999 photograph, Janine Balkin, R.N., demonstrates massaging techniques.

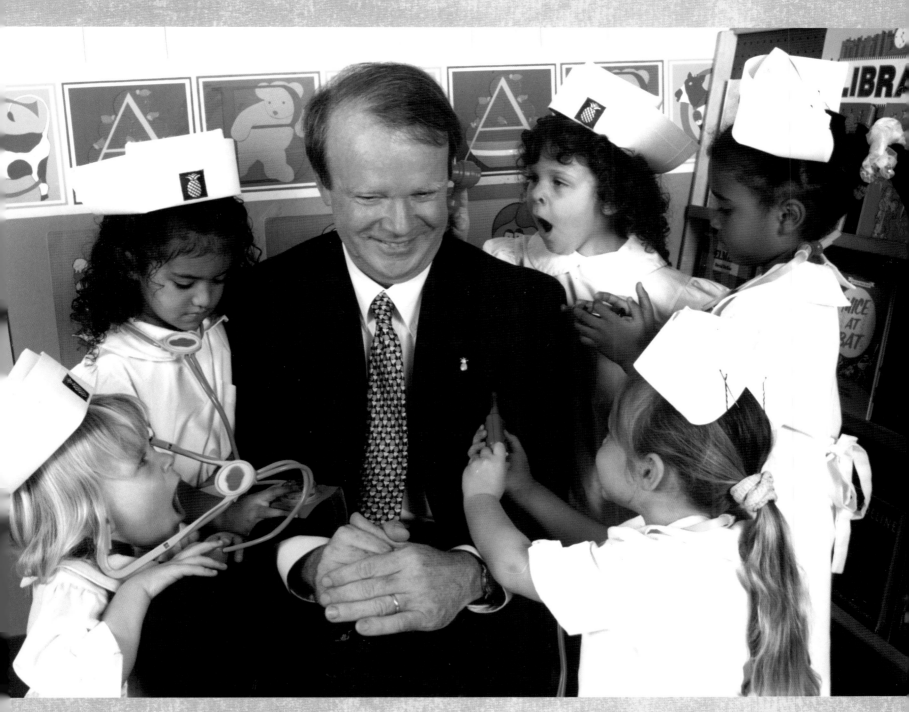

In the wake of financial pressures, Baptist Health maintained its focus on employees. Here, children of employees instruct CEO Brian Keeley in the art of play. The organization's commitment to providing child care helped employees stay engaged and was an important tool in recruiting nurses.

Back to Basics

In the midst of the problems, Baptist Health did experience some high points, most notably the February 1999 opening of the new Mariners Hospital. The $18.5 million, 72,000-square-foot facility nearly tripled the size of the old hospital. It included 42 private patient rooms, seven private rooms in the Emergency Center and eight intensive care rooms. The building reflected Baptist Health's commitment to quality design. It came complete with a breezy open feel and walls decorated with pictures and wallpaper borders that featured images reflecting the Florida Keys. The staff and employees consulted on the construction, adding their own expertise. CEO Robert Luse, who had studied engineering, brought his keen eye for detail to the project. Nurses helped design the layout of the patient floors, ensuring that nursing stations were well located. "We were all heavily involved and that made it all the more meaningful. It was a collaboration," remembered Robert Luse. "When it opened, it really felt like our hospital."

Equally important, the new Mariners was built to last. The construction, while expensive, included safeguards to protect Mariners from hurricanes up to category five. "It was one of our new facilities that we were building to withstand storms," Chief Financial Officer Ralph Lawson said. "It may cost more in the short term but it will pay for itself if we can protect ourselves from hurricane damage and stay open in the wake of a major storm. We saw it as standing like the Rock of Gibraltar."

For many in the Florida Keys, the new hospital was the culmination of years of hard work and struggles. "When we had the ribbon-cutting ceremony, I remember feeling such pride," said Mariners Board Chairman Jay Hershoff. "The building was first-class. Baptist Health did not skimp on anything. It was such an accomplishment to complete the deal with Baptist and get the new hospital, which I have always described as the 'crown jewel' of the Upper Keys."

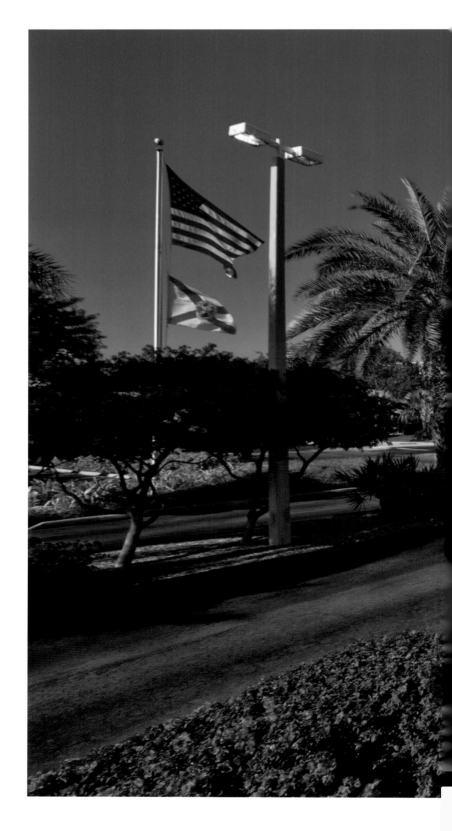

"*We were all heavily involved and that made it all the more meaningful. It was a collaboration. When it opened, it really felt like our hospital.*"

Robert Luse
Administrator, Mariners Hospital

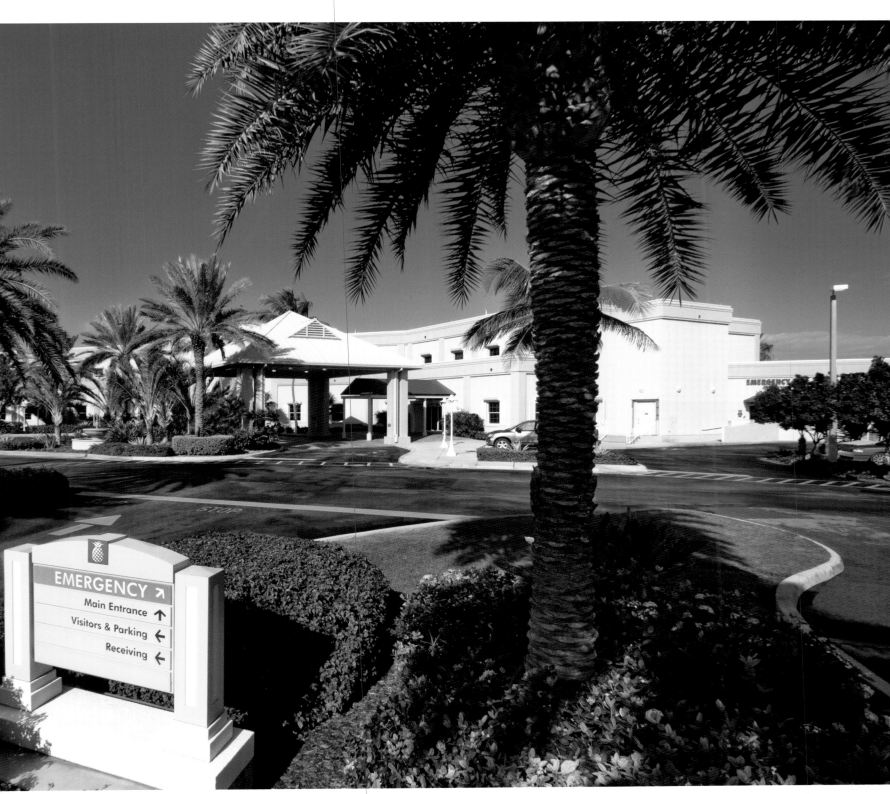

EMERGENCY ↗
Main Entrance ↑
Visitors & Parking ←
Receiving ←

In 1999, the new Mariners Hospital opened. With 42 patient rooms, an Emergency Center and intensive care rooms, it tripled the size of the old hospital.

With renewed focus, Baptist Health also concentrated on other areas. The organization, which was admired for its employee benefits, continued to meet the needs of its workforce. Despite the financial troubles, benefits, including holiday pay, on-call premium pay and weekend bonuses increased. Nurses were encouraged to further their education and take advantage of tuition reimbursements, flexible scheduling and scholarships. Employees were rewarded financially for money-saving suggestions. Baptist Health believed that satisfied employees were more efficient and better able to provide high-quality care. "It is simple," Mr. Keeley said. "We cannot afford to lose great employees."

By 2001, Baptist Health's financial picture turned around. The steps to narrow operations strengthened the bottom line and Baptist emerged a leaner and more efficient organization. "I am happy to report that the System's financial picture has improved dramatically after a devastating year in 1999, in which we, like healthcare providers around the country, struggled with reductions in Medicare reimbursement, changes in managed care, increases in uninsured patients and other challenges," Keeley wrote in Baptist Health's Report to the Community. "Fortunately, our incomparable team was able to pull together to overcome these obstacles."

In the wake of setbacks and recovery, Baptist Health looked to expand again. Mindful of the lessons of the past few years, however, administrators stayed close to Baptist Health's core business and engaged in what they deemed "controlled growth." South Miami Hospital began planning for its long-anticipated Medical Arts Building. Mariners opened its own Medical Office Building — the final step in fulfilling Baptist Health's commitment to the Upper Keys.

Baptist Health also added outpatient plazas, an undertaking that consistently proved strong. Their market need was apparent. The hospitals' Emergency Centers, particularly Baptist's, were still overcrowded. In 2001, the Baptist Hospital ER ranked as the second busiest in the county (behind Jackson Memorial Hospital) with more than 86,000 visits. South Miami and Homestead also saw increases in their ER patient visits. The medical plazas' urgent care centers were designed to draw some of the ER patients. To continue this effort, Baptist Health expanded Baptist Medical Plaza at Westchester at 8840 Bird Road, which had opened in 2000, and began building full-service Baptist Medical Plazas at West Kendall at 13001 North Kendall Drive, and Doral at 9915 N.W. 41st Street. The West Kendall location was an obvious choice. Its residents were familiar with

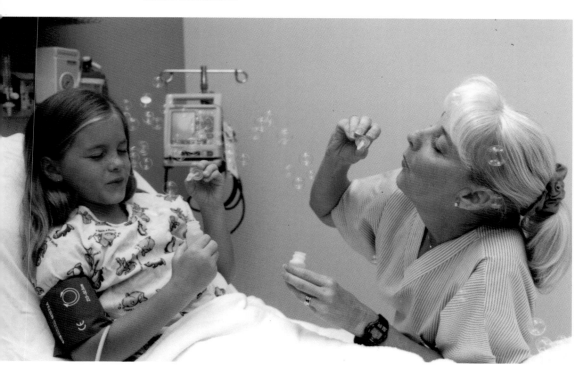

Linda Gaspeny, R.N., entertains a young patient at the new Mariners Hospital.

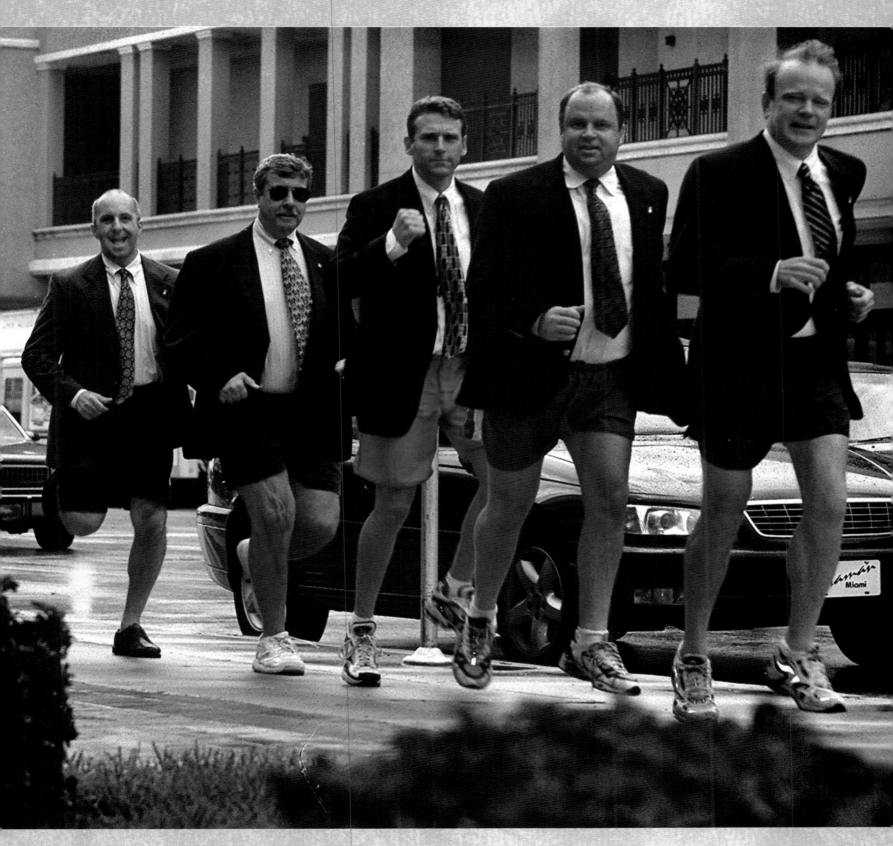

Employee benefits, including a comprehensive wellness program, are a hallmark of Baptist Health. In 2001, the organization's leaders participated in the local Corporate Run race to show the benefits of a healthy lifestyle. From left: Javier Hernandez-Lichtl, CEO of Baptist Health Enterprises; Robert Luse, CEO of Mariners Hospital; Bo Boulenger, CEO of Homestead Hospital; Wayne Brackin, CEO of South Miami Hospital; and Brian E. Keeley, CEO of Baptist Health.

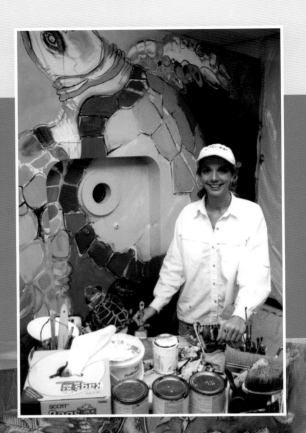

2002

Mariners Hospital...
LOOKING BACK

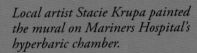

Local artist Stacie Krupa painted the mural on Mariners Hospital's hyperbaric chamber.

The hyperbaric chamber provides life-saving care for injuries such as those associated with scuba diving accidents.

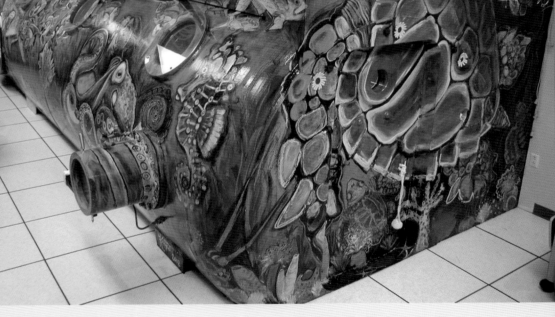

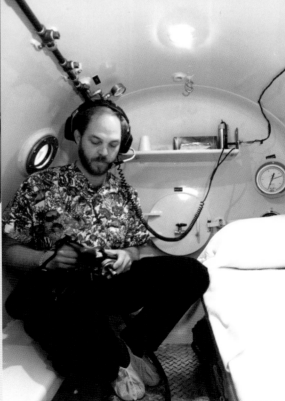

The Hyperbaric Chamber

In 2002, Mariners Hospital acquired a new 24-foot-long hyperbaric chamber — the only hospital-based chamber in the Florida Keys. Local artist Stacie Krupa worked six months on the nautically themed mural that decorated the chamber's exterior. Hyperbaric medicine is used to treat patients with decompression illness (commonly known as "the bends"), carbon monoxide poisoning, bone infections, wounds that won't heal and tissue damage from radiation. In the hyperbaric chamber, patients breathe 100 percent oxygen in a high-pressure environment. In 2009, patients received more than 530 hours of treatment in the hospital's hyperbaric chamber.

Baptist Hospital and had clamored for services closer to their neighborhood. The move to Doral was a bit riskier. It was Baptist Health's most northern venture and the area was farther away from its hospitals. But, the location was thoughtfully picked and well-studied. "Baptist Health decided to go into the Doral market because so many people in the community were traveling to Baptist and South Miami Hospitals for services," said then Baptist Outpatient Services CEO Javier Hernandez-Lichtl. "The Doral community has been underserved."

These expanding boundaries put the Baptist Health brand in more communities and neighborhoods. The pineapple became a familiar symbol to most South Floridians. And while they certainly recognized the Baptist Health brand, the full name, Baptist Health Systems of South Florida, was clumsy and confusing. In 2002, to simplify and streamline, the organization changed its name. The healthcare company's new moniker became Baptist Health South Florida. "There's no change to who or what we are," Mr. Keeley said. "It's just now we have a shorter, crisper and more memorable name."

In the next few months, with renewed vigor, Baptist Health would find a new and welcomed opportunity to partner with a hospital in the affluent city of Coral Gables.

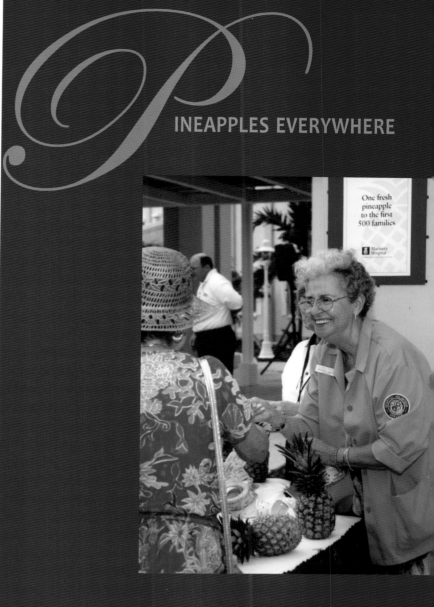

A Symbol of Hospitality

When Baptist merged with South Miami and Homestead Hospitals, Brian Keeley made one of his most important decisions — to designate the pineapple as the logo for Baptist Health. "We had been using Baptist Hospital's tower as our logo but as we grew with other hospitals it no longer fit," Mr. Keeley remembered. "I thought the pineapple — which was already at Baptist Hospital in the form of a fountain — was an easily recognizable symbol. With the merger and changes, we needed something that would make people instantly think of Baptist Health."

The pineapple symbolized hospitality in Renaissance Europe and early America. "Because of what it represented, the pineapple was a natural choice to show our commitment to service excellence," Mr. Keeley said. "What better way to say to our patients and visitors that they'll receive top-quality care and service in friendly and comfortable surroundings?"

In just 15 years, the pineapple has become one of the most recognizable brands in South Florida. "Our market research indicates eight out of 10 residents from Dade County and the Upper Keys connect the pineapple to Baptist Health," said Jo Baxter, corporate vice president, who has headed Baptist Health's marketing and public relations function for more than 30 years. "This is a remarkable achievement, especially when you consider the growth and diversity of the population since 1995. It's a memorable symbol for a healthcare organization. And our phenomenal caregivers fulfill its promise every day."

"*Our market research indicates eight out of 10 residents from Dade County and the Upper Keys connect the pineapple to Baptist Health. This is a remarkable achievement, especially when you consider the growth and diversity of the population since 1995. It's a memorable symbol for a healthcare organization. And our phenomenal caregivers fulfill its promise every day.*"

Jo Baxter
Corporate Vice President
Marketing & Public Relations

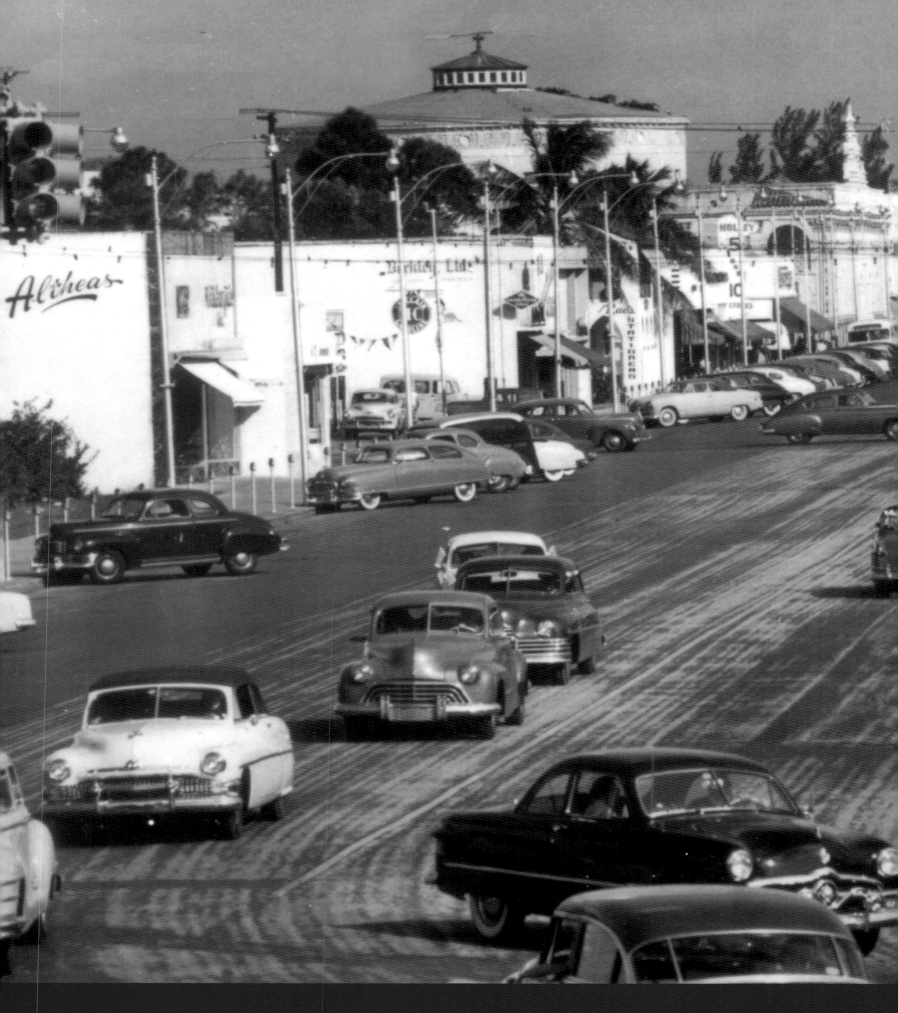

In the Heart of Coral Gables

Miracle Mile in Coral Gables, c.1950

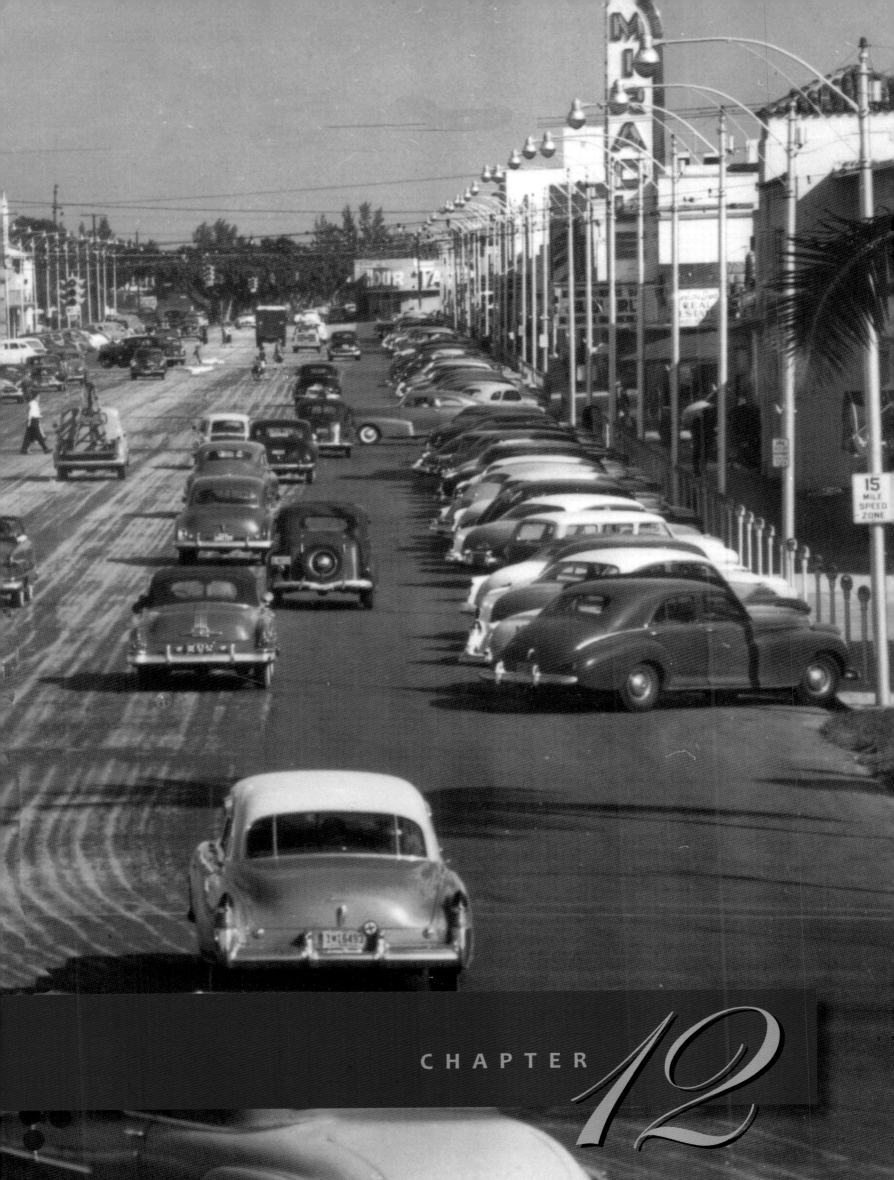

CHAPTER *12*

"The hospital can be likened to a human being in that it has a personality, responsibilities, accomplishments and the emotions of happiness and sorrow. ... Just as an individual desires the most modern and finest for himself, the hospital must keep abreast of medical advances. The modern practice of medicine requires a modern, up-to-date building completely supplied with the expensive and complicated modern medical equipment. With such facilities, this hospital and its personnel can render the patient the finest of medical service."

Mary Reeder
Director, Doctors' Hospital
1959

On May 10, 1948, a small crowd featuring local dignitaries such as Coral Gables Mayor Keith Phillips, University of Miami President Bowman Foster Ashe and John T. Macdonald, M.D., gathered on a wooden platform in the middle of a field near the University of Miami. The occasion celebrated the groundbreaking for Doctors' Hospital. The location would prove to be one of South Florida's most desirable addresses — the affluent City of Coral Gables.

At the time, the almost three-decades-old community was on the verge of explosive growth. Its population, which was just under 10,000 in 1945, would burgeon to nearly 20,000 by 1950. While Coral Gables already had staples of modernity, with a university and a lively new downtown shopping area called Miracle Mile, the future would bring more development and great change. Doctors' Hospital would sit amid this thriving center.

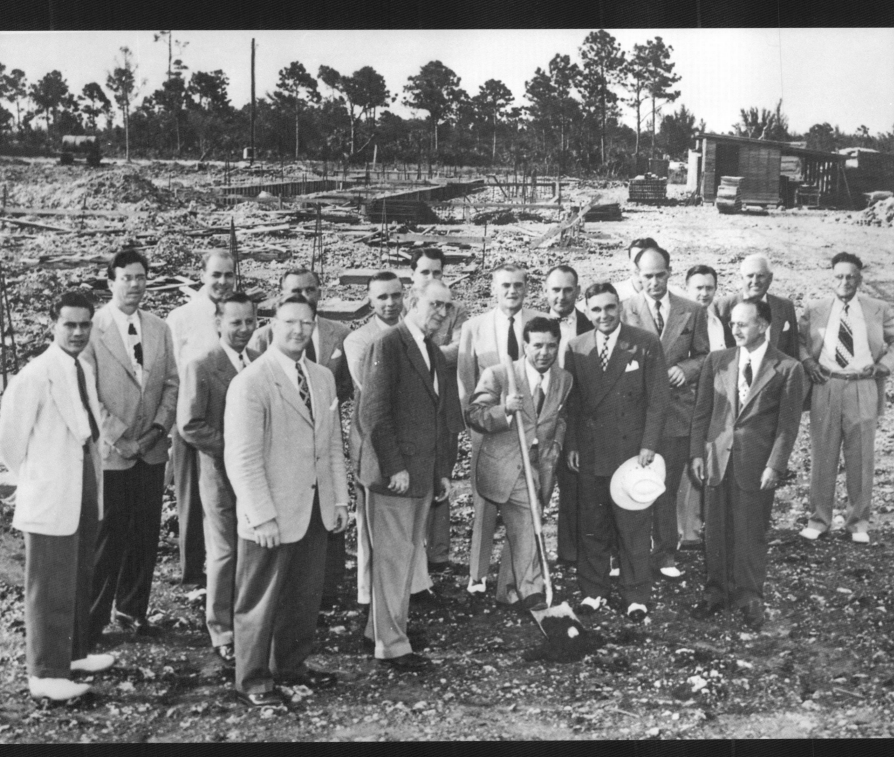

Groundbreaking for Doctors' Hospital, May 1949

A Familiar Start

The area that would become Coral Gables started out like other South Florida communities — a wilderness. It began as home to a collection of pioneers who eked out a life among palmettos, Indians, hurricanes and mosquitoes.

As more and more people discovered the tropical climate, development followed. One of the early arrivals was a 13-year-old boy just out of a New England prep school. George Merrick and his family came to South Florida in 1899 from Duxbury, Massachusetts, where his father was a minister. Merrick's parents, Solomon and Althea, had just suffered the loss of their four-year-old daughter and hoped the move to a warmer climate would soothe their souls. Sight unseen, the Merricks purchased a 160-acre homestead.

The initial years were difficult. The land was rocky and the area isolated and remote. But with the minister's ethos of hard work and perseverance, the family turned it into a working grove. The first crop was guava, which generated a small income. By 1907, Solomon Merrick had developed more profitable grapefruit groves.

The success allowed the intellectual son to leave the rigors of agriculture for college. George Merrick enrolled at Rollins College in Winter Park. Then, in 1909, he started law school in New York. The law was his father's idea, not his. Merrick was a dreamer and gifted writer and wanted to pursue writing full time. He wrote his father asking for permission to quit law school.

Before a decision could be made, Solomon took ill. George returned to Miami to help with the family's thriving groves, now named the Coral Gables Plantation. Ever the dutiful son, George worked the land. When Solomon died in 1911, George ran the operation independently. He purchased more land and planted more grapefruit, turning the enterprise into the largest vegetable and fruit producer in the area.

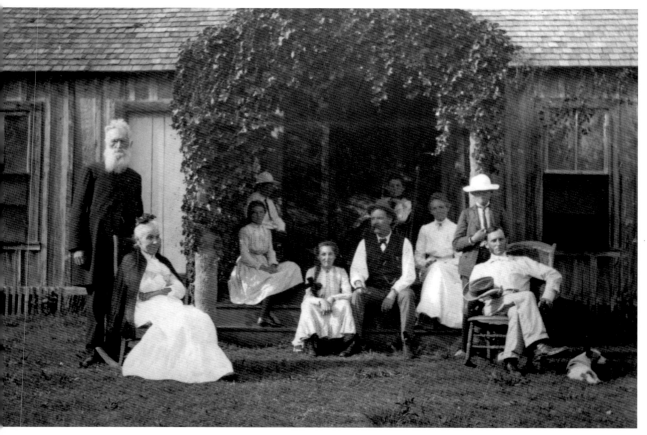

Members of the Merrick and Fink families gather in front of the Merricks' cabin on the site of today's Merrick House in Coral Gables. (Left to right) Grandpa and Grandma Fink, Medie Merrick, Ethel Merrick, William Fink (Althea's brother) and his wife Belle (behind), Althea Merrick, H. George Fink and Solomon Merrick.

George Merrick returned to Miami to help with the family's thriving groves, now named the Coral Gables Plantation. Ever the dutiful son, George worked the land.

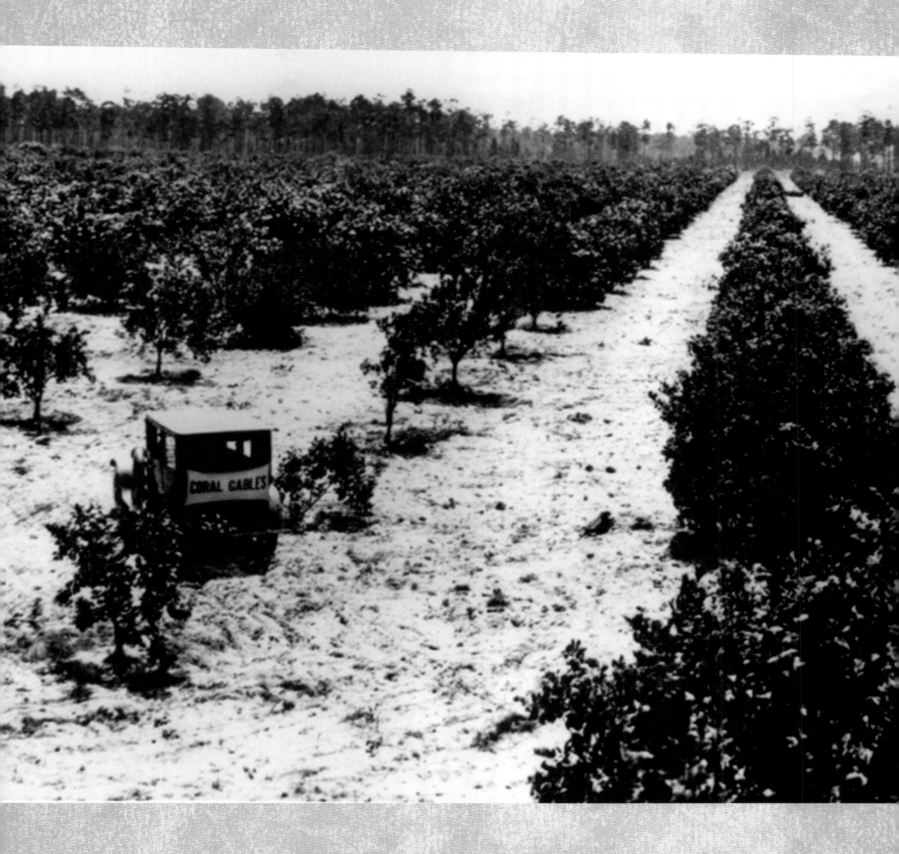

He also pursued other interests. As the city around him grew, Merrick became interested in real estate. He dreamed of building a planned community on the family's huge holdings. He read books about development, visited other communities throughout the country for ideas, and studied the Garden City and City Beautiful Movements.

He developed a myriad of subdivisions around Miami, including North Miami Estates, MacFarlane and Riverside Heights. Using what he learned, Merrick then set his mind to creating an ideal community that reflected the best ideas in planned development. By 1921, he had acquired enough land around the original plantation to plot Coral Gables. He brought together a team to design the city. His artist uncle, Denman Fink, a well-known magazine illustrator, created the city's color palette and look, inspired by Spanish Mediterranean architecture. Merrick hired landscape architect Frank Button, fresh from his work in Chicago's Lincoln Park and Miami's Charles Deering Estate, to plot the wide streets and boulevards that would characterize the community. Finally, Merrick's cousin, architect H. George Fink, came aboard to design the buildings.

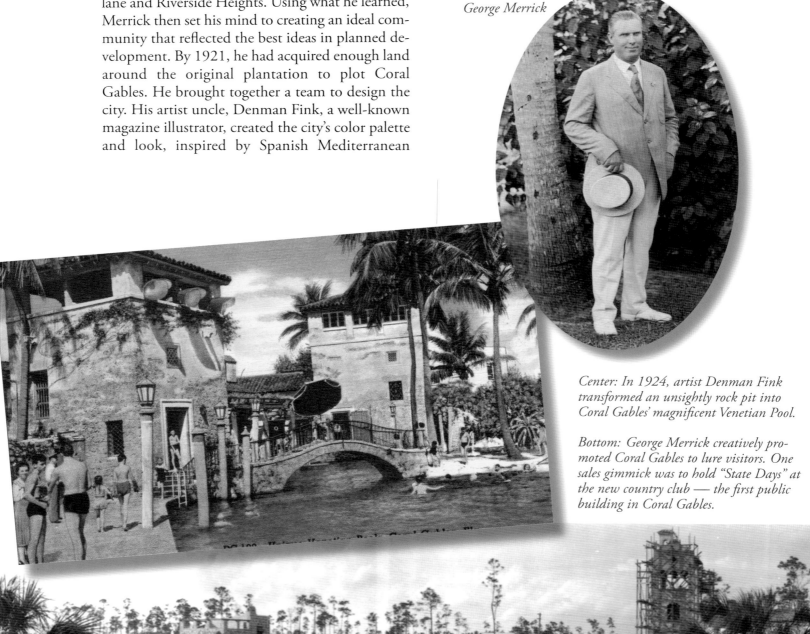

George Merrick

Center: In 1924, artist Denman Fink transformed an unsightly rock pit into Coral Gables' magnificent Venetian Pool.

Bottom: George Merrick creatively promoted Coral Gables to lure visitors. One sales gimmick was to hold "State Days" at the new country club — the first public building in Coral Gables.

A City Is Born

Merrick's plans and designs found a receptive audience. With Florida on the cusp of an unprecedented land boom, developments were popping up at a record pace. Merrick set the standard among the frenzy. A savvy marketer, he filled local newspapers with full-page advertisements celebrating the beauty of Coral Gables — the place, he wrote, "Where Your Castles in Spain Are Made Real!" With incentives such as fine china, he bused in would-be buyers to visit and hired a colorful auctioneer named "Doc" Dammers to sell lots at auction.

The promotional campaign was successful. On November 28, 1921, 5,000 people showed up in Coral Gables for the first day of sales. By 1923, Merrick had acquired more land and added a business section east of Le Jeune Road. He opened Granada Golf Course and the Country Club of Coral Gables. To handle the growth, Merrick added new members to his team — architects Walter DeGarmo, Martin Hampton and Louis Brumm, and designer Phineas Paist, who had worked on the famed Vizcaya mansion in Miami.

George Merrick's Coral Gables was now a full-fledged city, incorporated in 1925. Builders broke ground on a signature hotel, the Biltmore, educational leaders began planning the University of Miami and construction started on Ponce de Leon High School (today's Ponce de Leon Middle School). The prosperous conditions, however, would not last. On February 4, 1926, when Merrick stood with other dignitaries to lay the cornerstone for the university, the boom had already slowed. A major hurricane that struck Miami in September provided another blow, and within two years, the area was in the midst of a deep economic depression. Merrick poured all his vast wealth into trying to continue his dreams for Coral Gables, but the circumstances caught up with him. His development company went bankrupt and the dreamer was left penniless.

George Merrick and his wife left the city to open an upscale fishing camp in the Keys. But even without him, Coral Gables felt his influence. In 1937, the city adopted its first zoning code that followed Merrick's plans. By the time Coral Gables celebrated its 15th anniversary in 1940, Merrick was again formally embraced. The city he founded honored him at a dinner dance at the country club and gave him a life membership in the Coral Gables Chamber of Commerce. He died two years later, fully vindicated by the city's beauty and growth.

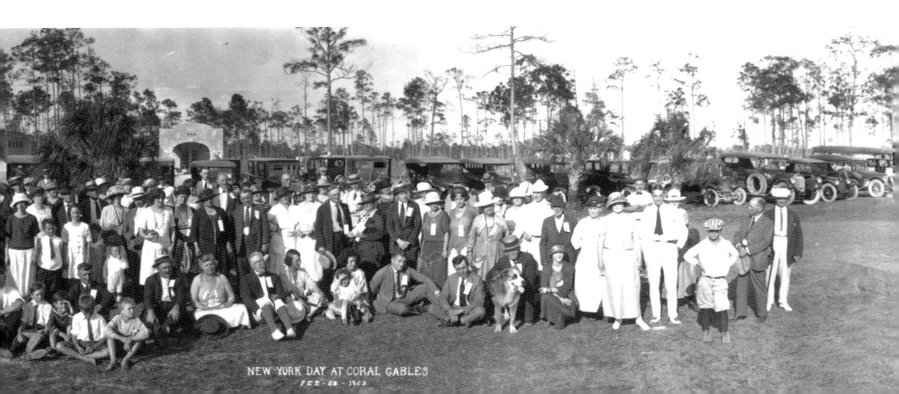

NEW YORK DAY AT CORAL GABLES
FEB-28-1923

The Challenges of Progress

In the wake of World War II, the city, like the rest of South Florida, enjoyed a renaissance. People came south to settle and new businesses opened. Coral Gables especially thrived. Soldiers used the G.I. Bill, a government benefit that provided returning veterans direct payment for college tuition, to enroll in the University of Miami. The school, which had fewer than 2,000 students in 1945, swelled to more than 5,000 by the 1946 fall term. They settled in neighborhood apartments or built small houses. The construction industry exploded with building permits at about $1 million a month by 1948.

With the surge in population came some challenges. The city's infrastructure struggled to handle all the growth. A proposed new high school, Coral Gables Senior High, moved from design to construction in hopes of relieving the crowding in class-rooms. Another big concern was hospital beds. At the time, only one hospital served the immediate area — University Hospital, a private facility of approximately 40 beds in the 3100 block of Douglas Road. Since 1931, two women, Lucille Bacon and Mary Reeder, had run the hospital. In 1947, it changed ownership and was renamed Coral Gables Hospital.

The upheaval left some physicians uneasy. The area already was vastly underserved by hospitals, and doctors wondered what would happen to their patients. Dade County had just over 1,000 hospital beds for a community that needed at least double the amount. The problem was especially acute in Coral Gables, whose population included full-time residents, University of Miami students and winter-time tourists.

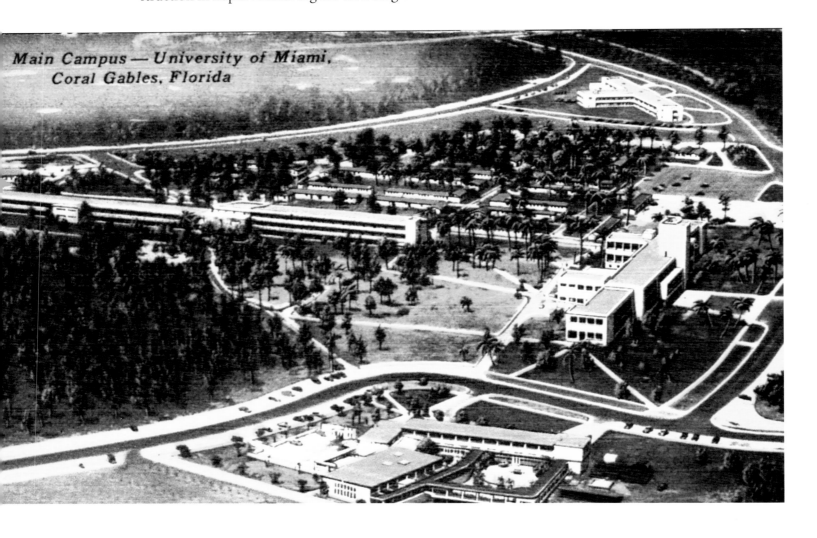

Main Campus — University of Miami, Coral Gables, Florida

A Hospital Is Born

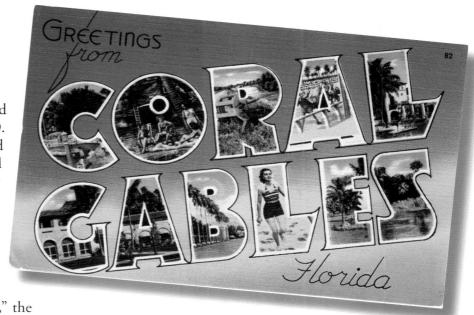

For John T. Macdonald, M.D., a renowned local surgeon, and three other physicians, A.D. Amerise, M.D., Joseph Lucinian, M.D., and Herbert Virgin, M.D., the problem sparked their interest and, ultimately, their involvement in a solution. The physicians met with Mrs. Reeder, a friendly face and experienced manager, and Edythe Harrison, a local nurse, about starting a new hospital to serve their patients. "People of the community who have given any thought to the need of a hospital must have spent quite a few sleepless nights," the prospectus for the hospital stated. "The Coral Gables area has been faced with the very real threat of gravely inadequate hospital facilities for any serious emergency or widespread outbreak of an illness."

The four men, joined by Mrs. Reeder, started by thinking small. They initially planned for a one-story, 28-bed hospital with only the barest essentials. Yet after working the numbers, they concluded such a small hospital could not be profitable. The group reached out to other doctors and professionals and decided to build a hospital with between 50 and 100 beds. Each new founding member of the group had to be approved unanimously by a membership committee.

To raise money for the proposed Doctors' Hospital, the group turned to each other and the surrounding community. The building was set to be funded by the sale of stock. Doctors who wanted to join the medical staff were required to buy at least $5,000 worth of common stock. An exception was made for returning veterans, who had to invest only $1,000. The initial offering raised $250,000. Hospital organizers also looked to the community. "For the community to profit by use of the hospital, it will be necessary for residents to actively support the financing of the institution," the prospectus read. Supporters could buy non-voting stock in the hospital to receive dividends or furnish rooms at a rate of $400. Fundraisers launched the campaign from the Coral Gables Chamber of Commerce office.

Residents got behind the hospital out of need and because of the stature of the leaders involved. Mary J. Reeder was a prominent figure in Dade County when she began organizing Doctors' Hospital. A native of Georgia, Mrs. Reeder came to South Florida in 1921. The next year, she put her nursing skills to good use by joining with two other nurses, Mary King and Elizabeth Brandon, to establish the 20-bed Edith Cavell Hospital, named for the famous British nurse martyred during World War I. The hospital, off S.E. Seventh Street, was one of several small neighborhood facilities, often opened in converted homes, which nurses operated to handle South Florida's growing population. Mrs. Reeder remained owner of the hospital when it moved to 642 N.W. Third Street and the name was changed to Riverview Hospital in 1923 and Riverside Hospital in 1928. For a short time, she also ran

Downtown Coral Gables, c.1940

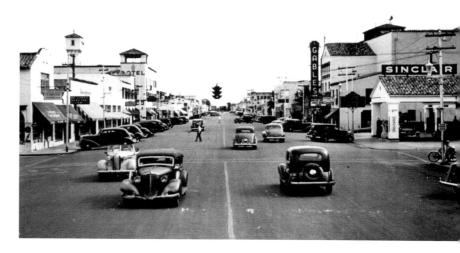

Victoria Hospital, located at 930 N.W. Third Street, under the name Victoria Hospital Operating Company, and worked there as an operating room supervisor. In 1931, Mrs. Reeder and Lucille Bacon took over University Hospital, where they worked with many local doctors.

Beyond her professional life, Mrs. Reeder was a fixture in South Florida's social and charitable circles. In 1929, she married local businessman Clifford Reeder, who served as a city commissioner and mayor of Miami in the 1930s. The couple settled in Coconut Grove and Mrs. Reeder proudly fulfilled the role of mayor's wife. She became active with the Red Cross, and the Florida Society of Crippled Children and Adults, and was a founding member of the Soroptimist Club.

With skill and grace, Mrs. Reeder moved between her professional image and her role as a "lady" of the era. For those who worked with her, she was competent and poised. "She was a quiet and determined lady," remembered James Vaughn, M.D., a local physician. "She would smile at you and then usually get what she wanted." Her personality was engaging and, although she was a leader, she never managed autocratically. "Perhaps her greatest accomplishment … was her ability to make people happy," wrote Joseph McAloon, who succeeded her as administrator at Doctors'. "She once told me that, like Will Rogers, she had never met a person she really didn't like. Conversely, I do not think that there was ever a person who met Mrs. Reeder who did not like her."

Like Mrs. Reeder, the doctors brought prestige and focus to the process of building a hospital. Dr. John Macdonald, a gynecologist and surgeon, was the group's unofficial leader. Tall and slim with a warm smile, he had an unwavering belief in the need for the hospital and the doctors' role in meeting it. His steely determination pushed the group forward. "Dr. Macdonald contemplated the fast growing population of the community and became alarmed at the scarcity of hospital facilities, daily

With skill and grace, Mrs. Reeder moved between her professional image and her role as a "lady" of the era. For those who worked with her, she was competent and poised.

growing more acute and hopelessly inadequate for the future. Many others had realized this situation and done nothing to correct it," James McShane, M.D., an early member of the hospital staff, wrote in 1951. "He met with several of his colleagues who similarly had foresight and planned a modern hospital, conceived, planned, financed, erected, managed by doctors under the great American tradition of private enterprise."

Another founding member, Dr. Virgin, chaired the building and architectural committee. He negotiated with the University of Miami to purchase five acres on University Drive. Although the hospital had no formal relationship with the university (its medical school did not open until 1952), the founders did envision collaboration. "The University of Miami welcomed us to this location and has done everything in its power to encourage and expedite our building," the hospital's prospectus stated. "While no such arrangements have been made or definitely contemplated, the proximity of the hospital and the University makes it natural for the two institutions to aid each other in medical research and instruction, thus adding to the prestige of both and elevating the caliber of medical service available to the public."

Facing page: In the mid 1950s, Mary Reeder was secretary of the Florida Hospital Association. She is shown here with John F. Wymer Jr. (right), administrator of Good Samaritan Hospital in West Palm Beach, and Pat Groner, executive director of Baptist Hospital in Pensacola.

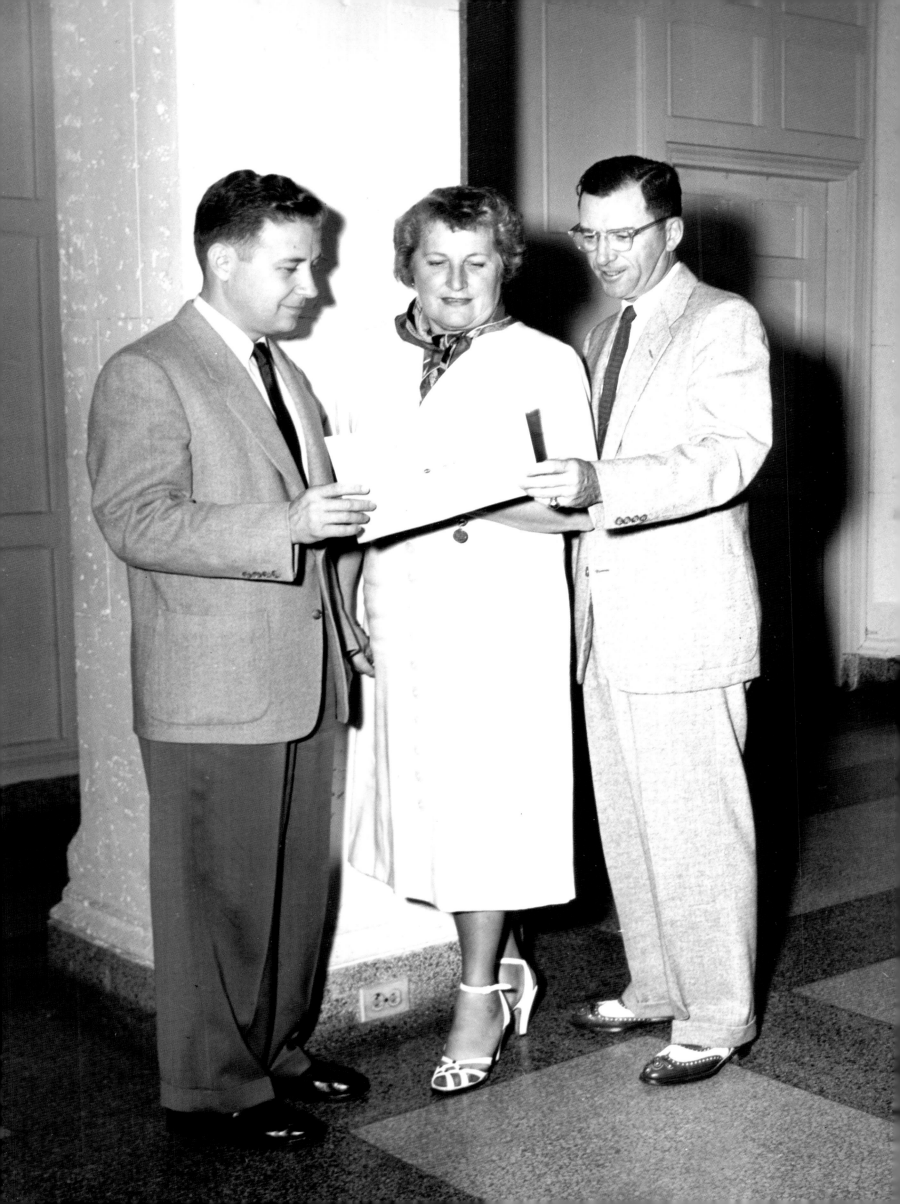

A Push for More

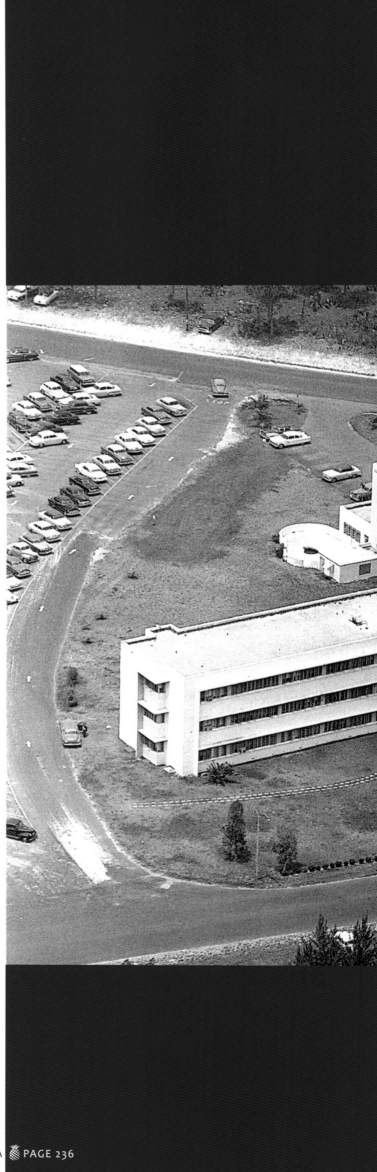

On February 27, 1949, the community got a first-hand view of what had been developing near the university. More than 500 visitors attended an open house at the two-story, 98-bed and 24-bassinet, $700,000 Doctors' Hospital. The day's activities were even broadcast by the Coral Gables radio station. Visitors marveled at the building, appreciated the soft pastel-colored walls and warm feel, and took pride in having a new hospital in their own community. Less than a week later, on March 3, 1949, Doctors' Hospital admitted its first patient — Marion Edwards, a Pan American Airways mechanic. Within the first two days of opening, physicians delivered two babies, admitted 21 patients and performed six operations. By the time the hospital completed 18 months of operation, physicians cared for about 500 patients a month and treated between 95 and 150 patients a month in the Emergency Room. They also delivered 1,200 babies.

The doctors who practiced at the hospital were among its staunchest advocates. The staff was close-knit. Many lived in the area and socialized with each other. They also found the environment sensitive to their own needs, and this was no accident. Doctors' Hospital was designed by physicians. In fact, the building was developed in rough sketches by a committee of four doctors, a superintendent of nurses and the wife of one of the doctors who could use a T-square and triangle.

The result was a practical design. The nurses' stations were centrally located in each wing. Specialists had input into the plans for their areas. Obstetricians consulted on the obstetrical wing and pediatricians influenced the nursery. Surgeons helped plan the large operating rooms, which measured 20 by 22 feet. Cabinets, accessible from each side, sat between them. "…Doctors' Hospital is not a hospital designed by architects who sometimes have little conception of surgical, medical and nursing procedures," Dr. Virgin wrote at the time. "It was designed by the doctors themselves and meets all the…requirements for facilities and services."

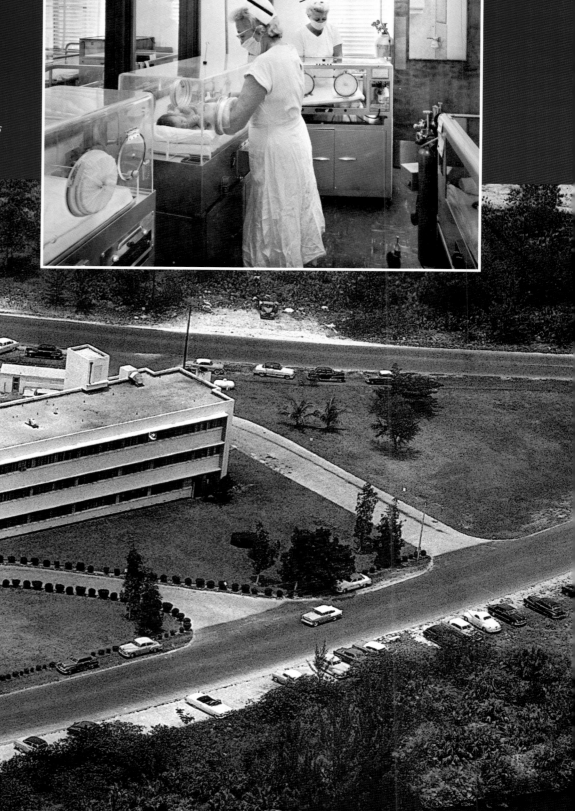

Right: Doctors' Hospital's maternity ward was a busy place.

Below: Doctors' Hospital's original building was two stories. The third floor was added in 1953.

$\mathcal{B}$y the time the hospital completed 18 months of operation, physicians cared for about 500 patients a month and treated between 95 and 150 patients a month in the Emergency Room. They also delivered 1,200 babies.

By the early 1950s, it was clear that Doctors' Hospital would need more space. Here, a surgical nurse reviews the schedule for a busy day.

As predicted, the hospital also benefited from its proximity to the University of Miami. The university's growth and developing medical school not only increased the patient base but also provided a pool of skilled employees. The hospital found itself amply served by returning veterans and their wives. Many of the nurses were married to servicemen who were attending the University of Miami on the G.I. Bill. Other nurses served with some branch of the military during the war and worked at Doctors' after their tenure.

From its influence in the community to the number of patients, Doctors' Hospital was a success. By 1951, admissions reached more than 6,000, with more than 1,600 maternity cases. Unfortunately, in the middle of the push forward, one of the key players died. On April 3, 1951, founding member and past Board Chairman Dr. Macdonald died at the hospital he helped create. In May, the hospital dedicated its surgical pavilion in his honor. "Today Doctors' Hospital stands as a great memorial to his ideals, his selfless devotion, his community spirit and untiring leadership," Dr. McShane said at the dedication ceremony. "He has left us great trust but keeping in mind his principles, although deprived of his great assistance, the Board of Directors of Doctors' Hospital is dedicated to maintaining [its] growth and development…as he visualized it for the future."

The first move toward the future was a $450,000 addition in 1953. The original architects had planned the two-story structure with expansion in mind. Its steel frame was topped in a way that made an additional story easy and cost effective. The new floor brought the bed total to 154 and added a new maternity and pediatrics setup. The improvements helped the hospital keep up with a thriving community and its demand for more services.

Four years later, the hospital took another important step — it was sold to the nonprofit Dr. John T. Macdonald Foundation. The foundation, created in 1953 after Dr. Macdonald's death, had been formed "to promote health and physical well-being, to alleviate suffering and to maintain and provide means for scientific research." It initially supported everyday hospital operations. By purchasing Doctors', the foundation could dramatically shape its future. While the transfer of ownership did not change the hospital's management, it did affect Doctors' tax status, making grants and government programs more accessible.

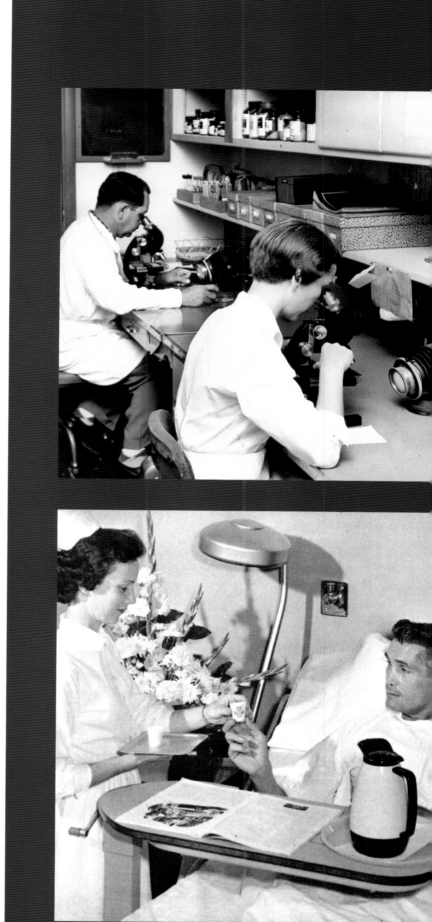

The hospital's services included a laboratory and extra attention by dedicated nurses.

A Mecca for Patients in South Dade

The first order of business with the new not-for-profit status was, not surprisingly, expansion. Hospital leaders hoped to increase Doctors' size with an ambitious $1 million wing. More than 230,000 people now lived within five miles of the hospital. Its occupancy rate averaged 92 percent. The hospital employed more than 400 workers with an annual payroll exceeding $1.2 million. The medical staff had doubled from opening day to more than 120.

Construction began in February 1959, just as the hospital was about to celebrate its 10th anniversary. The new three-story wing opened on December 6, 1959. An elaborate dedication ceremony, complete with the mayor of Coral Gables, the hospital's first patient and live television coverage, marked the occasion. The addition offered impressive features. It provided more operating and recovery rooms, a new clinical laboratory and pharmacy, air-conditioned rooms equipped with baths, piped-in oxygen and electronically operated beds. Some rooms even had televisions. Most importantly, the expansion brought the hospital's bed total to 225 with 44 additional bassinets. It made Doctors', in the words of one local newspaper, "a mecca for patients from throughout South Dade County."

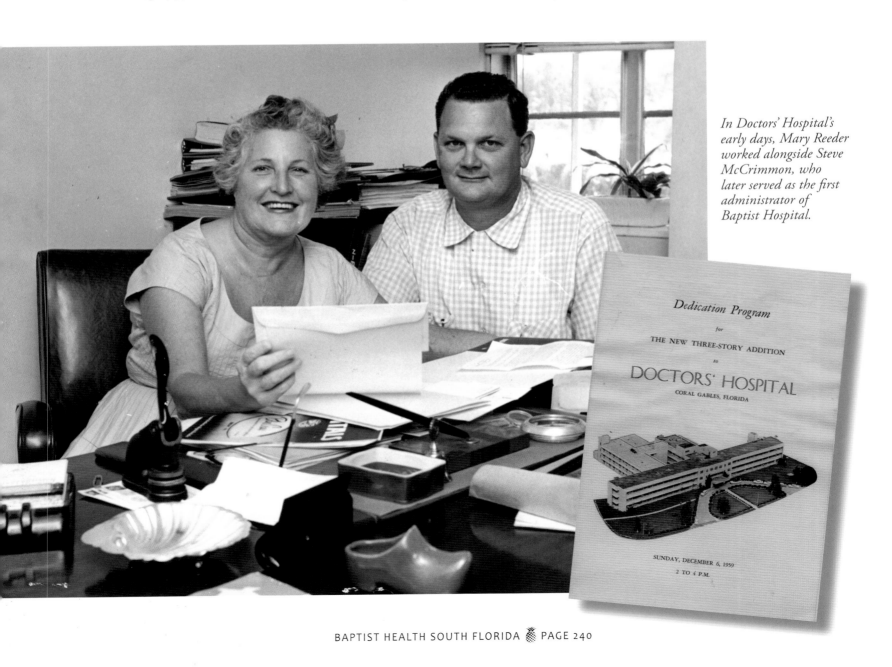

In Doctors' Hospital's early days, Mary Reeder worked alongside Steve McCrimmon, who later served as the first administrator of Baptist Hospital.

Dedication Program for THE NEW THREE-STORY ADDITION to DOCTORS' HOSPITAL CORAL GABLES, FLORIDA

SUNDAY, DECEMBER 6, 1959 2 TO 4 P.M.

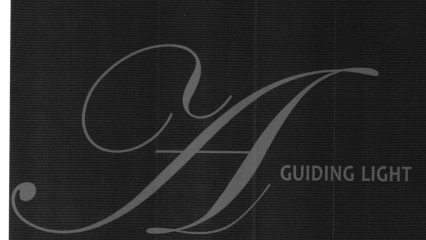

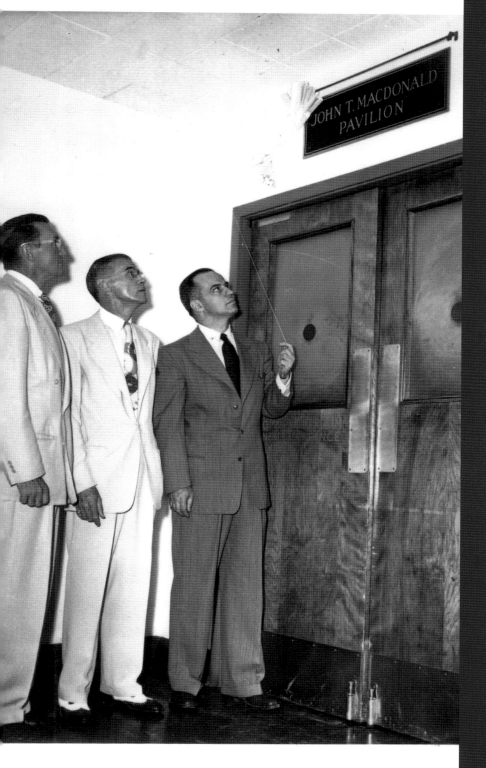

Mercier Brugler (right) unveils a plaque honoring his uncle, the late Dr. John T. Macdonald. With him is the Rev. David J. Davis of Plymouth Congregational Church and Dr. James K. McShane. The hospital dedicated a wing in the memory of Dr. Macdonald.

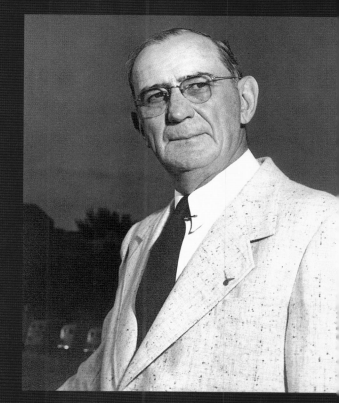

John Tremper Macdonald, M.D.

John Tremper Macdonald, M.D., was Doctors' Hospital's guiding light. Dr. Macdonald was born in Philadelphia in 1885. He graduated from the University of Pennsylvania and the Medico-Chirurgical College of Philadelphia. After service in World War I as an officer with the 78th Division, Dr. Macdonald began practicing in Norristown, Pennsylvania. In 1934, he came to South Florida, where he could work and pursue his other love — boating.

In 1938, he was appointed flight surgeon for Pan American World Airways and, six years later, medical director of Pan Am's Latin American Division. He became an authority on tropical diseases and helped protect the health of the airline's employees.

In addition to his work with Pan Am, Dr. Macdonald built a thriving practice in South Florida, where, like other physicians, he often struggled with the lack of hospital facilities. Typical of his no-nonsense approach, he surveyed the problem and acted. Friendly and approachable, he poked and prodded others to join an effort to build Doctors' Hospital.

In the indefatigable push for the hospital, he never lost his human touch. Peering down from the brim of his felt hat, Dr. Macdonald would speak warmly about his boat or ask about a family member. He was "a great doctor with a great heart," the Pan Am World Airways newsletter eulogized upon his death in 1951.

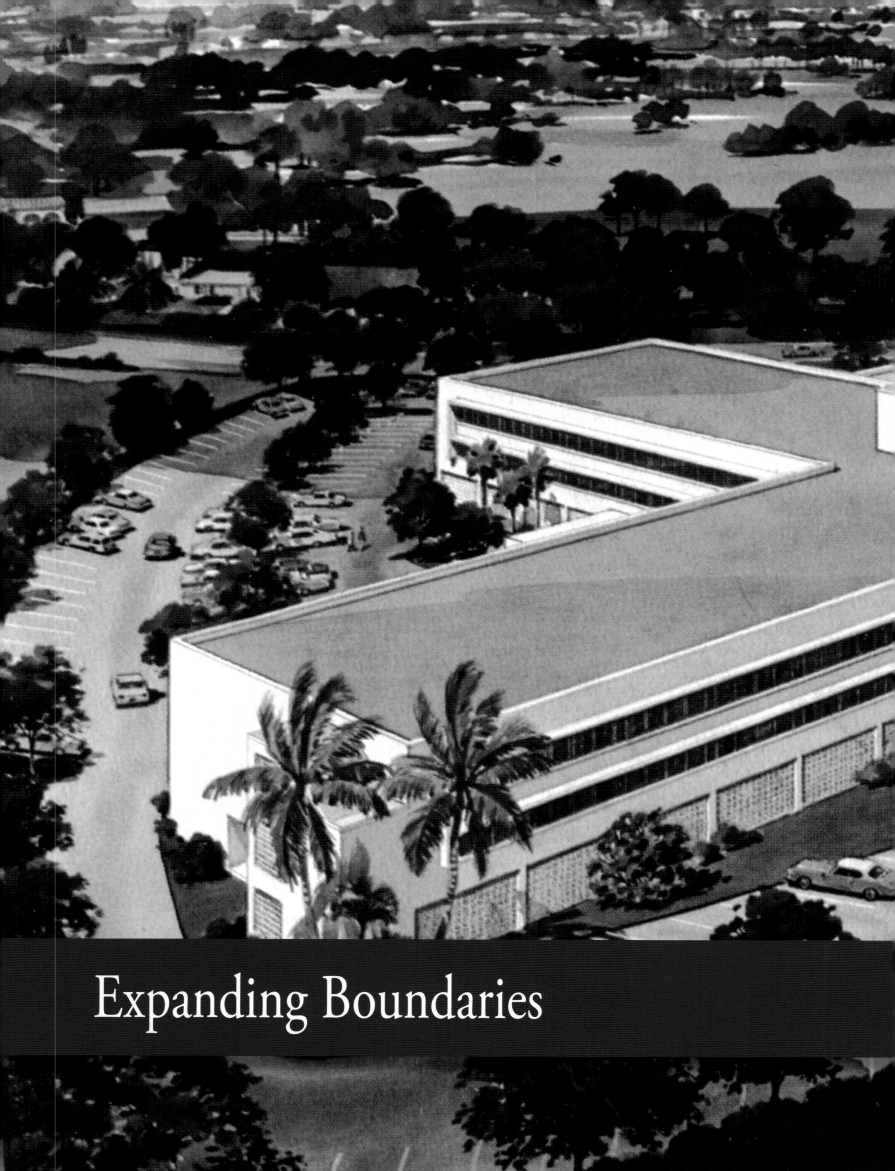

Expanding Boundaries

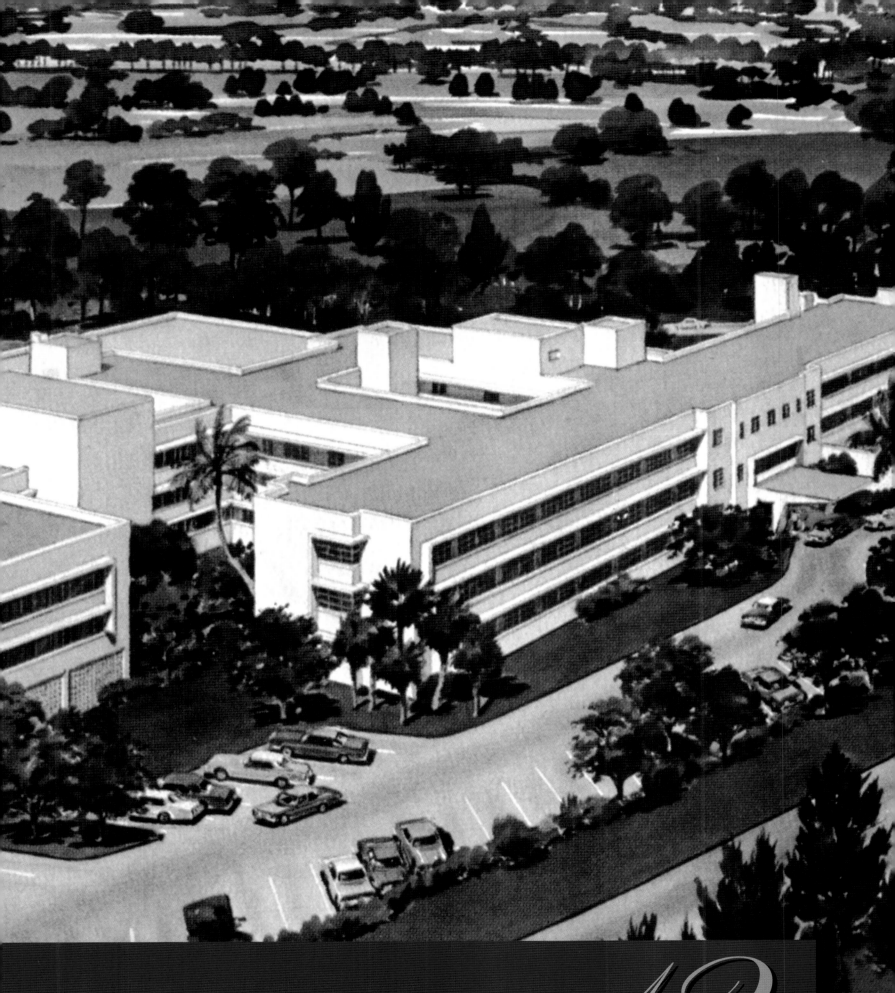

CHAPTER *13*

"The most important change is the coming together of our hospitals in the spirit of working together. While we still have spirited debates, there is more teamwork throughout Baptist Health than ever before."

Brian E. Keeley
President and CEO, Baptist Health Systems
1995

By 1962, the Doctors' Hospital Board of Trustees recognized that even with the new wing, the hospital was still too small. The 1960 openings of South Miami and Baptist Hospitals offered residents more choices, but the added supply of beds could not keep up with the demand. The area had changed dramatically and the booming population brought more and more patients through Doctors' Hospital's doors. As a result, doctors often had to wait for beds before they could admit patients.

In response to the space problems, the Board appointed a Long-Range Planning Committee to study the issue and make recommendations. This was not an easy task. When the hospital first opened, the surrounding land was mostly undeveloped. In the years since, the University of Miami had expanded and houses and apartments dotted the landscape. The committee had to find a way to grow the hospital in limited space. Doctors' occupied approximately 4.6 acres — a small footprint considering the increasing needs.

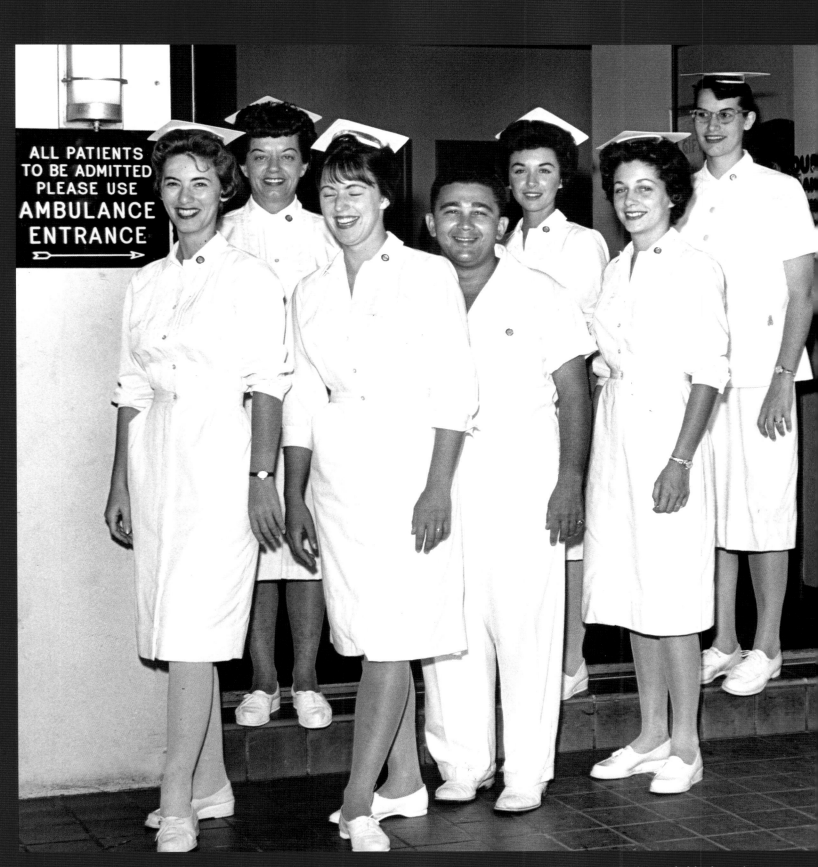

Nurses at Doctors' Hospital provided high-quality care. As a result of the hospital's success, it quickly outgrew its location.

A Mandate to Grow

As the hospital considered its next step, the woman who had shepherded Doctors' from its first days retired. Although she remained close to the hospital and employees after her tenure, Mary Reeder left her post at the Doctors' helm in 1964. To replace her, the Board tapped Joseph McAloon, who most recently had led Memorial Hospital in Hollywood, Florida. A native of Massachusetts, Mr. McAloon had a master's degree in hospital administration from Northwestern University. Before his time at Memorial, Mr. McAloon worked in hospital administration in Massachusetts and was a consultant in Florida.

With years of experience, McAloon brought business acumen to Doctors' Hospital. He had earned a reputation for his no-nonsense approach and was known for his close attention to finances. Longtime employees good-naturedly remember that he would reuse Christmas cards in order to save money. Joking aside, he spent money only when absolutely necessary and always put patient care first. "I believe that the hospital has an obligation to provide the very best possible care to each patient while keeping charges to the absolute minimum," he said later. "The patient, after all, ultimately pays all expenses."

One of Mr. McAloon's priorities was to sort through the expansion issue. For three years, hospital leaders and committee members had weighed the options during more than 100 meetings. They hired a consultant to conduct an area population and economic survey. The results, McAloon reported, "revealed a marked shortage of beds in the hospital service area and further indicated that the bed shortage would be extremely acute and even hazardous by 1970." The mandate for expansion became clear, with two conditions: that the hospital acquire more land and that the expansion add seven or more stories. With enthusiasm, Doctors' began negotiating with the neighboring University of Miami to purchase 1.19 acres.

In November 1965, the City of Coral Gables Zoning Board unanimously approved Doctors' seven-story expansion proposal. The hospital needed one more step — endorsement by the Coral Gables City Commission. Adding politics into the equation was problematic. Neighboring residents protested the plan and raised concerns about both the height of the building and its setbacks on the property. Following a lengthy meeting, the City Commission sent the hospital back to the drawing board.

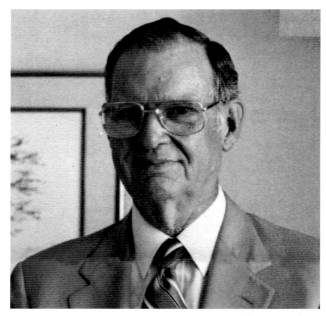

Joseph F. McAloon

Facing page: Doctors' Hospital front entrance, c.1960

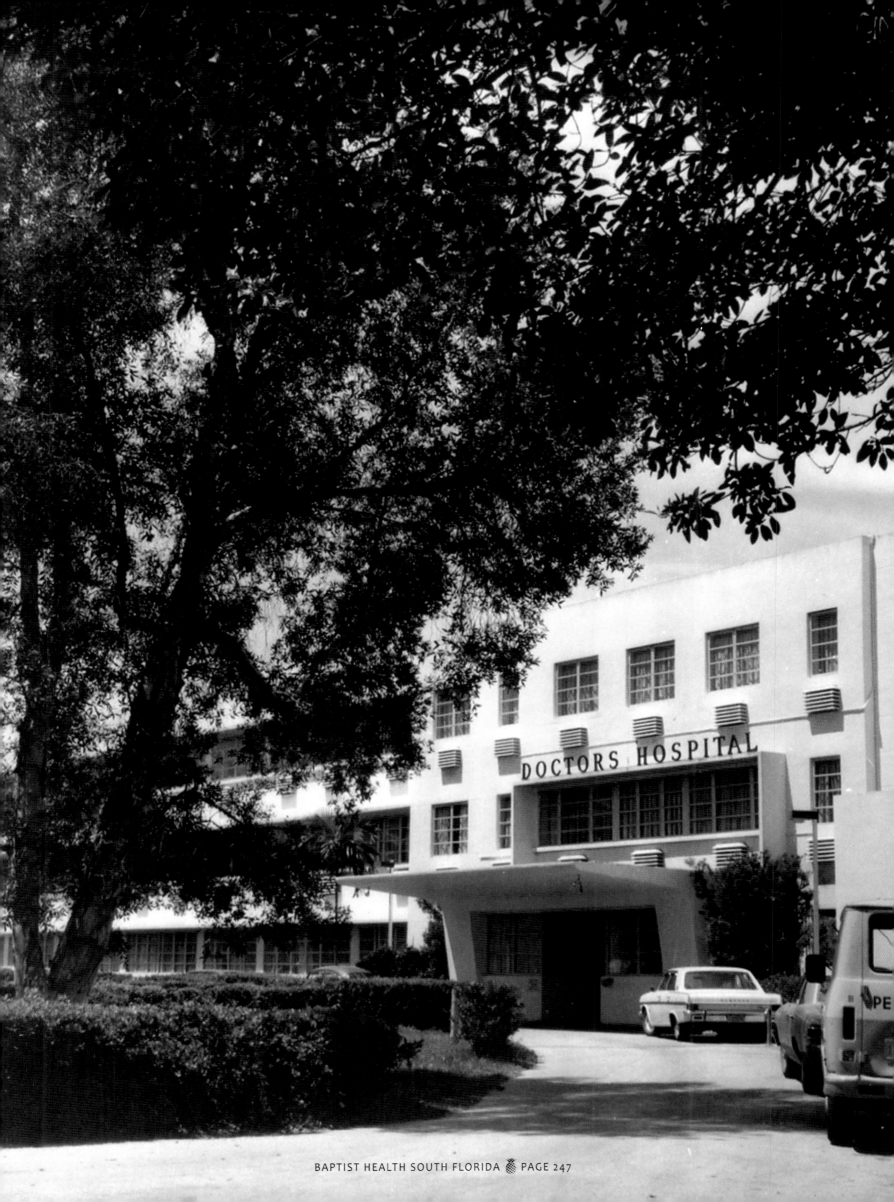

A Tale of Two Hospitals

Doctors' leaders were disappointed. "It has been a most frustrating process as almost every avenue of approach we pursued has ended up as a dead-end street," Mr. McAloon said. Local physicians who had developed the hospital had deep ties to the community and wanted to remain in Coral Gables. The constraints of space and city politics, however, made it a challenge. After "much soul-searching," as Mr. McAloon described it, hospital leaders signed a purchase agreement for 20 acres on S.W. 72nd Avenue between Miller and Bird Roads. The location, McAloon wrote, would "afford a plant which will be much more efficient than anything that could be built on the present hospital site."

Just as the leadership team was set to start the long process of building a new hospital, the political tides shifted. In April 1967, two Coral Gables city commissioners who had voted against the Doctors' proposal lost their seats. The hospital's potential move out of Coral Gables had been an important subtext in the election. By not re-electing the commissioners, the residents seemed to have affirmed their support of Doctors' Hospital. As a result, hospital leaders renewed their quest to remain in Coral Gables. The issue came down to emotions and money. "There is absolutely no doubt in my mind that, from a strictly objective unemotional viewpoint, the construction of a completely new hospital facility on 72nd Avenue would be the direction of choice," McAloon said in September 1967. "Such a project would permit the construction of a completely modern medical complex devoid of any restrictions or compromises."

But the administrator realized that many of the doctors objected to leaving Coral Gables. "There was certainly a strong effort to move the hospital because our location was so restrictive and we had no parking," remembered Norman Kenyon, M.D., who joined Doctors' in 1965 and later joined the Board. "Many members of the medical staff, however, were dead set against it. They considered themselves part of Coral Gables and did not want to move away from their community."

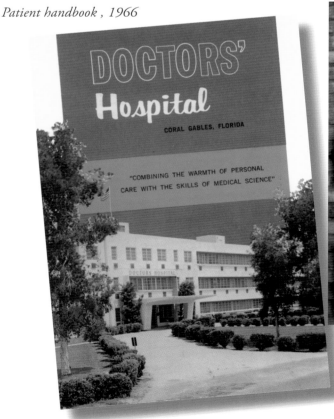

Patient handbook , 1966

In 1966, Doctors' Hospital honored Mary Reeder (far right) for her role as its first administrator. Pictured with Mrs. Reeder are civic leaders Belle and Frank Inscho.

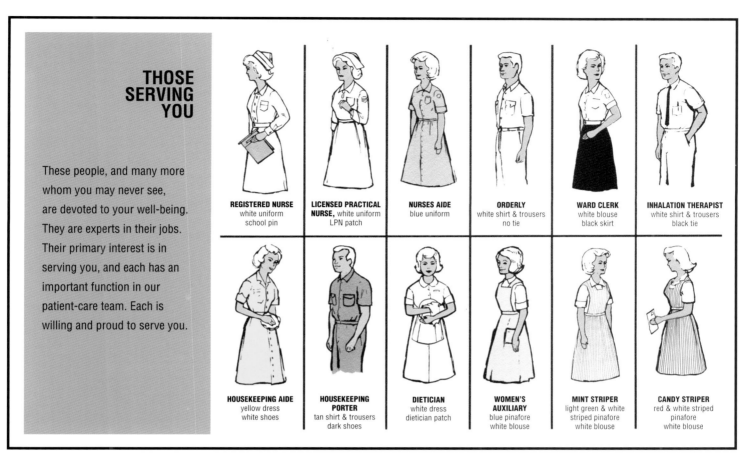

THOSE SERVING YOU

These people, and many more whom you may never see, are devoted to your well-being. They are experts in their jobs. Their primary interest is in serving you, and each has an important function in our patient-care team. Each is willing and proud to serve you.

REGISTERED NURSE	LICENSED PRACTICAL NURSE,	NURSES AIDE	ORDERLY	WARD CLERK	INHALATION THERAPIST
white uniform school pin	white uniform LPN patch	blue uniform	white shirt & trousers no tie	white blouse black skirt	white shirt & trousers black tie

HOUSEKEEPING AIDE	HOUSEKEEPING PORTER	DIETICIAN	WOMEN'S AUXILIARY	MINT STRIPER	CANDY STRIPER
yellow dress white shoes	tan shirt & trousers dark shoes	white dress dietician patch	blue pinafore white blouse	light green & white striped pinafore white blouse	red & white striped pinafore white blouse

This hospital brochure, c.1965, shows the different caregivers at Doctors' Hospital.

In the end, the leadership team recommended that Doctors' expand and renovate its existing facility. Just as it had done in 1965, the hospital plans came before the City Commission for review. "If the commission doesn't approve the new plan, I don't know what we'll do," McAloon told the newspaper. "We'd rather expand at our present site, but if the city doesn't approve these plans, we would certainly consider moving west."

This time around, however, the plan enjoyed broader support. After collaborating with the city and the University of Miami, architects and officials tweaked the design, while maintaining its scope. "It was a masterpiece of compromise for the good of the community," Commissioner W. Keith Phillips Jr. said. The open process even impressed former critics. "In my opinion the hospital has done all it can possibly do to make the new plan practical," said Commissioner Joe Murphy, who originally opposed the hospital's expansion.

In June 1968, the City Commission approved the expansion. But nearby residents brought law-

suits against Coral Gables and the John T. Macdonald Foundation, challenging the plan. The legal action slowed the momentum and forced Doctors' leaders to reconsider. As a result, the leadership team changed directions. They decided to build a new hospital on the property off 72nd Avenue and abandon plans to renovate the Coral Gables hospital. The idea was to run the two sites simultaneously and possibly phase out the Coral Gables campus in a few years.

Revisiting the idea of moving west, away from Coral Gables, stirred deep feelings, especially among the medical staff. As called for by the by-laws, members of the Foundation, the caretakers of Doctors' Hospital, had the final say about the plan. In an emotionally charged meeting on May 12, 1969, several doctors pleaded with the group to remain in Coral Gables at all costs. In a short meeting a month later, the Foundation rejected the relocation plans. Doctors' Hospital's future was now in the hands of the courts and everyone awaited the outcome of the lawsuits.

Changing Plans

The residents' protests were successful and the courts overturned the city's zoning approval. The ruling forced Doctors' to revamp its design yet again. The new, more modest proposal called for a three-story, L-shaped addition on the southwest side of the property. The expansion, estimated to cost nearly $8 million, would add approximately 75 beds, giving the hospital 300 beds. In May 1971, the City Commission approved the project.

One final round in the courts remained after residents again sued to stop the hospital expansion. A year later, the Third District Court of Appeals refused to rehear the case. The long battle to shape the hospital's future was finally resolved. "We believe at this time that all litigation over our plans to build this addition is finished," Mr. McAloon said in August 1972.

On December 4, 1972, community leaders, government officials, physicians and area residents gathered at Doctors' Hospital for the addition's groundbreaking. Those present erupted with applause when L.W. Dowlen, M.D., medical staff president; Joseph McAloon, administrator; and Frederick Poppe, M.D., chairman of the Board for the John T. Macdonald Foundation, shoveled dirt for the ceremonial beginning of construction. In the audience was Mary Reeder, the original force behind the hospital. Hospital founder A.D. Amerise, M.D., was there as well — though not quite so close. Dr. Amerise was a patient at Doctors' but managed to view the festivities from his third-floor window.

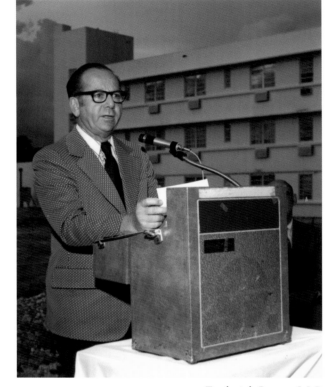

Frederick Poppe, M.D.

By September 1974, phase one of the project was complete. Construction had progressed smoothly, even moving ahead of schedule. In addition to the added patient rooms, the renovation expanded the X-ray department and added a clinical laboratory and Emergency Center. A second phase, including a new operating room suite, pharmacy, medical records room, medical library, physical therapy department, gift shop and doctors' lounge, was set to begin by 1976.

While Doctors' supporters embraced the new era, they also deeply mourned the passing of an earlier one. On June 28, 1976, Mary Reeder died at the hospital so close to her heart. Then, on December 31, 1976, Dr. Amerise died. In a half-year, Doctors' Hospital lost two of its original faces. The hospital community recognized their contribution by dedicating a new CT scanner in their honor.

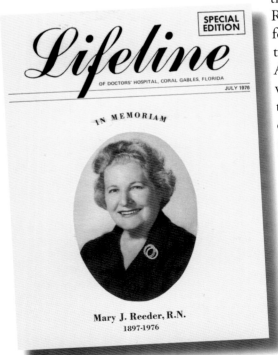

Lifeline

OF DOCTORS' HOSPITAL, CORAL GABLES, FLORIDA

SPECIAL EDITION

JULY 1976

IN MEMORIAM

Mary J. Reeder, R.N.
1897-1976

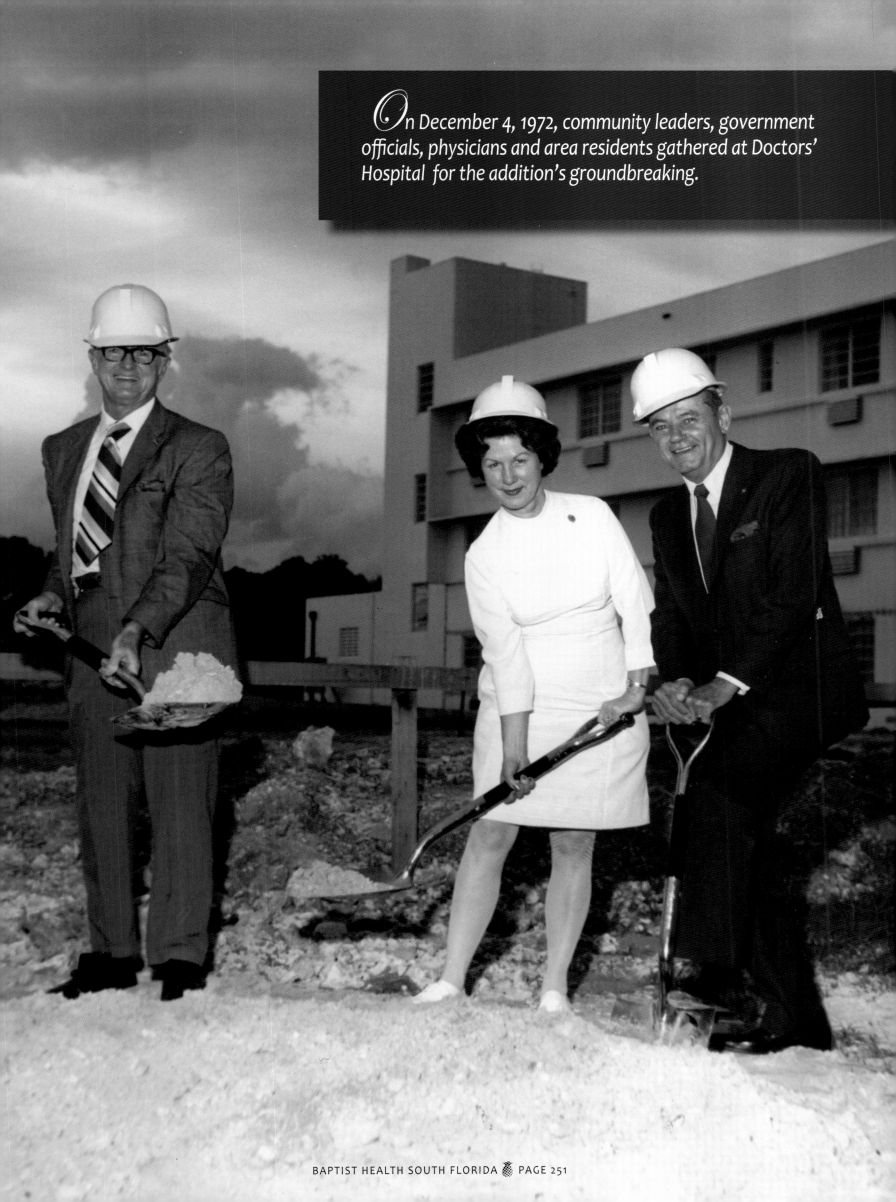

On December 4, 1972, community leaders, government officials, physicians and area residents gathered at Doctors' Hospital for the addition's groundbreaking.

Moving Forward

As the hospital celebrated its 30th anniversary, the expansion was nearly complete. Workers put the finishing touches on the cafeteria, doctors' lounge, medical records room, gift shop and hospital chapel, as well as the clinical areas such as the surgery unit and a new cardiovascular laboratory. The physical plant, often the source of controversy, had been improved and upgraded. Certainly, the results were not perfect. Many still yearned for more space, but Doctors' Hospital had weathered the questions of how to grow and progress by staying true to its roots. The founders had wanted a hospital in Coral Gables. After three decades of push and pull, negotiations and demands, their legacy remained intact.

For Doctors', the next years were about moving forward and adapting, especially to changes in insurance. Like other local hospitals, Doctors' was adjusting to the first stages of managed care and limits on Medicare reimbursements. The idea of containing costs was nothing new. The frugal Joseph McAloon had advocated for cost containment long before it became a catchword in the hospital industry. Doctors' strived to become a model of efficiency. Engineers regulated the air conditioning system to shut off unused areas, switched to fluorescent lights and controlled the water flow in hospital bathrooms. The moves prevented waste and the savings were passed on to patients. Annual surveys consistently showed that Doctors' rates were among the lowest of all South Florida hospitals.

In early 1985, amid an increasingly challenging healthcare environment, Joseph McAloon retired. For 13 years, he had made morning rounds each day, stopping by the nurses' stations to make sure everything was running smoothly. The old-school manager was 67 years old and felt it was time to travel, play golf and visit his grandchildren. As Mr. McAloon reflected on his career, he lamented the changes in his more than 30 years as a hospital administrator. "It used to be that the patient was the main concern," he told *The Miami Herald*. "Now we have to worry about Medicare, malpractice suits, HMOs, cost containment."

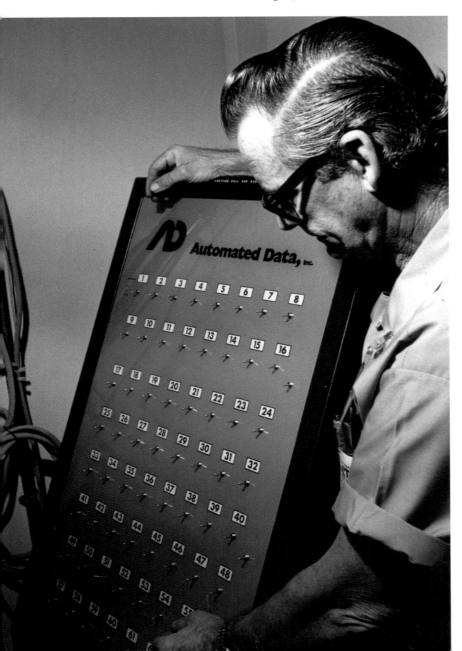

The administrators of Doctors' Hospital were fiscally conservative. The hospital was among the first in the area to install a computer to control the air conditioning, saving nearly $6,000 a month.

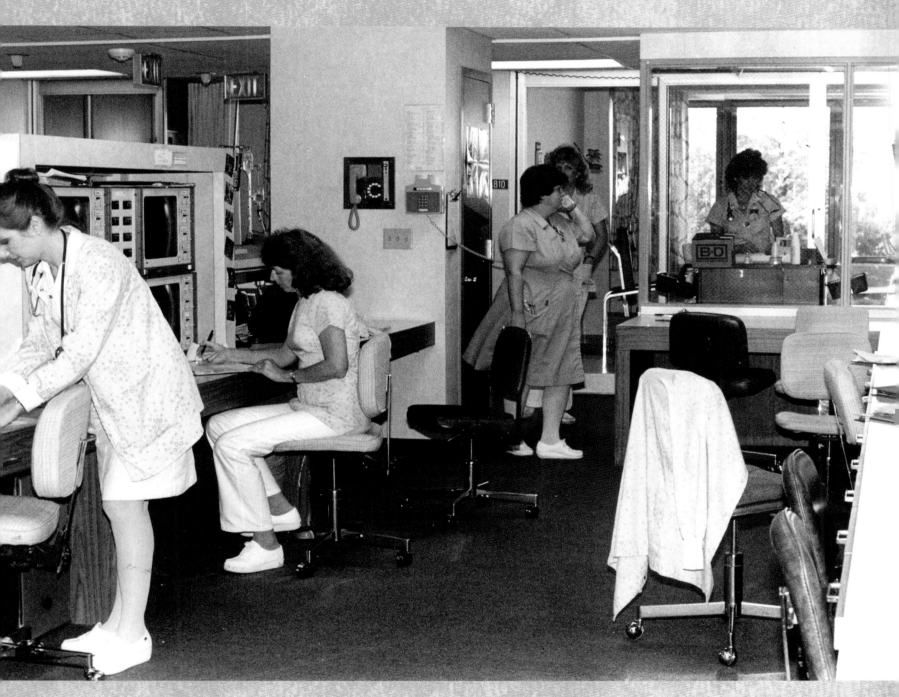

"It used to be the patient was the main concern. Now we have to worry about Medicare, malpractice suits, HMOs, cost containment."

Joseph F. McAloon
Administrator, Doctors' Hospital

With the question settled of whether to relocate, Doctors' Hospital focused on its role in Coral Gables. The nurses in the critical care area (left to right), Toni Nastasi, R.N., Mary Ann Bruce, LPN, Carol Horovitz, R.N., and Critical Care Supervisor Georgiann Peterson, R.N., provided 24-hour care to the sickest patients.

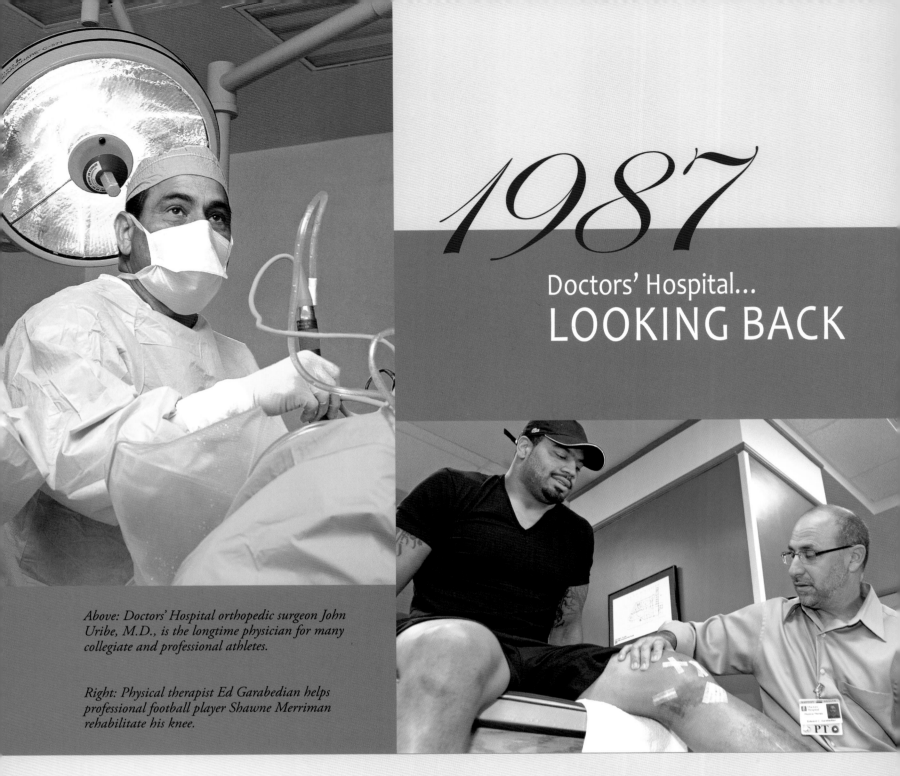

Above: Doctors' Hospital orthopedic surgeon John Uribe, M.D., is the longtime physician for many collegiate and professional athletes.

Right: Physical therapist Ed Garabedian helps professional football player Shawne Merriman rehabilitate his knee.

Sports Medicine

On a typical day, elite athletes walk through the halls of Doctors Hospital. They may be track stars, basketball or football players, or tennis champs. They come to Coral Gables for the hospital's renowned Center for Orthopedics & Sports Medicine. Since 1987, when orthopedic surgeon John Uribe, M.D., set up his practice, Doctors Hospital has provided world-class care to professional and amateur athletes. Through word of mouth, the Center's reputation has spread from Olympic sprinters in the Caribbean to professional football players from around the country. Doctors Hospital is the official sports medicine provider for the Miami Heat, Florida Panthers, Florida International University and the Orange Bowl game.

The hallmark of the Center is its comprehensive, state-of-the-art approach to treating orthopedic and sports injuries. Physicians trailblazing and testing new surgical techniques consult with trainers and physical therapists to create individualized patient care plans. At least half the program's patients are regular active people of all ages. The surgeons also use the latest technology, including robot-assisted surgery and minimally invasive procedures, to help their patients recover. With years of experience, they have refined the care to ensure a quicker return to normal activities.

To succeed McAloon, the Board tapped William Comte, who had been assistant director at Naples Community Hospital. Comte, 32 years old, had a simple directive — to broaden the services offered at Doctors' Hospital. Soon, the hospital added a Diabetes Treatment Center and a Health & Fitness Institute to encourage patients to be personally responsible for their own health. In 1987, the hospital opened a cardiac catheterization laboratory and developed a sports medicine program that would ultimately attract elite athletes from around the world. Two years later, the hospital resumed maternity care. Once the hospital's crowning jewel, the obstetrics unit had closed during the 1970s in a cost-cutting move. Doctors' planned to reopen the service with a new, thoughtful design. Using the concept of single-room maternity care, known as labor-delivery-recovery-postpartum (LDRP), Doctors' would allow women to stay in the same room, one that resembled a bedroom at home, through the entire experience. The family-oriented approach would reduce stress and anxiety, and create a comforting and comfortable environment in which to give birth. "We intend to differentiate ourselves in the market by offering a very progressive concept in obstetrics," Comte said.

In the midst of this expansion, the hospital formed a limited partnership with neighboring Larkin General Hospital, a 112-bed facility at 7031 S.W. 62nd Avenue. Officials believed the alliance would take advantage of each hospital's strengths. Doctors' could use Larkin's psychiatric unit, for example, while Larkin could use Doctors' physical therapists and sports medicine program. More importantly, the partnership would give the two hospitals strength in numbers. "To thrive in today's healthcare market, hospitals will have to be involved with health systems," Comte said as he announced the agreement. "It will be more and more difficult for community hospitals to stand alone."

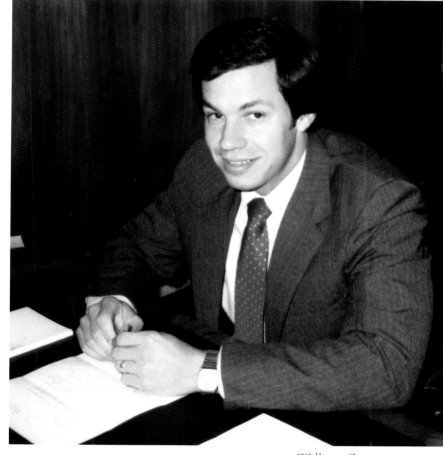

William Comte

"*To* thrive in today's healthcare market, hospitals will have to be involved with health systems. It will be more and more difficult for community hospitals to stand alone."

William H. Comte
Executive Director, Doctors' Hospital

A New Partner

Mr. Comte's words proved prophetic. Despite its partnership with Larkin, the hospital needed more money and support to meet the needs of the modern patient. Doctors' won approval in 1988 from the City Commission to build a much-needed parking garage and physician office building, but lacked the $5 million to build them. In an era when big for-profit companies were buying hospitals and infusing them with capital, Doctors' found a source and opportunity. In 1991, the hospital began negotiating with HealthSouth Rehabilitation Corporation, an Alabama for-profit company that owned 88 rehabilitation centers and acute-care facilities in 24 states. "We needed to survive," remembered Karl Smiley, M.D., a medical staff leader. "The company was offering us a way to keep going during a time when things were very difficult."

After 10 months of negotiations, in January 1992 HealthSouth purchased Doctors' Hospital. The deal also included majority interest in Larkin General Hospital. For Doctors', the sale was necessary if not universally welcomed. The player — whom to sell to — was less an issue than the sale itself. During the process, Baptist Health expressed interest in purchasing Doctors'. At the time, Baptist Health was just beginning its strategy of expansion. "We made a presentation to the Board," remembered Chief Financial Officer Ralph Lawson. "But I think it was a question of timing. We didn't have the experience yet of running a chain of hospitals and the Board really found a better deal with HealthSouth." It boiled down to Doctors' having capital needs and HealthSouth meeting them.

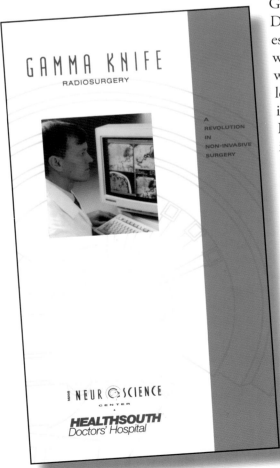

With the deal complete, HealthSouth announced its plans. The company would not make any employee or health services changes, but would renovate the hospital. "This is a very well-financed company and we expect to spend at least $25 million to improve both hospitals [Doctors' and Larkin]," said Richard Scrushy, HealthSouth chairman. "We see strong potential in these hospitals, but right now we think they can be offering better services." Those services included the long-awaited garage and physician office building.

The push ahead, however, met familiar opposition — Doctors' neighbors. A group of nearby residents formed Save Gables Zoning in an effort to stop the expansion, taking their case to the city despite the hospital's efforts to discuss the new construction's appearance. After Coral Gables refused to reconsider the permit, the residents sued. In the midst of the debate, construction began in November 1992. Two months later, the court halted the project, ruling that the city did not properly advertise public hearings on the project.

The court's action sparked public hearings, emotional debate and counter suits. The hospital argued that the garage and offices were desperately needed in light of the growth of outpatient services and competition from other hospitals. "We can only meet the changing needs here in the Gables by keeping pace," said Doctors' Administrator Arthur Tedesco. Tedesco had replaced William Comte, who became regional vice president for HealthSouth.

In April 1994, after more than a year of complicated legal wrangling, the lawsuits were settled in a confidential agreement. The tenuous peace allowed the project to be completed. In addition to the parking garage and medical office building, the hospital added other services, including the first Gamma Knife radiosurgery program in Florida, a high-tech, minimally invasive method to treat brain tumors and other abnormalities in the brain.

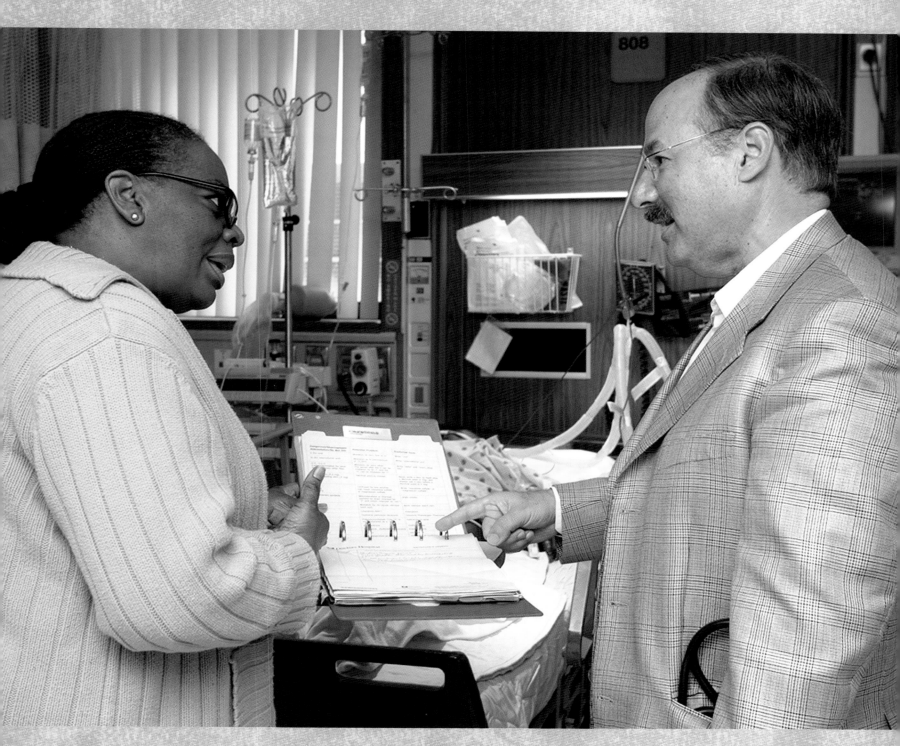

Longtime nurse Barbara Florence, R.N., confers with Richard Levine, M.D.

Despite the growth, pressure on the for-profit hospital mounted. The impact of managed care and declining reimbursements and the increasing financial problems for the parent company left Doctors' Hospital struggling. In 1998, the hospital lost $2.4 million, and a year later $2.3 million. HealthSouth took steps to cut back, including shutting down maternity care. "You have to take a hard look at your product line and concentrate on those that are viable and growing," said Lincoln Mendez, the hospital's chief executive in 1999.

While the sale to HealthSouth began with promise, the relationship deteriorated. Many felt that the parent company, involved in so many facilities throughout the United States, could not focus on the needs of a single hospital in Coral Gables. "I think there was some discontent," Dr. Smiley remembered. "The company was based in Alabama and certain things weren't taken care of — new equipment and infrastructure needs. HealthSouth put money into areas that made money but other parts were left unattended. They had to answer to shareholders so what happened reflected that."

As early as 2001, HealthSouth considered selling Doctors'. By unloading the hospital, the company could focus on its primary specialty — rehabilitation centers. Initial talks with the University of Miami, a natural partner given its close proximity, fell through because the two sides could not come together financially. The idea of a sale took on greater urgency in 2003. HealthSouth had been rocked by scandal, criminal accusation and financial turmoil. Several company leaders had pleaded guilty to fraud and falsifying records. Chief Executive Richard Scrushy, facing his own legal woes, had been fired and ultimately ended up in prison.

On the brink of collapse, HealthSouth had no choice but to sell Doctors' Hospital. "The deal was really one of necessity," Mr. Mendez said. "It became a business call."

Doctors' Hospital drew several suitors. The University of Miami, with the hopes of relieving overcrowded Jackson Memorial Hospital, again expressed interest. Other competitors emerged including Mercy Hospital, Baptist Health and a group of doctors aligned with OrthoNeuro, a North Carolina firm. By August 2003, with the financial strength of the bid as the sole criterion, Baptist Health purchased Doctors' Hospital for $115 million.

Having explored acquiring Doctors' Hospital before, Baptist Health was enthusiastic about the move. "We knew a lot about the hospital and its service area," Mr. Lawson said. "It was never a question about if we should buy it, it was when." Doctors' Hospital fit perfectly within the larger organization. "It was a community hospital with strong ties to the area. We thought it brought a lot to the table," Mr. Keeley said. "It offered some specialized services — orthopedics and the Gamma Knife. We also recognized that it was terribly undercapitalized and we could really grow the hospital."

Some physicians and employees at Doctors' Hospital were uneasy about Baptist Health. "I think there was a little grumbling about control in the beginning," Dr. Smiley remembered. "But I think it quieted once Baptist started making improvements and employees were reassured about their jobs."

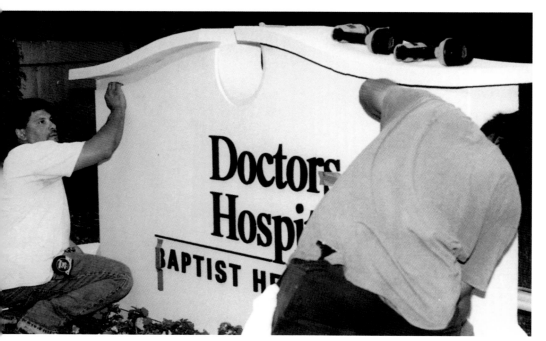

In 2003, Doctors Hospital became a part of Baptist Health. The name — minus the apostrophe — stayed the same.

With an efficiency practiced in previous mergers, Doctors Hospital became part of Baptist Health. Workers synchronized the computer systems, personnel policies and even signage. "The night of the closing was amazing," Lincoln Mendez said. "We were all in a room talking and all of a sudden a crew came in and put up a new sign with the Doctors Hospital name and the Baptist Health pineapple. Where did they come from? The transition went smoothly."

Within a year, due to Baptist Health's financial backing, Doctors added 55 employees, including 40 nurses dedicated to direct patient care. The organization also committed $20 million in capital projects over two years, including new operating room equipment, diagnostic tools and an exterior paint job. "What we've been able to do with Baptist is elevate our services, and compete across the board," Mr. Mendez said. Baptist Health brought an organizational strength, a focus on quality healthcare and the ability to put resources where they were needed. "There is no doubt that with all the improvements and growth, the wisdom of selling to Baptist Health has been reaffirmed," Dr. Kenyon said.

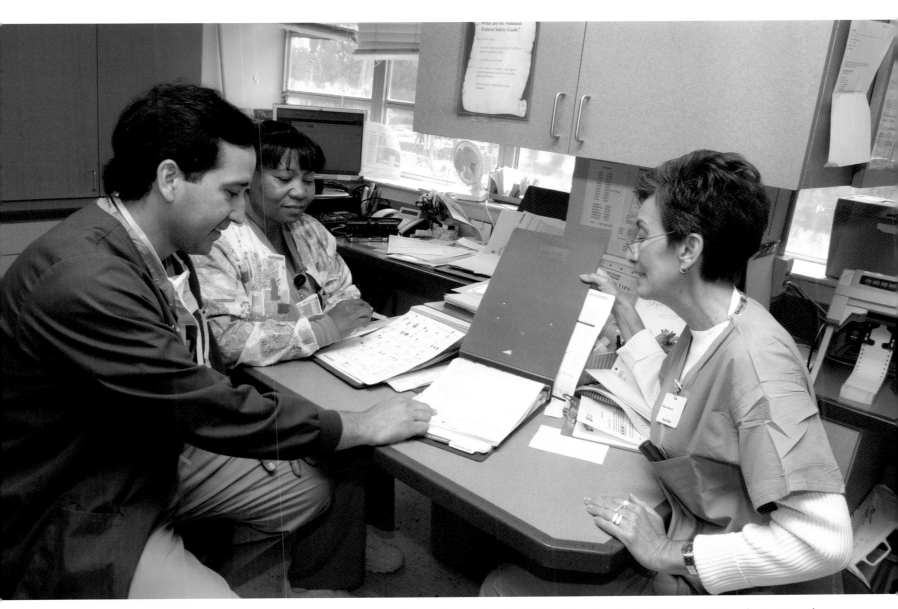

Left to right: Jose Davila, M.D., Beverley Davis, R.N., and Foundation Board member Bonnie Blaire review a chart. Ms. Blaire visited Doctors Hospital as part of Baptist Health's Shadow a Nurse Day.

New Directions

As Baptist Health added Doctors into the fold, it made another important strategic decision — to build a new Homestead Hospital. For several years, Baptist Health leaders had pondered the future of Homestead Hospital. In 2000, Baptist Health had negotiated with the Public Health Trust, which oversees Jackson Memorial Hospital in Miami, about a possible public/not-for-profit partnership to run Homestead Hospital. The two sides were not able to hammer out an agreement.

Baptist Health leaders were on their own to decide the hospital's future. The aging building, although repaired after Hurricane Andrew, needed considerable improvements. It was too small and outdated to meet the demands of modern medicine. After weighing the cost of renovations, Baptist Health, at the urging of Board Chairman George Cadman III, decided to build a new hospital at a new site — the first new full-service hospital facility in Miami-Dade in three decades.

Without a doubt, they were encouraged by Homestead's changing demographics. In the years since the hurricane, the area had become one of South Florida's fastest growing. Young people were flocking south, drawn by available land and reasonable home prices. Patient volumes were steadily climbing and the number of babies born at Homestead Hospital had increased 50 percent since 1997, reaching 1,300 by 2001. More than 33,000 visits to the Emergency Room were logged annually.

Considering the potential growth of Homestead, Baptist Health finalized plans for a 300,000-square-foot hospital on more than 60 acres on the north side of Campbell Drive (S.W. 312th Street) in full view from Florida's Turnpike. "This is very good news for the people of Homestead and south Miami-Dade County," said Bo Boulenger, the hospital's CEO at the time of the announcement. "The new hospital will be three times larger than the current one, which will allow us to incorporate new services and enhance the quality of care we provide."

In 2005, Baptist Health marked the 10th year of its merger with South Miami, Homestead and Mariners Hospitals. The decade had been marked

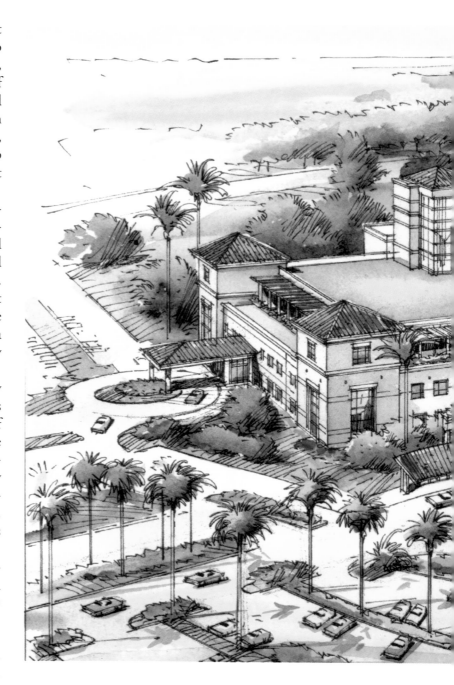

by growth. In addition to the hospitals, Baptist added Medical Plazas in Palmetto Bay, Coral Gables, Westchester, West Kendall and Doral. With 2,000 affiliated physicians and more than 10,000 employees, revenues exceeded $1 billion. And on the horizon was more growth. "The years ahead," Brian Keeley said in 2005, "are going to be filled with as many achievements as the years past."

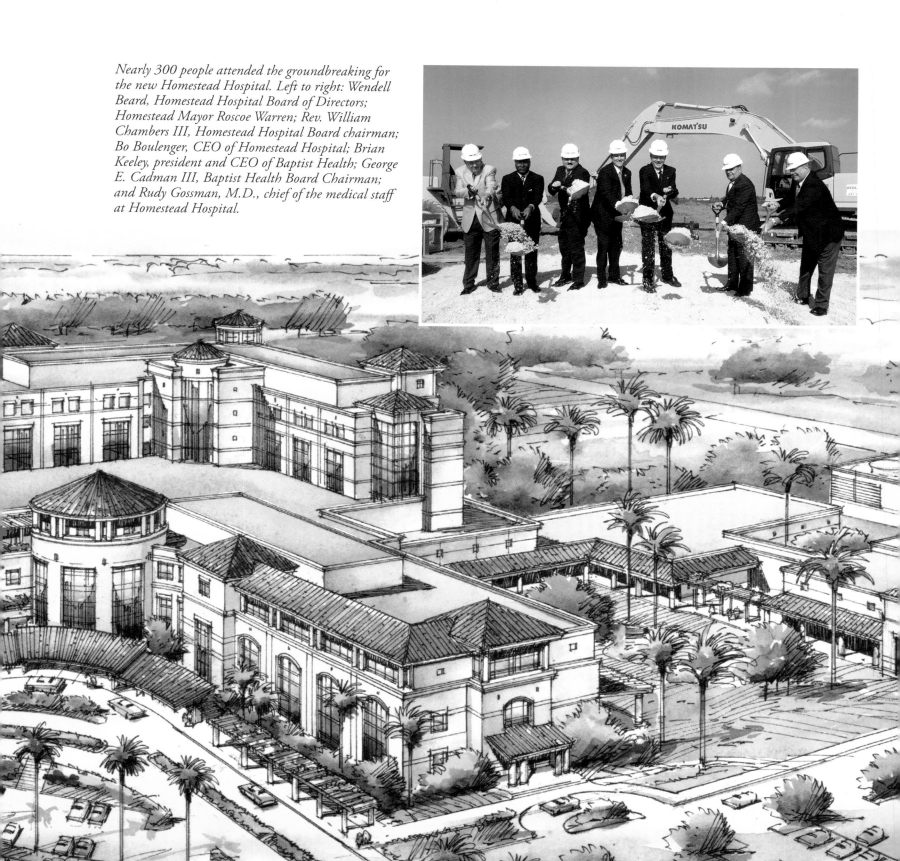

Nearly 300 people attended the groundbreaking for the new Homestead Hospital. Left to right: Wendell Beard, Homestead Hospital Board of Directors; Homestead Mayor Roscoe Warren; Rev. William Chambers III, Homestead Hospital Board chairman; Bo Boulenger, CEO of Homestead Hospital; Brian Keeley, president and CEO of Baptist Health; George E. Cadman III, Baptist Health Board Chairman; and Rudy Gossman, M.D., chief of the medical staff at Homestead Hospital.

"This is very good news for the people of Homestead and south Miami-Dade County. The new hospital will be three times larger than the current one, which will allow us to incorporate new services and enhance the quality of care we provide."

Bo Boulenger
CEO, Homestead Hospital

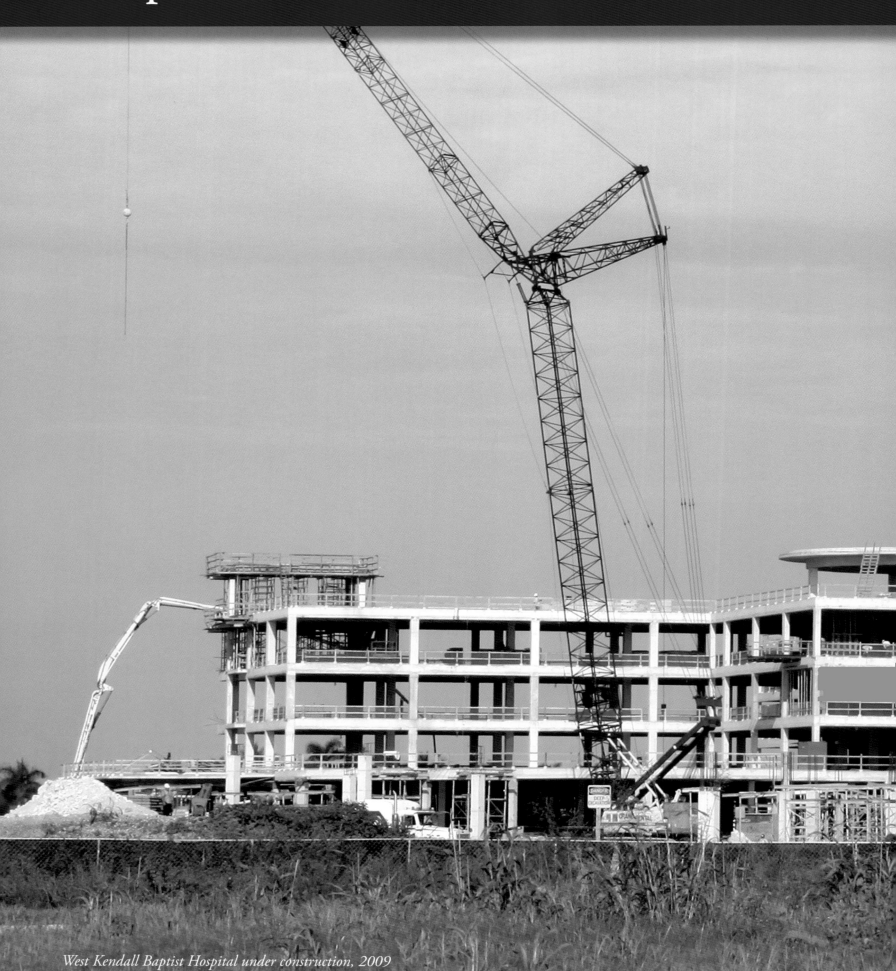

Baptist Health of Tomorrow

West Kendall Baptist Hospital under construction, 2009

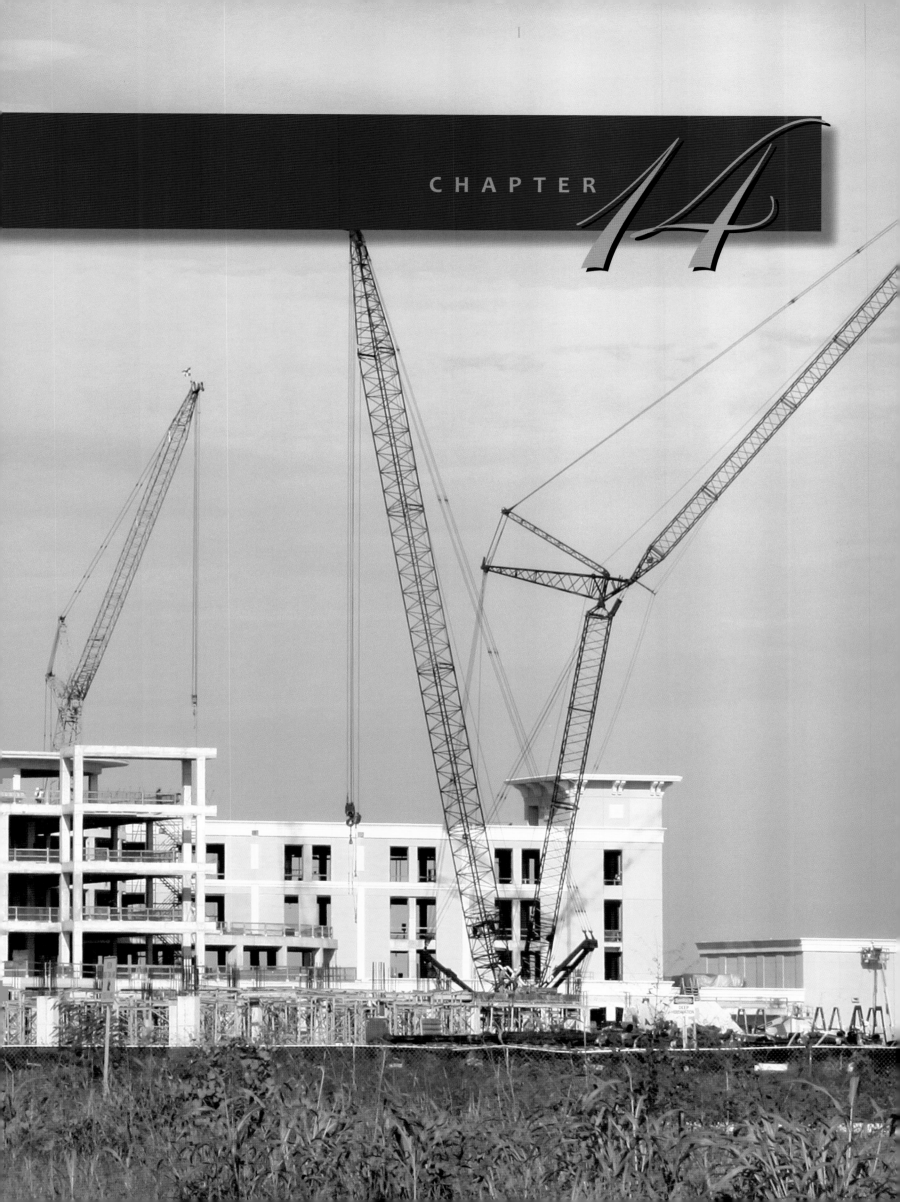

CHAPTER *14*

"We don't plan for the next five or 10 years. We plan for the next 50 years. Baptist Health has always focused on the long term. We think generational. We make decisions that will ensure our continued success for many years down the road."

Brian E. Keeley
President and CEO, Baptist Health South Florida
2010

By mid-2007, Baptist Health's achievements included the eagerly anticipated opening of the new Homestead Hospital. After three years of construction, the $135 million, five-story facility was complete. With 21st century technology and plenty of natural light, soothing colors and open spaces, the hospital looked more like an upscale hotel. "It's a prototype for the future," said Homestead Hospital CEO Bill Duquette, who assumed the leadership role in the fall of 2006 after Bo Boulenger was tapped to head Baptist Hospital. "The entire hospital is built with the patient in mind — from the large private rooms to the wireless network. I consider it the Taj Mahal of hospitals."

Architects also designed the building to withstand category five hurricane conditions. Two high-powered generators — similar to those used in power plants — were installed in an elevated concrete structure. The exterior shell was made of eight-inch-thick concrete panels. The half-inch-thick laminated windows withstood tests of 155-mile-per-hour winds. "The standards we've put in place will help protect patients and staff and ensure the building is around for a very long time," said Tom Tulloch, corporate vice president for construction management.

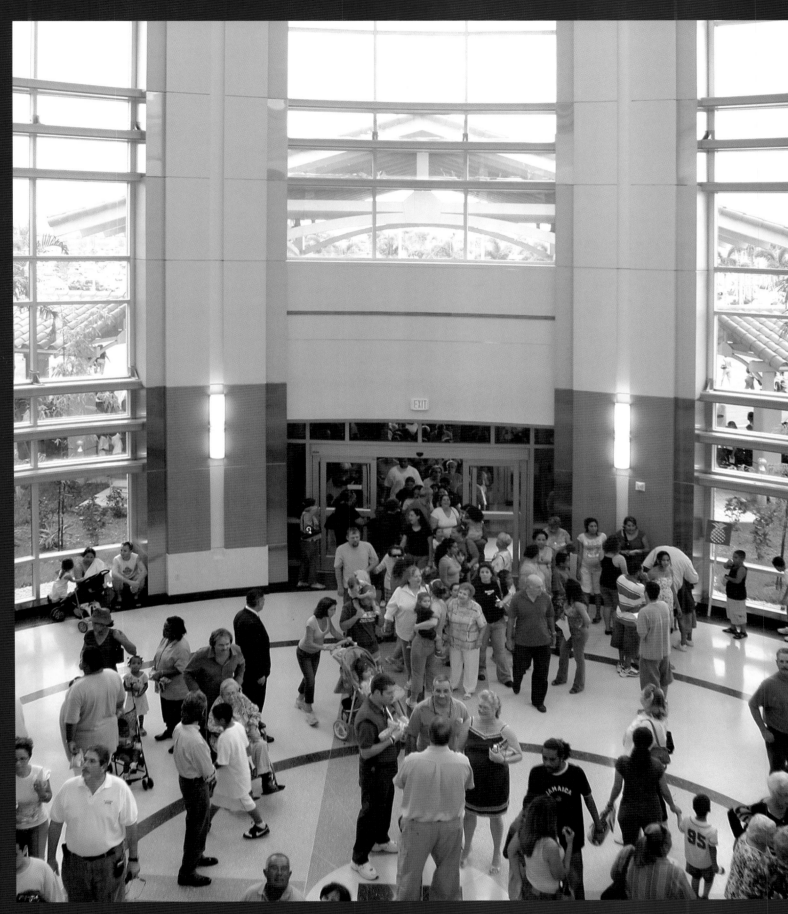

The new Homestead Hospital is an impressive building, complete with an atrium that allows for plenty of natural light.

Moving Day

As workers put the final touches on the new hospital, employees planned for the move. The process was complicated. Staff needed to be trained at the new hospital, which included an unfamiliar layout and different equipment and technology. Patients had to be transferred safely. "We spent a lot of time on just how to move," Duquette remembered. "We had to coordinate everything and, most importantly, ensure the well-being of the critically ill patients during the transition."

Administrators chose Sunday, May 6, as moving day. Hospital staff discharged as many patients as possible and loaded the remaining 104 in ambulances. Police barricaded the streets as the ambulances drove in a caravan the fewer than four miles to Homestead Hospital's new home. Residents watched the procession and cheered. The precision planning paid off. Administrators hoped to complete the move in four hours and accomplished the feat with 15 minutes to spare. "On the day we moved, it was a community event," said Chief Nursing Officer Gail Gordon, R.N. "We had police redirecting traffic and doctors handing out water to the crowd. There was really a sense that Baptist Health was doing something to serve Homestead."

In return, the community embraced the hospital. At a public open house a few weeks before the move, attendance reached 7,000 — 5,000 more than expected. "I think that at the event I understood what this hospital really meant. The entire community wanted to be there," Duquette said. "Everything about the residents' response, from the open house to the cheering crowds on moving day, reaffirmed Homestead's appreciation for Baptist Health's investment."

The investment came despite the calculated impact on the bottom line. The new hospital was projected to lose $35 million over the first five years. With the economic downturn and a high population of uninsured residents, the actual losses were much greater — reaching more than $20 million per year. "When we made a decision to build the hospital, we went in with our eyes open," Baptist Health CEO Brian Keeley said. "We knew that the hospital was the lifeblood of the city and our Board of Trustees understood its importance. We wanted to show our faith in the area and its people." The new hospital also supported Baptist Health's faith-based, not-for-profit mission. "We brought compassionate medical care to an underserved community," Keeley said. "A for-profit company would never have built a new hospital for Homestead. We don't have to answer to shareholders so we can direct our assets from our profitable operations to Homestead. It is a case of our margin driving our mission."

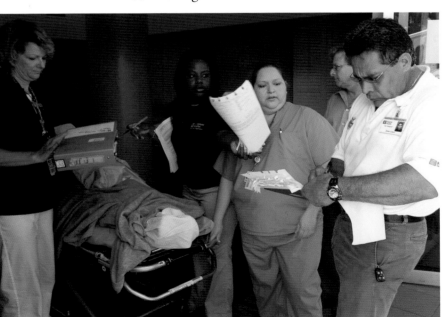

Moving patients from the old building to the new location required months of planning. On moving day, employees worked together to ensure a smooth and safe transition.

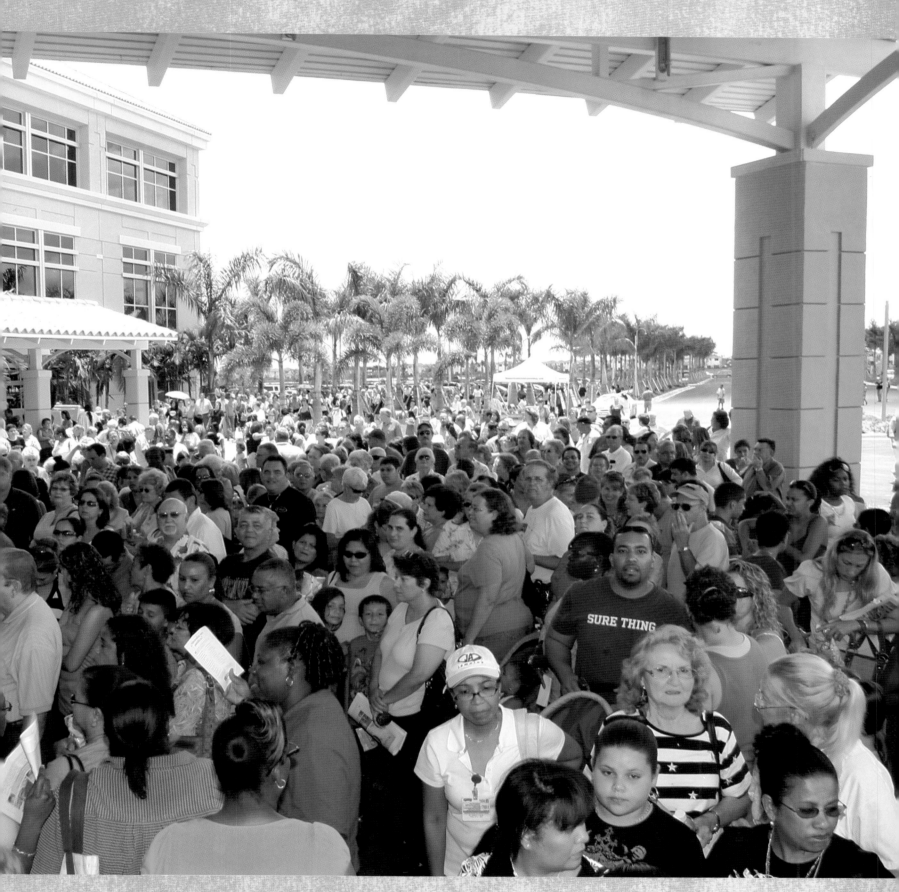

The Homestead community embraced the new hospital. At a public open house a few weeks before the move, more than 7,000 people attended.

Looking West

In 2008, Baptist Health celebrated a groundbreaking for another new hospital, one that had been contemplated for nearly a decade. West Kendall Baptist Hospital would rise on 30 acres at S.W. 96th Street and 162nd Avenue. "We realized that this was one of the fastest growing areas in Miami-Dade County," said Chief Strategic Officer Ana Lopez-Blazquez. "Many of the residents came to Baptist Hospital for care, often traveling 45 minutes in traffic. We knew the need was there."

Baptist Health filed a letter of intent with state regulators in February 2003. The application included 4,337 letters of support from residents. "It is clear that the community is behind our effort to bring healthcare services closer to them," Mr. Keeley said at the time. After navigating through regulatory and zoning processes, Baptist Health finally received the go-ahead. Scheduled to open in 2011, the $200 million, four-story hospital will include 133 beds, four operating rooms, maternity care, diagnostic services, an Emergency Center expected to handle 45,000 visits annually, and an adjacent, four-story medical office building.

West Kendall Baptist Hospital will be "green" — reflecting the latest in environmentally conscious design. The hospital will feature energy-efficient lighting, recycled materials, native plants and eco-friendly paints, tiles and accessories. It is expected to be the first hospital in Miami-Dade County to earn LEED certification (Leadership in Energy and Environmental Design) by the Green Building Council, a nonprofit group that promotes environmentally friendly buildings. "This is part of our environmental commitment throughout the organization," said George Foyo, chief administrative officer, who leads Baptist Health's green initiatives. "We want to be the role model for sustainability for hospitals across the country. West Kendall Baptist Hospital helps us meet this goal."

The hospital will also focus on primary care. Through an academic affiliation with Florida International University's Herbert Wertheim College of Medicine, West Kendall Baptist will house an accredited family practice residency. "This is an exciting and natural fit," said Javier Hernandez-Lichtl, CEO of West Kendall Baptist Hospital. "By teaching tomorrow's primary care doctors, we are really serving the community's needs. We will have a tremendous synergy with FIU, combining Baptist Health's tradition of high quality and service with the cutting-edge practices of a teaching facility." Hernandez-Lichtl is chief academic affiliation officer for Baptist Health and associate dean of the FIU medical school. More than 100 Baptist Health physicians are also on the medical school's faculty, with several heading departments.

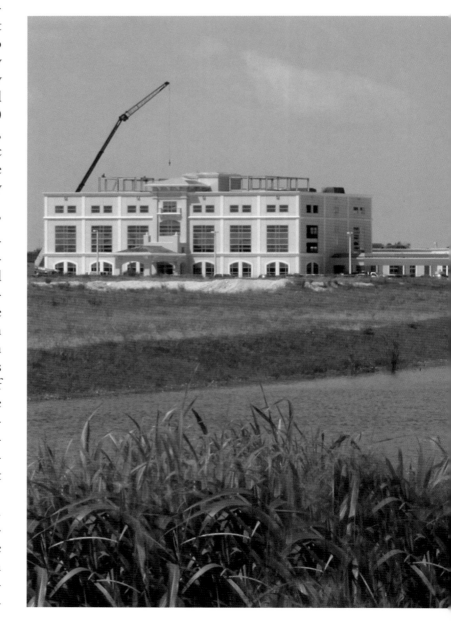

"*This is an exciting and natural fit. By teaching tomorrow's primary care doctors, we are really serving the community's needs. We will have a tremendous synergy with FIU, combining Baptist Health's tradition of high quality and service with the cutting-edge practices of a teaching facility.*"

Javier Hernandez-Lichtl
CEO, West Kendall Baptist Hospital

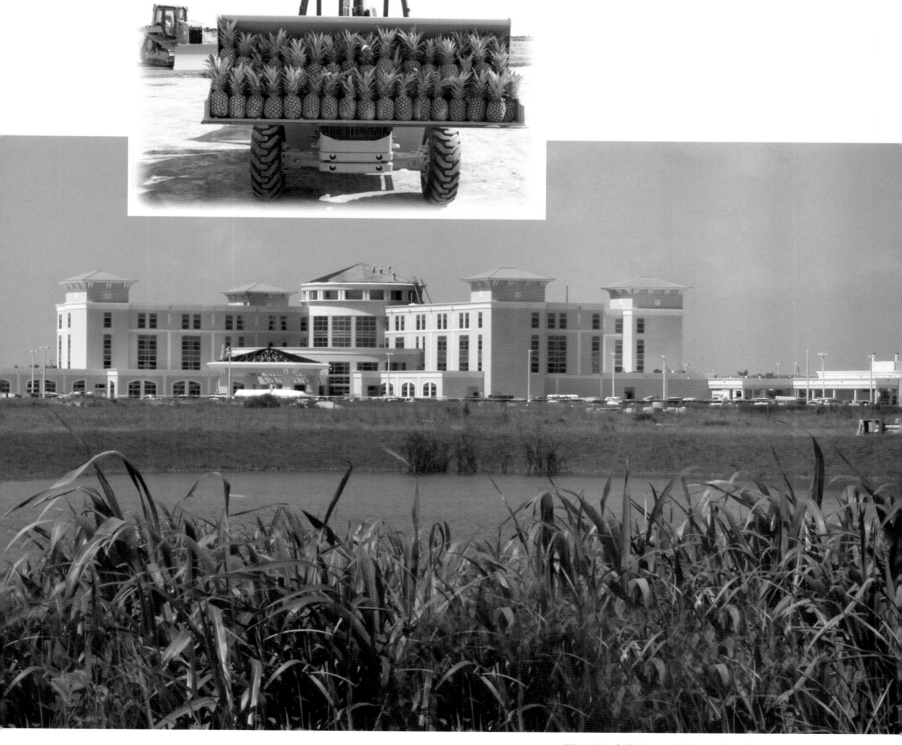

West Kendall Baptist Hospital under construction

Far right: In June 2010, Baptist Hospital's Yvonne Barbato, R.N., cared for Lucinda Long during Baptist Children's Hospital's ninth Day of Smiles. Doctors and other hospital staff volunteered their expertise to correct cleft lips and palates, drooping eyes, scars, burns and other deformities.

Right: Rufina Tinoca (left) received free cataract surgery, enabling her to go back to work as a baker. Her eyesight had gotten so bad she could barely see her own grandchildren.

Bottom: Joel Levin, M.D., repaired a cleft lip as part of the 2010 Day of Smiles.

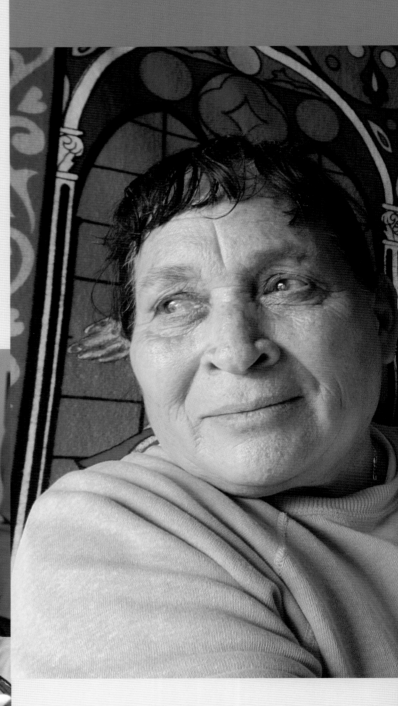

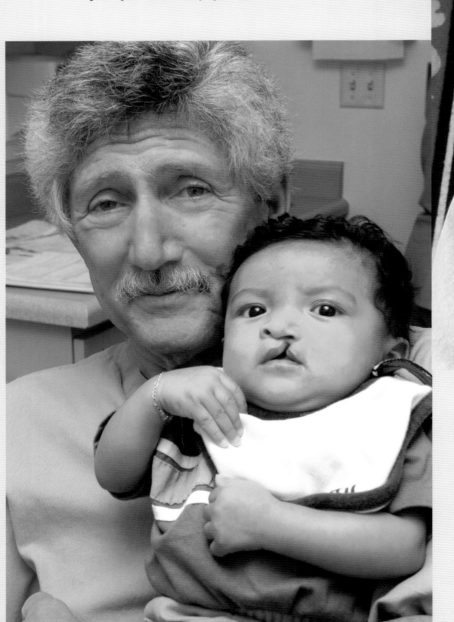

Baptist Health South Florida...

CHARITY CARE PROGRAM

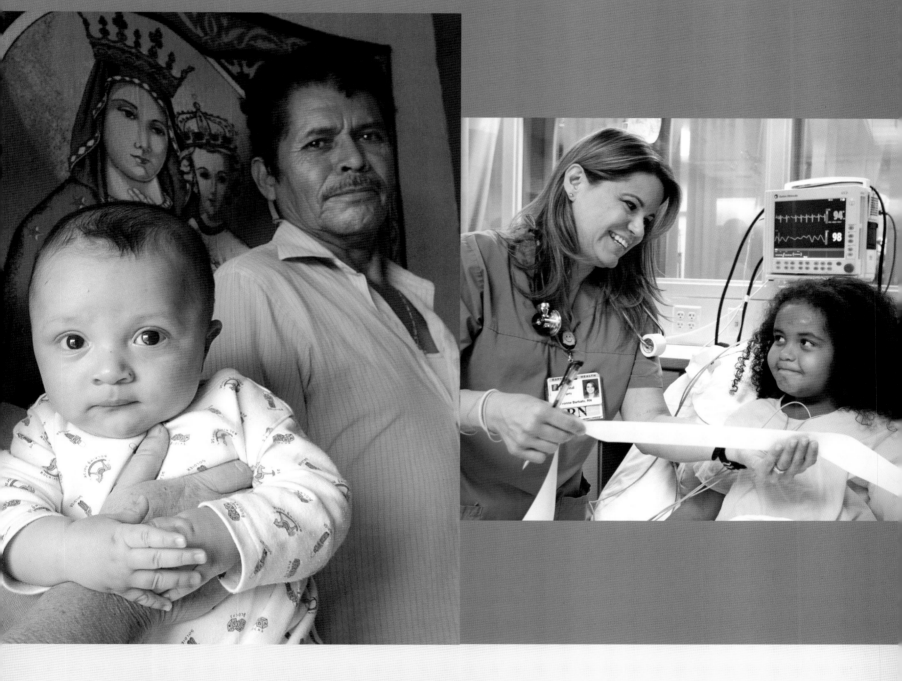

Helping the less fortunate is part of Baptist Health's not-for-profit mission. Baptist Health hospitals give free or reduced-fee care to uninsured patients who qualify. In addition, Baptist Health supports several South Florida clinics for the poor, including the Good Health Clinic in Tavernier, the Good News Care Center in Florida City, the Open Door Health Center in Homestead and the South Miami Children's Clinic. The clinics offer primary care or specialty care to residents who qualify. Clinic patients receive free care at Baptist Health hospitals. Baptist Health also sponsors hundreds of free or low-cost medical screenings and health education programs. In 2009, Baptist Health provided more than $215 million in charity care and other community benefits. "Our charity care policy reflects our desire to give back generously to the communities we serve," said Brian Keeley. "We have a long history of giving compassionate care to all and we remain deeply committed to this principle."

Looking North

Beyond West Kendall, Baptist Health expanded into other neighborhoods. Baptist Medical Plazas opened at Miami Lakes (2006), Tamiami Trail (2007) and Country Walk (2008). The formula — high-quality care with an emphasis on customer service in neighborhood centers — continued its remarkable success. "Our model works," said Patricia Rosello, CEO of Baptist Outpatient Services. "We offer convenience to patients away from the crowded hospitals and we wow them with our service. They keep coming back." The numbers tell the story. In 2004, the diagnostic side of Baptist Outpatient Services performed 144,313 tests and procedures. By 2008, with the addition of more centers, the number had jumped to 206,299. Urgent care visits increased from 66,274 in 2006 to 90,812 in 2008.

In April 2009, Baptist Health took its outpatient strategy north, beyond the county line, with the opening of Baptist Medical Plaza at Coral Springs. A second outpatient facility in Davie opened in May 2010 and locations in Pembroke Pines, Plantation and Weston are in the planning stages. The centers marked Baptist Health's first foray into Broward County. "It is a bold move for us," Rosello said. "We know it's a bit out of our comfort zone, a bit on the fringe. At the same time, the expansion of outpatient services is important financially. And while there's some competition in the area, we believe the residents will welcome us, recognize that we offer something unique and appreciate our commitment to quality care and service."

The expansion into untested territory does bring some risks. "We are broadening our boundaries. We are not in areas where our name is identified with a longstanding hospital," Rosello said. "We will see if our brand is as good as we say it is."

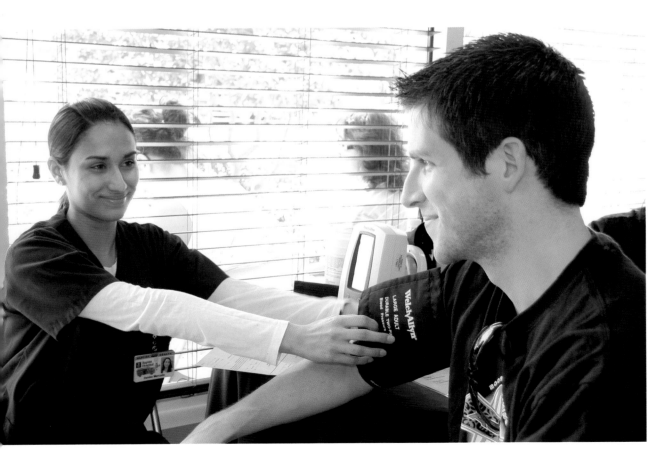

Left: Baptist Medical Plaza at Coral Springs marked the organization's first entry into Broward County. At the community opening, Denise Mercado, R.N., takes a visitor's blood pressure.

Facing page bottom: Maria Pilar Martinez, M.D., medical director of women's imaging at the Baptist Health Breast Center

Right: The map shows Baptist Health's expansion into Broward County. Medical Plazas are in Coral Springs and Davie with Pembroke Pines opening soon. Plans are under way for locations in Plantation and Weston as well.

Below: Opening of Baptist Medical Plaza at Tamiami

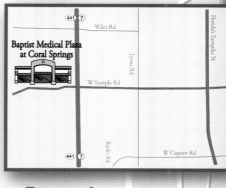

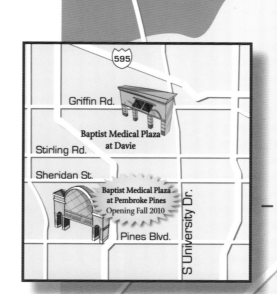

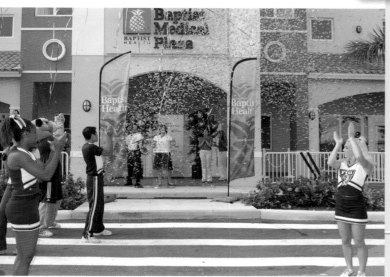

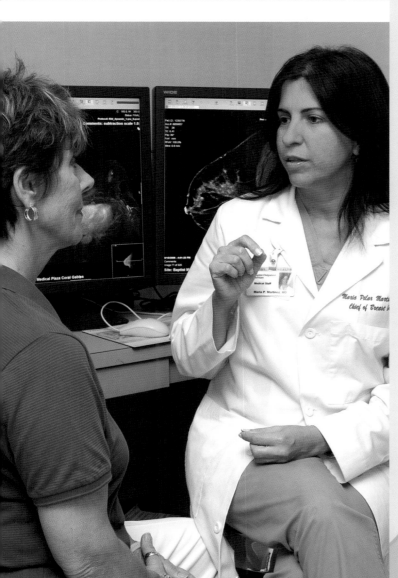

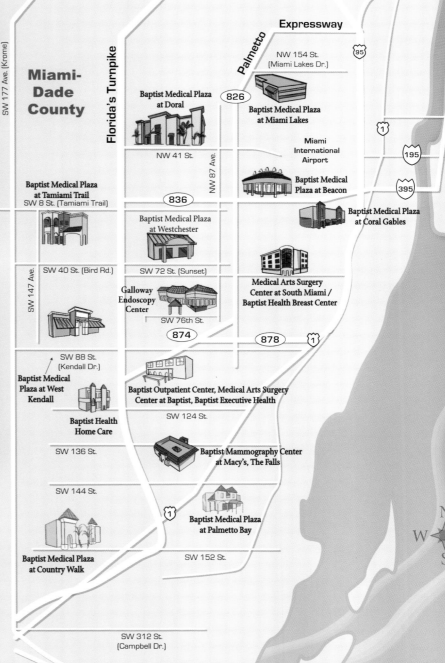

Looking Abroad

The Baptist Health brand has found success internationally. Because of South Florida's cultural diversity and location, the area is a natural draw for foreign patients seeking healthcare. Both South Miami Hospital and Baptist Hospital treated international patients before the merger. With the growth of Baptist Health, the international program has developed into one of the largest in the United States.

Today, Baptist Health's international program treats nearly 12,000 patients a year from dozens of countries — primarily from Latin America and the Caribbean. "South Florida is a multicultural area," said George Foyo, Baptist Health's chief administrative officer. "International patients find the environment friendly and welcoming, and give high marks for patient satisfaction."

A multilingual staff of more than 50 employees coordinates the details of patients' visits. Representatives schedule medical tests and appointments, help with travel arrangements and transportation, counsel family members and coordinate insurance benefits. "Our employees understand that seeking treatment away from home can be unsettling. We provide international patients unparalleled personal attention and service by handling all the details," said Michael Stein, corporate vice president of International. "Our program is one of the leading hospital-based centers in the country because of our commitment to exceptional service."

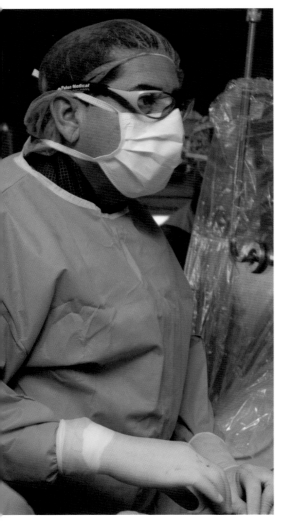

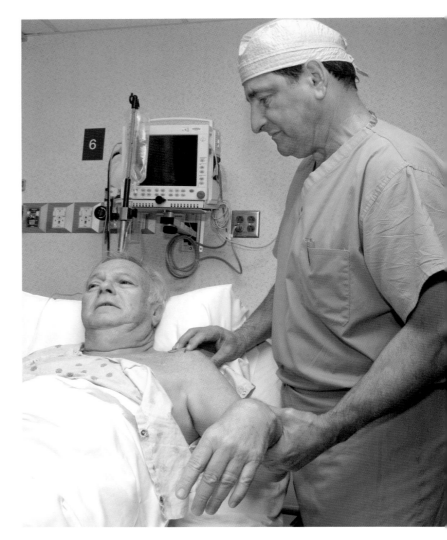

Above: John Uribe, M.D., of Doctors Hospital's Center for Orthopedics & Sports Medicine, is an international leader in the field of orthopedics and sports medicine. The team at Doctors Hospital, including Harlan Selesnick, M.D., Keith Hechtman, M.D., John Zvijac, M.D., Thomas San Giovanni, M.D., as well as other orthopedic specialists, treats patients from around the world.

Left: International patients come to Baptist Cardiac & Vascular Institute for its innovative approach to treating cardiovascular disease. Ramon Quesada, M.D., the Institute's medical director of interventional cardiology, uses minimally invasive techniques to repair structural problems in the heart.

Baptist Health South Florida...

ON THE HONOR ROLL

Baptist Health has been lauded widely for its workplace environment. The organization supports employees with progressive policies such as family-friendly hours, a comprehensive wellness program and professional development. "Our employees are the 'heart and soul' of Baptist Health," CEO Brian Keeley said. "We believe in treating them well and offering innovative employee programs. They are our most valued asset." Baptist Health's many awards include:

- 100 Best Companies to Work For: FORTUNE magazine (1998, 1999, 2003-2010)

- Most Diverse of FORTUNE 100 Best Companies to Work For (2010)

- 100 Best Places to Work in Healthcare: Modern Healthcare magazine (2008-2010)

- 100 Best Companies for Working Mothers and Working Mother Hall of Fame: Working Mother magazine (1989, 1991-1996, 1999-2002, 2004-2010)

- Best Employers for Healthy Lifestyles: Platinum Award to Baptist Health from the National Business Group on Health (2005-2010)

- Corporate Health Achievement Award: American College of Occupational and Environmental Medicine (2010)

- Great Workplace Award for having a productive and engaged workforce: Gallup (2009)

- 100 Most Wired Hospitals and Health Systems: Hospital & Health Networks (1999, 2001-2003, 2005-2009)

- Best Florida Hospital Workplace (Large Hospital): Florida Hospital Association (2009)

- Sustainable South Florida Award: Inaugural award to Baptist Health for environmentally friendly practices from the Greater Miami Chamber of Commerce (2009)

- Excellence in Healthcare Award: South Florida Business Journal honored Baptist Health South Florida in the hospital category (2009)

- Gold Medal for an Organization: Miami Today Gold Medal Awards (2009)

- Top Five Nonprofit Companies for Female Executives: National Association of Female Executives (2007-2009)

Proudly showing off their Fortune 100 Best Companies to Work For shirt are (left to right) Susie Simmonds, R.N., Deborah Espana, operating room tech, and Shirley Anderson, R.N. Baptist Health has earned this award 10 times.

Baptist Health South Florida...

Reaching Out

Baptist Health employees volunteer for a variety of community organizations. They help build homes for Habitat for Humanity, refurbish schools, beautify parks, feed the homeless and participate in United Way events, among other projects. They also give medical screenings and first aid to athletes competing in the Special Olympics and organize the American Cancer Society's Relay for Life on the campuses of Baptist and Homestead Hospitals. "Baptist Health employees are tremendously dedicated and caring people, volunteering their time, efforts and passion almost every weekend to improve the quality of life in our community. It's just the Baptist Health way," said Phillis Oeters, vice president of Community and Government Relations.

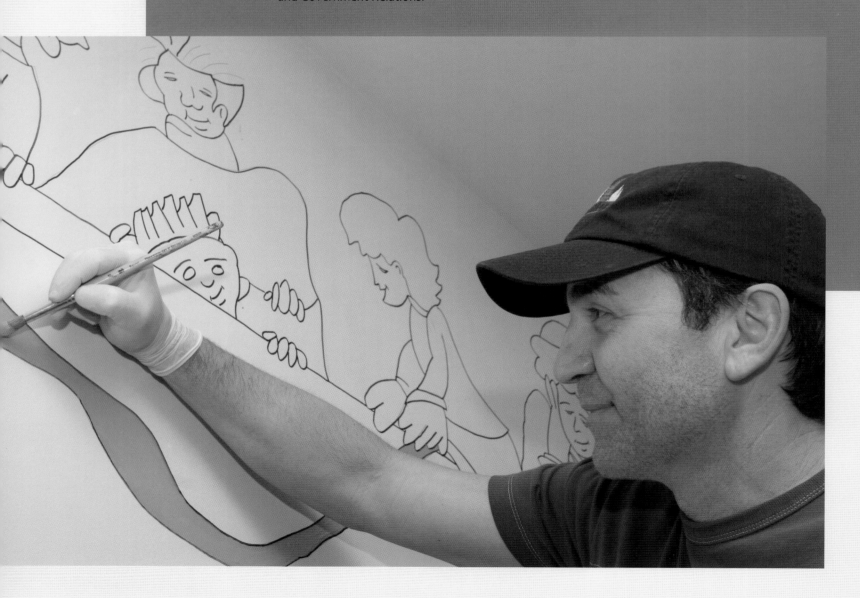

Right: Homestead Hospital's Xohan Lafont takes part in a Baptist Health day at the Habitat for Humanity development in South Dade. Baptist Health has sponsored more than 20 Habitat homes.

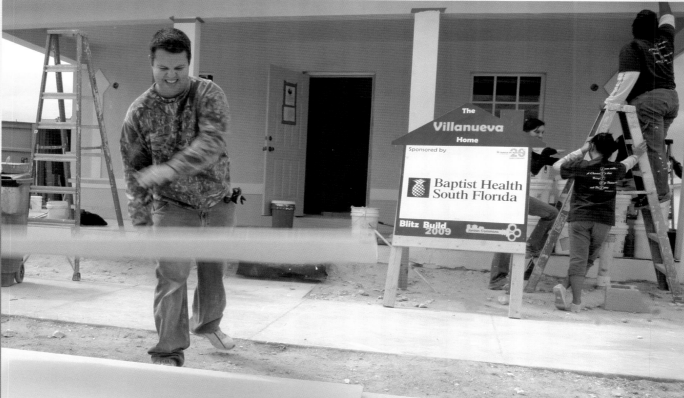

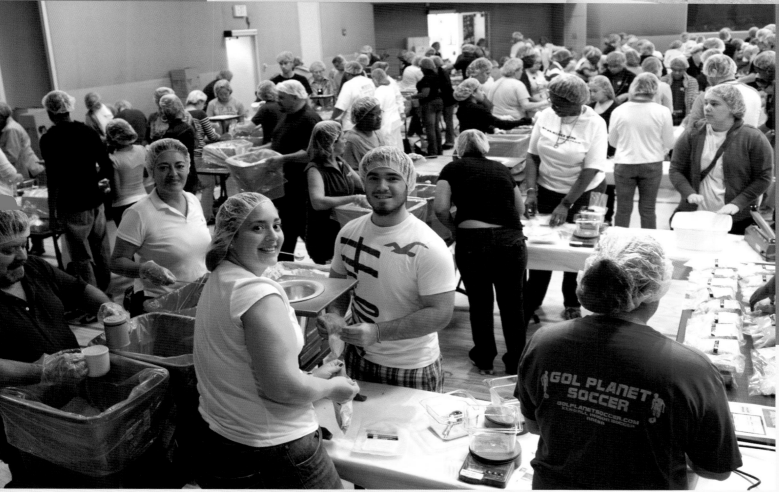

Above: Nearly 4,000 Baptist Health employees, physicians, Board members, family members and friends spent four days packaging more than one million meals that went to children in Haiti, victims of the devastating January 2010 earthquake. Volunteers worked two-hour shifts at stations set up in the auditorium at South Miami Hospital. They scooped rice, dehydrated vegetables, soy nuggets and vegetarian chicken flavoring into boxes containing six meals.

Facing page: Doctors Hospital's Paul Mungo, R.N., paints a mural at a Homestead elementary school in 2009 as part of Baptist Health's involvement with Hands on Miami.

Looking Ahead

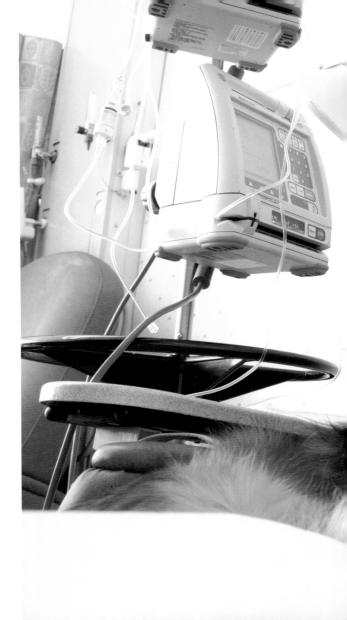

With planned expansion, growing markets and a strong financial foundation, Baptist Health looks to the future. The organization will continue to focus on its primary mission — providing outstanding medical care.

As it has done in the past, Baptist Health will evolve to accommodate the changing community. "We have to grow and strategize, especially as economics and healthcare reform dictate," Mr. Keeley said. "We will not, however, expand for expansion's sake. Our desire is not to simply get bigger and bigger. We will add services carefully, with foresight and financial discipline."

As the challenges of tomorrow unfold, Baptist Health's culture — an emphasis on customer service, dedicated physicians, engaged employees and a deeply rooted tradition of caring for the community — will guide the way. "Our future will be marked by the same principles and core values that we have had since our beginnings," Brian Keeley said. "We will focus on our faith-based mission to provide the highest quality of care to the patients we serve."

Above: Baptist Health's Regional Cancer Program includes the latest diagnostic and radiation therapy, clinical trials for new treatments, a variety of surgical procedures, as well as education and support. In this photograph, Sukie, a pet therapy dog, visits patient Nidia Villegas.

Left: Nicholas Lambrou, M.D., uses the da Vinci Surgical System to perform gynecologic surgery. The team at South Miami Hospital's Center for Robotic Surgery, under the leadership of Ricardo Estape, M.D., medical director, is among the most experienced in the state in using the robot to treat cancers and other conditions.

Right: Homestead Hospital's Julie Brandt, R.N., cradles a baby on the hospital's maternity floor. Baptist, Homestead and South Miami Hospitals offer a full range of maternity services. Baptist and South Miami Hospitals also have Level III Neonatal Intensive Care Units to care for the tiniest and sickest babies.

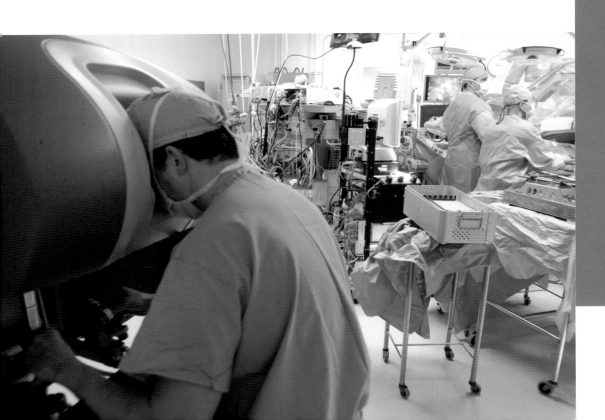

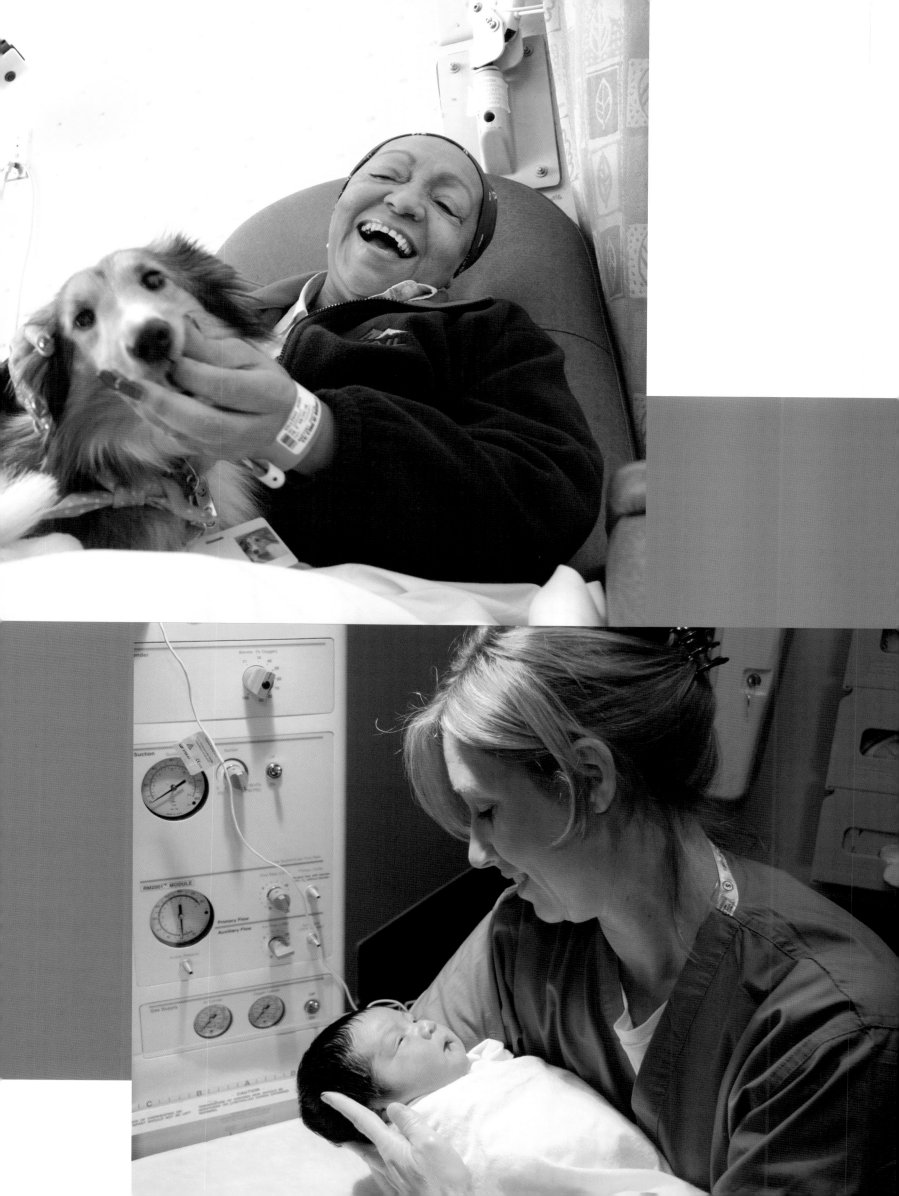

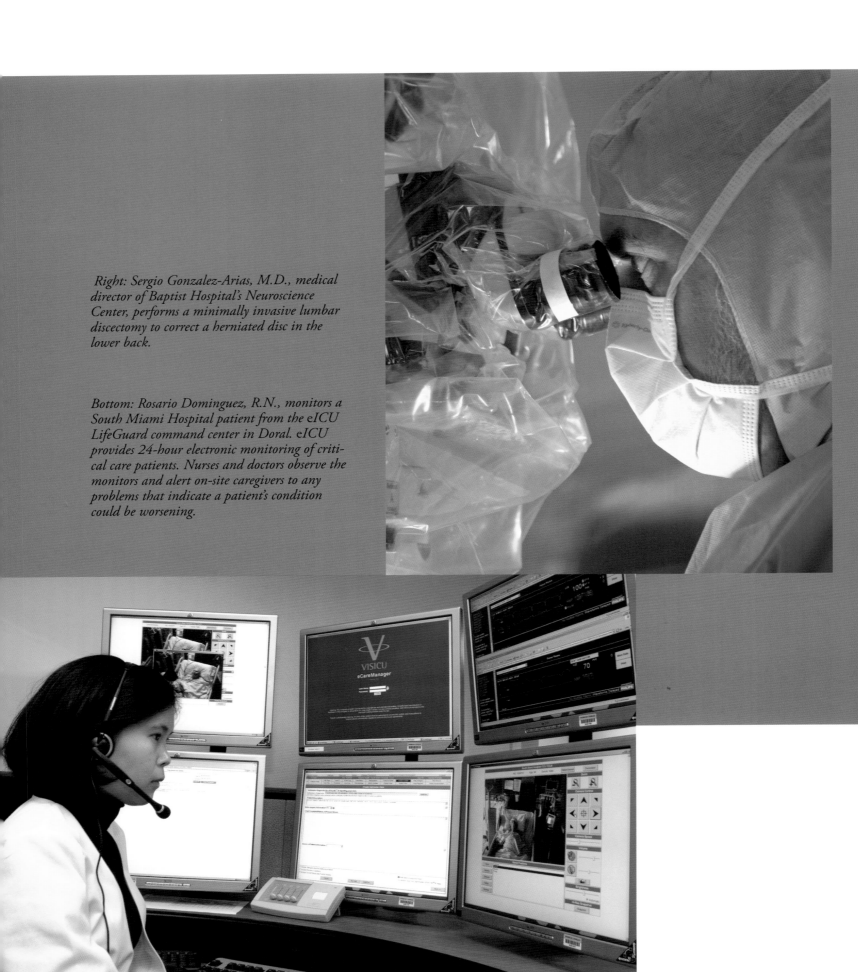

Right: Sergio Gonzalez-Arias, M.D., medical director of Baptist Hospital's Neuroscience Center, performs a minimally invasive lumbar discectomy to correct a herniated disc in the lower back.

Bottom: Rosario Dominguez, R.N., monitors a South Miami Hospital patient from the eICU LifeGuard command center in Doral. eICU provides 24-hour electronic monitoring of critical care patients. Nurses and doctors observe the monitors and alert on-site caregivers to any problems that indicate a patient's condition could be worsening.

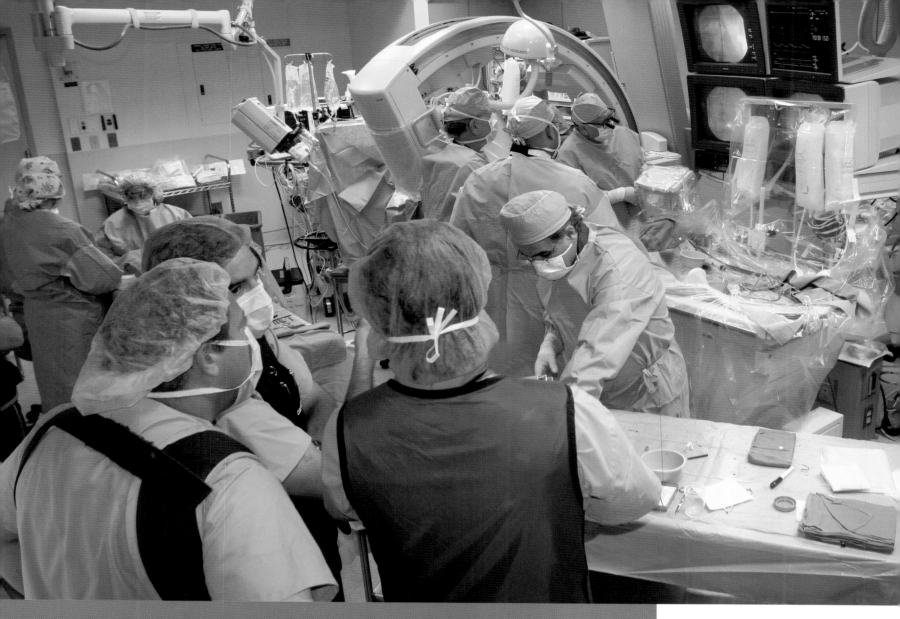

Above: Barry Katzen, M.D., and the team at Baptist Cardiac & Vascular Institute use state-of-the-art technology for minimally invasive procedures.

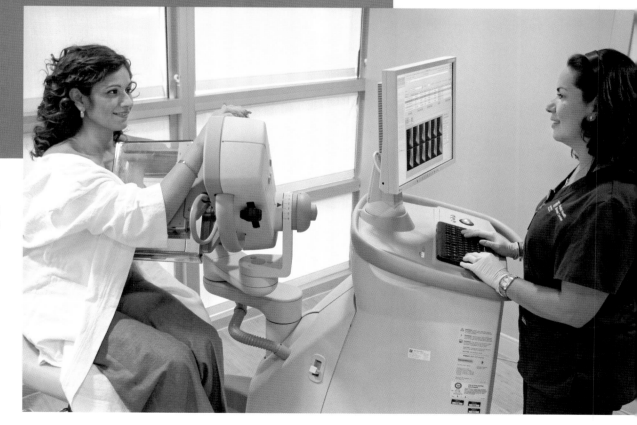

Right: Esther Gonzalez, a technologist at the Baptist Health Breast Center, performs a positron emission mammogram.

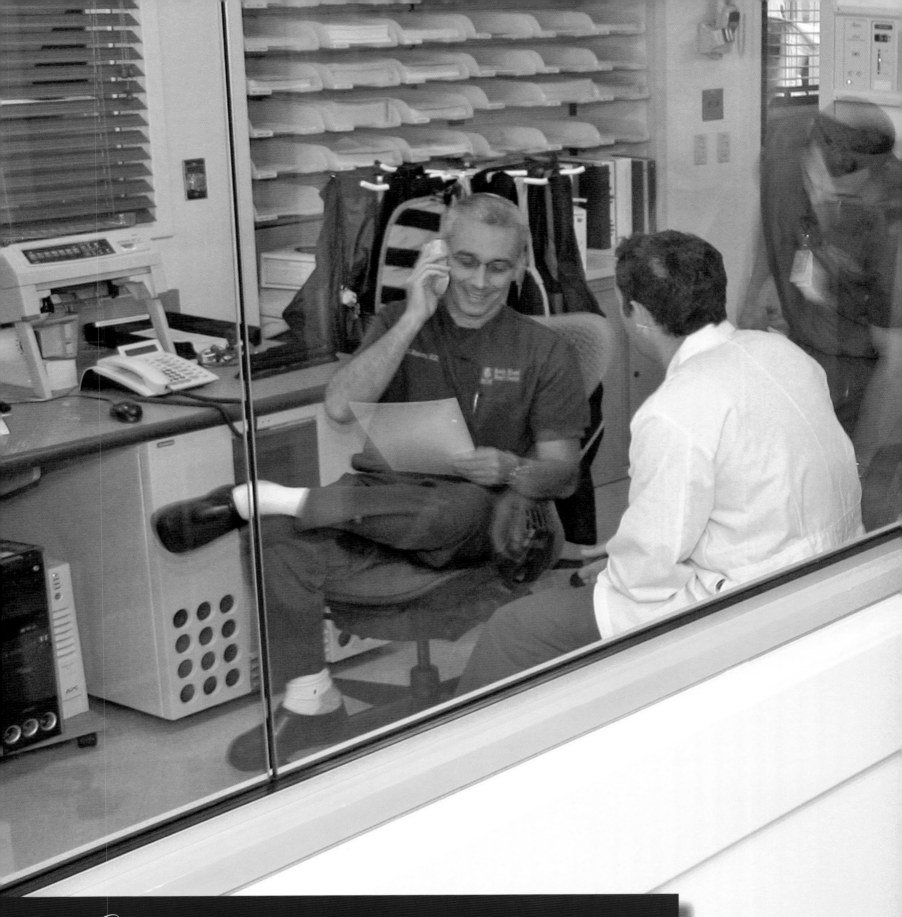

" *Our future will be marked by the same principles and core values that we have had since our beginnings. We will focus on our faith-based mission to provide the highest quality of care to the patients we serve.*"

Brian E. Keeley
President and CEO, Baptist Health South Florida
2010

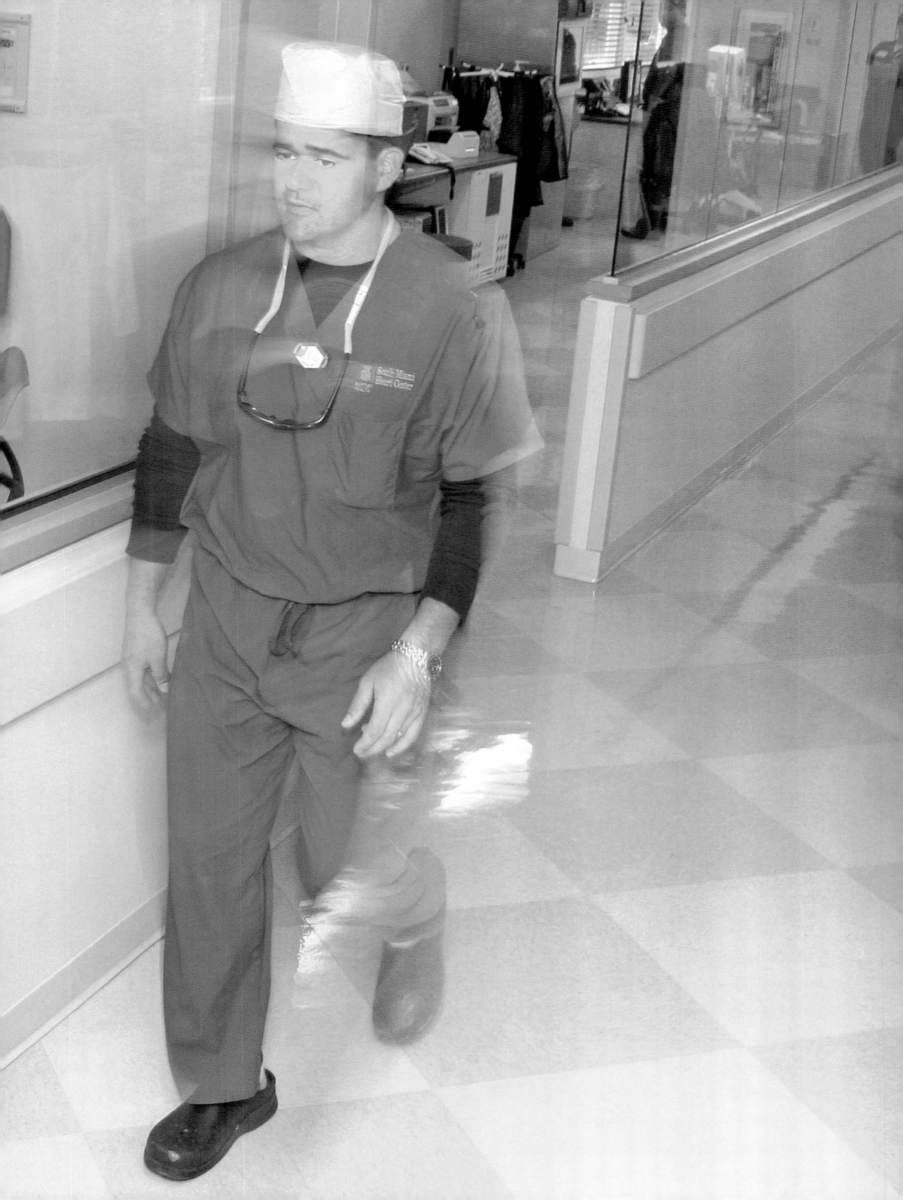

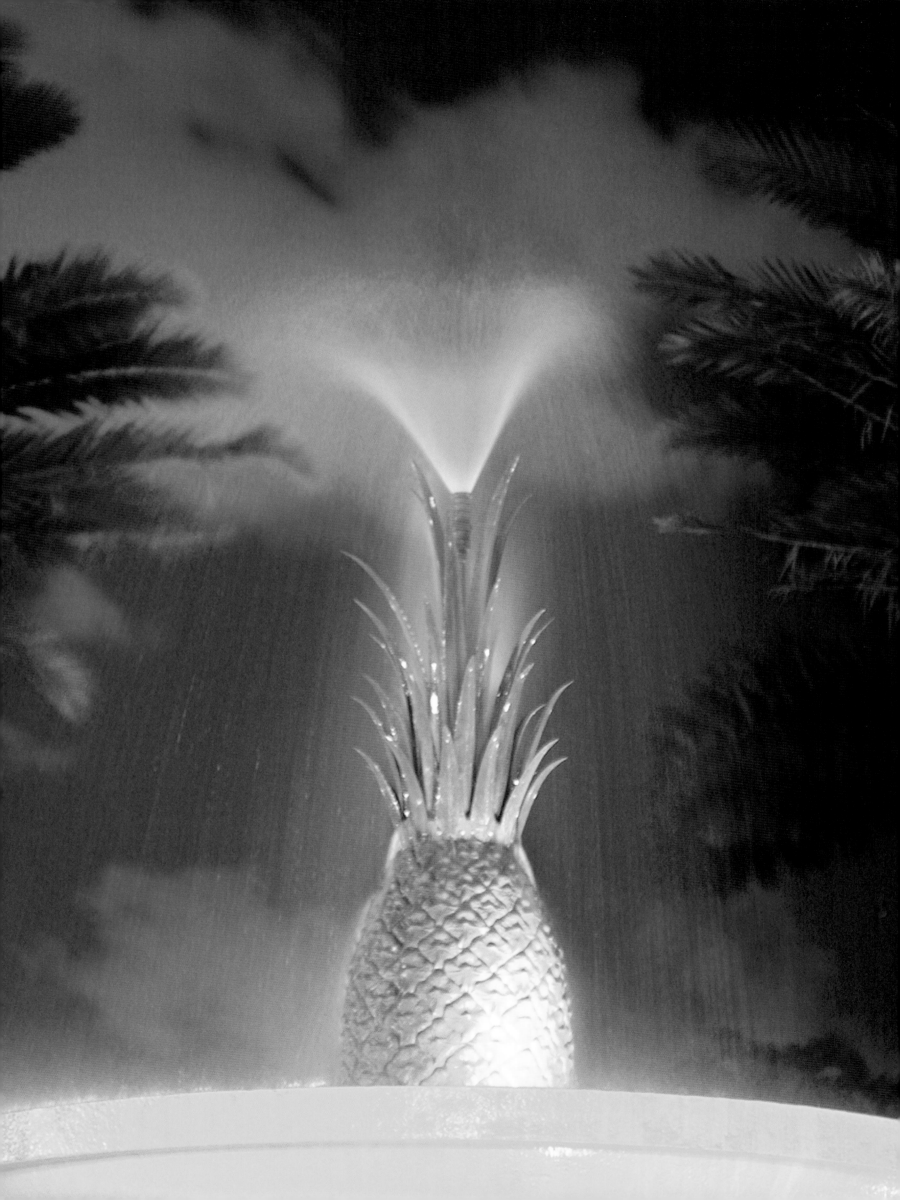

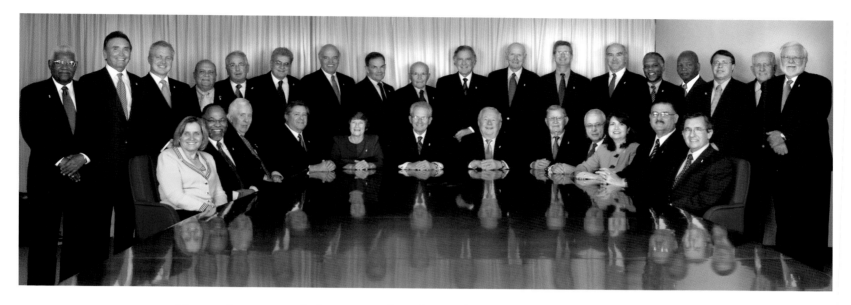

Baptist Health South Florida Board of Trustees

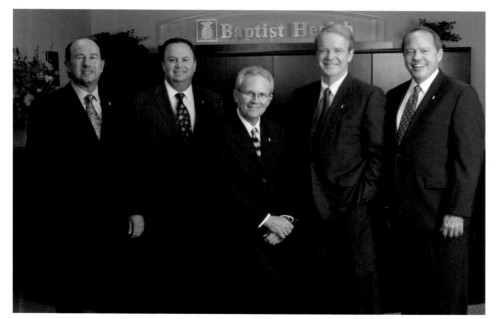

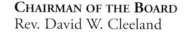

From left: George W. Foyo, D. Wayne Brackin, Rev. David W. Cleeland, Brian E. Keeley and Ralph E. Lawson

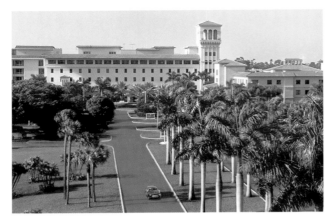

BAPTIST HOSPITAL OF MIAMI

Chairman of the Board
Calvin H. Babcock

Chief Executive Officer
Bo Boulenger

Board of Directors
Orlando L. Bajos
Mark Caruso, M.D.
Elizabeth Diaz de Villegas
Eugene Eisner, M.D.
Charles M. Hood III
Rev. Dr. Gary Johnson
S. Lawrence Kahn III
Manuel Lasaga
María Camila Leiva
Charlie Martinez
Paul D. May
Joseph P. McCain, DMD
Rev. Tom Thompson
Rev. Dr. William W. White
William W. Wilson III

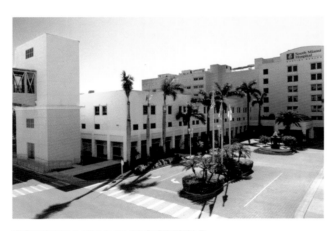

SOUTH MIAMI HOSPITAL

Chairman of the Board
The Hon. Judge Robert L. Dubé

Chief Executive Officer
Lincoln Mendez

Board of Directors
Yvette A. Aleman
Yerby T. Barker

Robert G. Berrin
Barron Channer
George M. Corrigan
I. Allan Feingold, M.D.
Michael F. Graham, M.D.
James W. Harris
Alysa R. Herman, M.D.
Elizabeth M. Hernandez, Esq.
Nathan B. Hirsch, M.D.
Orlando J. Leon, M.D.
James W. Loewenherz, M.D.
Hans C. Mueller
Guillermo L. Pol, M.D.
Rev. Dr. Marcos A. Ramos
Ian M. Reiss, M.D.
Domingo C. Rodriguez, Esq.
Robert J. Shafer Jr.
Karent Sierra, DDS
W. Peter Temling
Joseph A. Traina, M.D.
Leonard J. Zwerling, M.D.

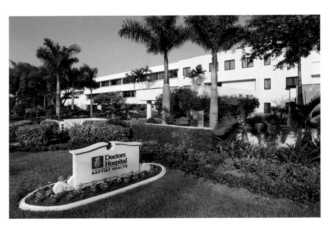

DOCTORS HOSPITAL

Chairman of the Board
Norman Kenyon, M.D.

Chief Executive Officer
Nelson Lazo

Board of Directors
Mario A. Almeida-Suarez, M.D.
Dick Anderson
James T. Barker
James Carr
Carlos Garcia
George C. Kakouris
George F. Knox
Miriam Lopez
Martha S. Pantin
Jay Perkins
Ramón E. Rasco, Esq.
Ronald A. Shuffield
Roberta Stokes
Patricia Thorp
Sats Tripathy
Lisa Guerrant White

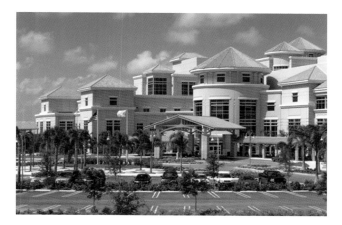

HOMESTEAD HOSPITAL

Chairman of the Board
Rev. William L. Chambers III

Chief Executive Officer
William M. Duquette

Board of Directors
Willie Carpenter
Maria C. Garza
Herbert H. Greene, M.D.
David E. Hallstrand, M.D.
Barbara Hanck
Jeanne F. Jacobs, Ph.D.
John P. Maas, Esq.
Ramon F. Oyarzun
M. Johanna Paterson
Steven S. Sapp
Maria Costa Smith
Rene W. Taylor
George R. Tershakovec, M.D.

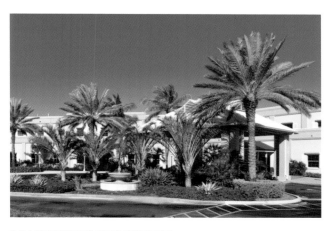

MARINERS HOSPITAL

Chairman of the Board
Jay A. Hershoff, Esq.

Chief Executive Officer
Rick Freeburg

Board of Directors
Bette Brown
Elisa M. Brown-Soltero, M.D.
William Dickinson
William H. Gilbert Jr.
Robert M. Gintel
Gerald Hirsch
David P. Johnson
Stanley Margulies, M.D.
Joy C. Martin
Charlen Regan
I.E. Schilling

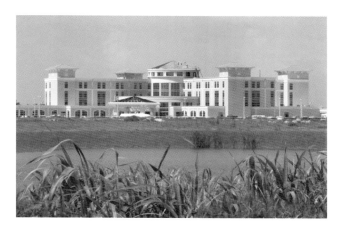

WEST KENDALL BAPTIST HOSPITAL

Chairman of the Board
Tony Alonso

Chief Executive Officer
Javier Hernandez-Lichtl

Board of Directors
Wendell R. Beard
George E. Cadman III
Rev. David W. Cleeland
Rev. Otto Fernandez
Armando J. Ferrer, Ph.D.
Ann E. Pope
John A. Rock, M.D.
Aida Shafer

BAPTIST HEALTH SOUTH FLORIDA

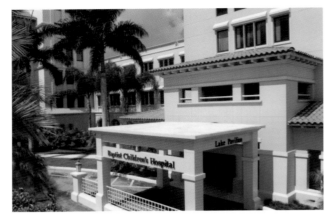

BAPTIST CHILDREN'S HOSPITAL

Administrator
Randall Lee

Executive Committee
Marta I. Blanco
Adriana Castro, M.D.
Arcenio Chacon, M.D.
Maura Cintas, M.D.
Doured Daghistani, M.D.
Alfredo Fernandez, M.D.
Jonathan Fields, M.D.
Michael Finer, M.D.
Norman Goldberg, M.D.
Gail Gordon, R.N.
Andrew B. Kairalla, M.D.
Pam Larcada, M.D.
Guillermo Llosa, M.D.
Francisco Medina, M.D.
Nina Sanchez, M.D.
Juan Sola, M.D.
Phuket Tantivit, M.D.
Tony Tavarez, M.D.
Ernesto Valdes, M.D.

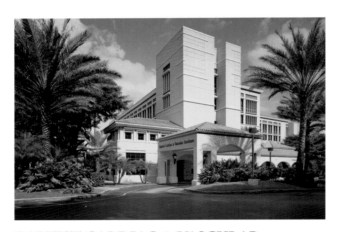

BAPTIST CARDIAC & VASCULAR INSTITUTE

Founder and Medical Director
Barry T. Katzen, M.D.

Administrator
Carol Mascioli

Board of Managers
Barry T. Katzen, M.D.
Manuel Lasaga
Ramon Lloret, M.D.
Niberto L. Moreno, M.D.
Alex Powell, M.D.
Ramon Quesada, M.D.
Ignacio Rua, M.D.

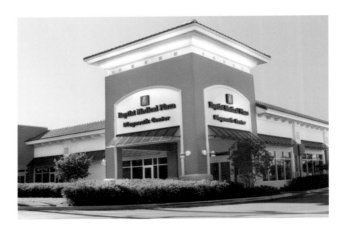

BAPTIST OUTPATIENT SERVICES

Chairman of the Board
Roberta Stokes

Chief Executive Officer
Patricia Rosello

Board of Directors
Tony Alonso
George E. Cadman III
James Carr
Rev. David W. Cleeland
The Hon. Judge Robert L. Dubé
Joyce J. Elam
Gretchen Goslin
Charles M. Hood III
Rev. Dr. Gary Johnson
Martha S. Pantin
Ann E. Pope
Ronald A. Shuffield
Paul S. Soulé
Lee Stapleton, Esq.
Sats Tripathy
J. Scott Weston

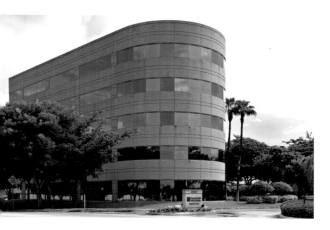

BAPTIST HEALTH ENTERPRISES

Chairman of the Board
James Carr

Chief Executive Officer
Ana Lopez-Blazquez

Board of Directors
Tony Alonso
George E. Cadman III
Rev. David W. Cleeland
The Hon. Judge Robert L. Dubé
Joyce J. Elam
Gretchen Goslin
Charles M. Hood III
Rev. Dr. Gary Johnson
Martha S. Pantin
Ann E. Pope
Ronald A. Shuffield
Paul S. Soulé
Lee Stapleton, Esq.
Roberta Stokes
Sats Tripathy
J. Scott Weston

BAPTIST HEALTH FOUNDATION

Chairman of the Board
James W. Harris

Chief Executive Officer
Stephen J. Parsons

Board of Directors
Richard T. Alger
Cira Almeida
Mario A. Almeida-Suarez, M.D.
Dick Anderson
George N. Aronoff
William A. Baldwin
Oscar Barbara
Yerby T. Barker
Rodney Barreto
Kerrin F.Bermont
Robert G. Berrin
Bonnie Blaire, Esq.
James W. Bokor
Joseph Bolton, Esq.
James Boruszak
Judi Bray
Elisa M. Brown-Soltero, M.D.
Joseph R. Buchanan, Esq.
Mita Burke
Robert Burstein
Barbara A. Calev-Moran
Miguel Cano
Thomas P. Carlos, Esq.
James Carr
Susan Carr
Gerald Case
Ray Castellanos
Joe A. Catarineau, Esq.
Mauricio Cayon
Victor E. Clarke
Agustin G. De Goytisolo
William Dickinson
Lani Kahn Drody
Denise King Ehrich
Eugene Eisner, M.D.
Tomas P. Erban
Theodore Feldman, M.D.
Manny S. Fernandez
J. Arturo Fridman, M.D.
Augusto J. Gil
Robert M. Gintel
Paul A. Gluck, M.D.
Leif Gunderson
Barry Halpern, M.D.
Kent Hamill
Barbara Hanck
Daniel Hanrahan
Carol R. Berry Helms
Agustin Herran
Jay A. Hershoff, Esq.

Gerald Hirsch
Nathan B. Hirsch, M.D.
Jacque Huttoe
Lane M. Jones
Thomas R. Jones Jr.
Barry T. Katzen, M.D.
Judith Katzen
Robert Kramer, Esq.
Rudy Kranys
Katrina Lavene
Cynthia Leesfield
María Camila Leiva
Victoria London
Bruce Wirtz MacArthur
Flora Mamakos
Charlie Martinez
Arva Moore Parks McCabe
Derek A. McDowell
Joanne J. McGregor-Ganus
Andrew J. Menachem
Niberto L. Moreno, M.D.
Patricia B. Mull
Thomas P. Murphy Jr.
Paula Owens
Omar Pasalodos, M.D.
M. Johanna Paterson
Jorge E. Perez, M.D.
Jay Perkins
Guillermo L. Pol, M.D.
Jose E. Portuondo, M.D
Ramón E. Rasco, Esq.
Mindy Rich
The Hon. Judge Bonnie Rippingille
Ron Robison
David Rosenbaum
Ruth Rosenberg
Audrey Ross
Jeff E. Rubin, Esq.
James F. Russell
Darren Salinger, M.D.
Gonzalo Sanabria
Joel H. Schenkman, M.D.
Betty Anne Schilling
Liz Schmier
Emery B. Sheer
Joel M. Shepherd
Paul S. Soulé
Patricia Stanley
James G. Stewart, M.D.
Rene W. Taylor
George R. Tershakovec, M.D.
Henry Tie Shue
Bill R.Tillett
Nick Waddell
Jeff B. Weiner
Warren Weiser
William W. Wilson III
Philip Wolman
Lloyd Wruble, DMD
Jerrold Young, M.D.

BAPTIST HEALTH SOUTH FLORIDA

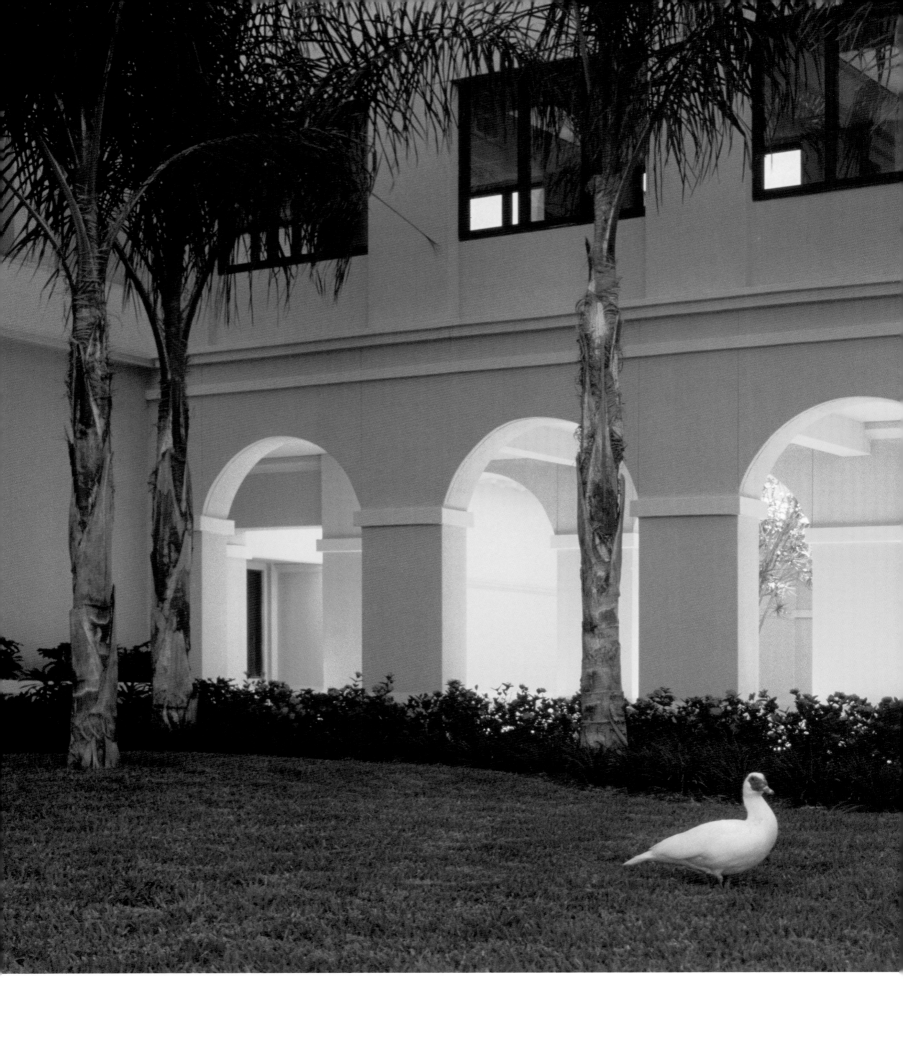

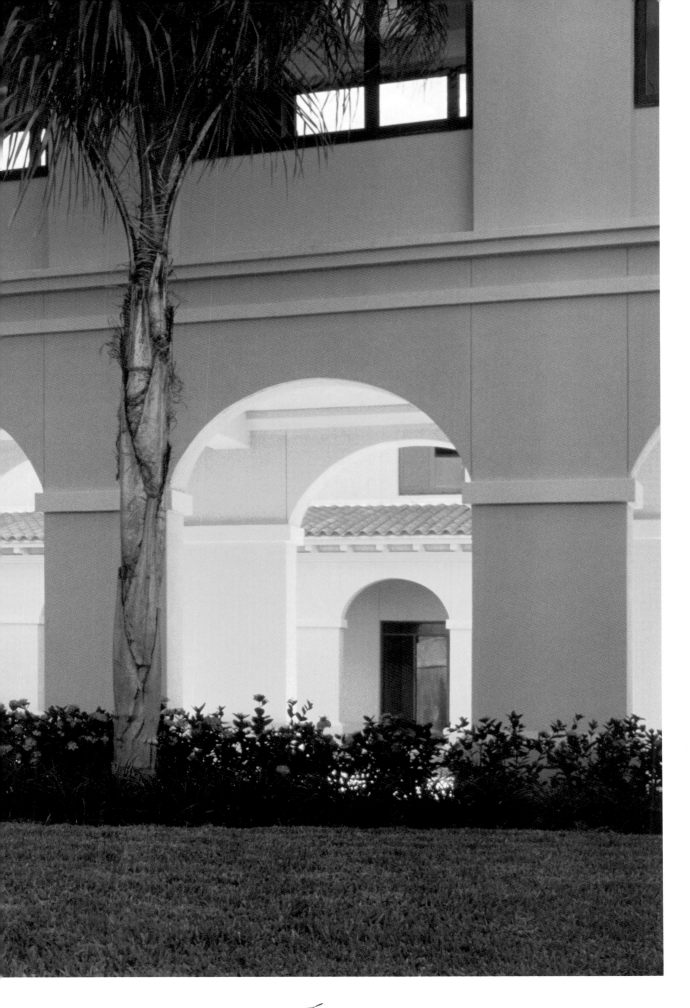

"*It* is one of the most beautiful compensations of life that
no man can sincerely help another without helping himself."

RALPH WALDO EMERSON
An excerpt from Baptist Hospital's
chapel dedication program, 1961

Index

Index

Acknowledgments

*M*any members of Baptist Health — Board members, employees, physicians and volunteers — contributed to *Baptist Health South Florida: A History of Caring for the Community*. From the beginning, Corporate Vice President of Marketing & Public Relations Jo Baxter brought more than 30 years of expertise to the project. Her vision, intimate knowledge and commitment to creating an institutional memory provided the framework for the book. The organization's publications produced under her direction, including *Resource* magazine and *Pineapple Press* (as well as its predecessor, *Vocal Chord*), offered much of the information used in this book. Baptist Health President and CEO Brian E. Keeley enthusiastically embraced the history and spent hours answering questions and sharing memories.

Wayne Brackin, Ralph Lawson, George Foyo, Ana Lopez-Blazquez, Bo Boulenger, Lincoln Mendez, Nelson Lazo, William Duquette, Rick Freeburg, Javier Hernandez-Lichtl and Patricia Rosello offered their time and thoughts and filled in gaps in information.

Past and present Baptist Health leaders, employees, consultants and physicians provided insights and material. They include Richard Alger, Trudy Armstrong, Robert Baal, Debbie Blaida, R.N., Diane Bolton, R.N., Norma Burke, Cindy Cancio, Jerry Case, Sol Colsky, M.D., Cheryl Cottrell, R.N., George Corrigan, JoAnn Crebbin, R.N., Barbara Dempsey, R.N., Charlotte Dison, R.N., the Honorable Judge Robert Dubé, Allan Feingold, M.D., Roberta Fismer, R.N., Gail Gordon, R.N., David Hallstrand, M.D., Barbara Hanck, Therese Havel, R.N., Jay Hershoff, David Horovitz, Helen Hudnall, R.N., Doug Jolly, Norman Kenyon, M.D., Christine Kinik, Howard Lerner, Joel Levin, M.D., James Loewenherz, M.D., Robert Luse, Melvin Mackler, M.D., Georgia Mayo, Cathy Miller, Deborah Mulvihill, R.N., Ramon Oyarzun, Charlen Regan, Domingo Rodriguez, Barbara Russell, R.N., Kyle Saxon, Charlotte Schmunk, Bernard Silverstein, M.D., Karl Smiley, M.D., Kathy Sparger, R.N., Michael Stein, James Stewart, M.D., Lee Streater, R.N., Joseph Traina, M.D., James Vaughn, M.D., Cira Villorin, Rick Wolfson and Lori Young.

Others who contributed include Bob Jensen, James Lyons II, Louise Lyons, Larry Wiggins and Jerry Wilkinson. Tracy Lovitt and Barbara Stephenson from the *South Dade News Leader* and Patty Murphy from *The Keynoter* shared photographs and newspaper clippings. *The Road to Somewhere* by Donna Knowles Born was an excellent source of information and photographs depicting Baptist Hospital. The Mariners Hospital Ladies Auxiliary kept detailed scrapbooks of the hospital's earliest days that helped trace the history.

Among those who reviewed files, scheduled interviews, provided contact information and photographs, and answered questions were Elsa Figueredo, Amanda Gonzalez, Shannon Johns, Linda Knudsen, Georgette Koch, Wendy Kornfield, Sheila Konczewski, Christine Kotler, George Lakis, Liz Latta, Vanessa Lopez, Barbara Moore, Patricia Otero, Mabel Rodriguez, Kelli Romano, Bethany Rundell, Anne Smith, Anne Streeter, Phyllis Teitelbaum, Tanya Walton and Denise Winston.

Writer and editor Patty Shillington worked tirelessly to help the book's readability and clarity. Arva Moore Parks, Adrienne Sylver and Dorothy Stein offered comments, suggestions and corrections. On the design and production end, graphic designer Rhondda Edmiston and her assistant, Sue Edmiston, combined their extraordinary talent with an eye for detail.

This book reflects the valuable role of everybody at Baptist Health. It is truly a collaborative effort.

Laura Pincus

What I like best about my nurse is...

She helps me get Better.

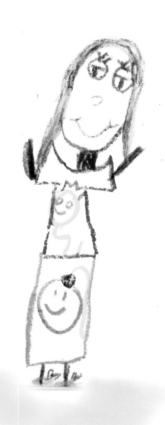

Illustration by Taylor Dennis
Baptist Children's Hospital, 2000

$\mathcal{W}$E ARE MADE WISE

NOT BY THE RECOLLECTION OF OUR PAST,

BUT BY THE RESPONSIBILITY

FOR OUR FUTURE.

GEORGE BERNARD SHAW

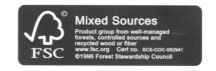